RETHINKING PARKINSON'S DISEASE

Also by John Coleman

Stop Parkin' and Start Livin':
Reversing the Symptoms of Parkinson's Disease

Shaky Past:
Life, Parkinson's Disease, Recovery, Winning against Impossible Odds!

Interview with John Coleman, ND:
How John Coleman Reversed his Own Parkinson's Disease Symptoms
(with Robert Rodgers PhD)

RETHINKING
PARKINSON'S
DISEASE

The definitive guide to the known causes of Parkinson's disease
and proven reversal strategies

JOHN C. COLEMAN

HYBRID
PUBLISHERS

Published by Hybrid Publishers

Melbourne Victoria Australia

© John Coleman 2020

First published 2020

 A catalogue record for this
book is available from the
NATIONAL
LIBRARY   National Library of Australia
OF AUSTRALIA

ISBN: 9781925736465 (p)
9781925736472 (e)

Cover design: Gittus Graphics www.gggraphics.com.au

CONTENTS

FOREWORD

"All truth passes through three stages. First, it is ridiculed. Second, it is violently opposed. Third, it is accepted as being self-evident."
— Arthur Schopenhauer, philosopher

I first met John Coleman when I presented a guest teaching session at the College of Naturopathy where he was studying. The session was on the importance of hydration in human health, a subject that has been of great interest to me for some years, and which had spawned a new company that offered some herbal and homoeopathic formulas which our research had shown to be effective to improve hydration state. John approached me at the end of the session and asked if I thought hydration would be important in Parkinson's disease, telling me that he had been diagnosed with PD. We sent John some formulas and, after some initial challenges getting the dose right, he reported that these formulas did, indeed seem to help. There began a 25-year association that culminates in me having the privilege of writing the foreword for his third published book.

Like me, John comes to his work as a scientist. Part of being a good scientist is constantly asking questions, forming hypotheses, testing them and adjusting them, until something that approaches a "truth" may be crafted. These truths are never absolute because some new idea, a new measurement tool or knowledge imported from another discipline may call the temporary truth into question, render it obsolete, or at least in need of modification. Another part of being a good scientist is collecting data, analysing it and using it to support or refute the null hypothesis. Thus science moves forward, mostly in baby steps, but sometimes in great leaps. However, when the advances come they are usually treated, as the Schopenhauer quote above says, at first with ridicule, then opposition and finally acceptance.

John's unique perspective on the disease that has been his burden, and our gift, has gone through the first two of those stages. I have watched him hold onto his truth in the face of all kinds of opposition from the conventional medical establishment and even some complementary practitioners. This book will, I hope, propel his body of work toward the third stage that Schopenhauer predicts, but I suspect there will still be a while before the self-evident nature of his reasoned approach becomes widely embraced. The perspectives and advice he offers come, not just from his own experience, but from thousands of PD sufferers who have made their way to his clinic. As the italicised "case notes" show, not all of these people have been in a place where they can take the advice on board and make the necessary lifestyle and thought process changes to allow their improvement. So, we see that at the level of the individual, as well as the broader medical profession, there has been resistance. And that is to be expected when a long-held belief, in this case in the irreversible, progressive nature of PD, is being challenged.

If you or someone you care for is suffering from the symptoms of PD, I commend you to take the time to read this, and John's previous books, and integrate his sensible and profound guidance for a healthy life and a recovery of wellness. He and many of his patients are living proof that it can be done.

Jaroslav Boublik PhD
2020

HOW TO GET THE BEST VALUE
FROM THIS BOOK

When we are diagnosed with Parkinson's disease, we are often bombarded with enormous amounts of information, most of it ranging from depressing to dire, with little or no advice about what we can do to feel better or become healthier.

When diagnosed in 1995, I was tempted, at first, to rely on acknowledged medical experts to give me answers to my questions and advice on how to relieve my symptoms, function better and feel more "normal". I was disappointed, as all I heard from these experts was that they did not know what caused Parkinson's disease, there was no hope of recovery and I could do nothing to help myself. Drugs were the only answer.

I had no access to the internet in 1995, but was still overwhelmed by the amount of information about Parkinson's disease that I found in books, studies, journals, research papers and statements from a variety of medical practitioners. My first task was to find the tiny seeds of positivity and hope amongst the huge pile of technical and experimental information I read.

These days, there are thousands of pages of information on the internet, books written by doctors, researchers and hopeful patients, fabulous amounts of research information available on sites like PubMed, and diagnosed celebrities telling their stories to entice us to give money to their foundations or charities.

It can all be really confusing.

This book is intended to reduce the confusion and give you, the person diagnosed with Parkinson's disease, the opportunity to explore options to improve your state of wellbeing. It also offers healthcare practitioners the opportunity to increase their knowledge base with information about causes and recovery from an author who has both experienced advanced Parkinson's disease himself and helped many others to reverse their symptoms.

You may be someone hungry for knowledge and wanting to know everything NOW! If so (and that is like me), start at the beginning and read through to the end, making notes or highlighting as you go.

However, if the thought of reading 440 pages and absorbing so much information is daunting, here are some ideas to make it easier.

Person with Parkinson's disease

If you want to begin your journey to better health now, start at **Section 3**, Chapters 12 through 16, and make the changes advised to your food choices, supplements, lifestyle and activities.

You will find it easiest to begin with food. Start with breakfast, get that right, then move onto your other meals. With food sorted, you will find it easier to begin supplementation (there are suggestions for the most important supplements) and activity.

Chapters 17 through 19 give details of other strategies that will help you improve your health. Work through those step by step, setting goals to adopt a new strategy each two weeks.

When you feel that you can manage the basic changes in this section, it is time for you to read Section 2 (WHAT CAUSES PARKINSON'S DISEASE?) and discover what has caused your symptoms. You can then adopt the strategies specific for the pathways that have led to your state of unwellness. Writing some notes about your family and life history will help and, if you need more clues, read Chapter 11 (FINDING THE AETIOLOGICAL PATHWAY) for help.

Healthcare practitioner

You already have many skills that can help a person with Parkinson's improve their state of health. However, if you want to understand the aetiology of symptom patterns, as I do, so you can advise and prescribe more effectively, but are time-poor, Section 2 (what causes Parkinson's disease?) is the place to start.

Chapters 6 through 10 include research from Western allopathic medicine and complementary/alternative medicine on the causes of neurodegeneration, plus my clinical experience of over twenty years. Chapter 11 gives some strategies for discovering aetiological pathways for those patients who present with complex and confusing symptom patterns.

Once you have knowledge of what has caused your patient's journey from good health to poor health, and broken through the camouflage of differential symptom diagnosis and polypharmacy, you can adopt or adapt the strategies in Section 3 to help your patent achieve the best possible health outcomes.

Section 1 is there for all those who want to know more about the history of Parkinson's disease and its treatment, common attitudes and some basic differences between the approaches offered by Western allopathic medicine and complementary/ alternative medicine. This section is for the adventurous and the curious, and may help patients and practitioners to understand why I needed to write this book.

I hope you will all read **Section 4** when you are ready to ponder the divide in health care throughout the Western World and consider your individual response to those challenges.

SECTION 1

PARKINSON'S DISEASE

What it is and standard treatment

CHAPTER 1

I USED TO HAVE PARKINSON'S DISEASE

I used to have Parkinson's disease. My symptoms were very severe – stage 4 on the Hoehn and Yahr Scale of disease severity.[1] There are only five stages on this scale and, at stage 5, we need full-time care, so stage 4 is very bad.

My diagnosis of Parkinson's disease was in early 1995 but, by late in 1998, I was free from all symptoms. This was not a "cure". I had recovered my health.

For nine years, following my diagnosis, I searched, studied and observed strategies that reduced my symptoms or didn't, or even made my symptoms worse, then wrote it all down in a manuscript called *Stop Parkin' and Start Livin'*, which was published in 2005.[2] Details of my story of recovery and search for meaning are found in "My Adventure with Parkinson's Disease" (Appendix 5) and *Shaky Past*.[3]

Research into Parkinson's disease treatment and illness processes, and my understanding of how to help people with Parkinson's become well, has expanded exponentially since 2005. It is time to bring our strategies for recovery into the 2020s. There is still no "cure" for Parkinson's disease and probably never will be. That is not relevant because we can become well. We can recover our health.

There are many books about Parkinson's disease. Some are written by doctors acknowledged by their peers as "experts" in Parkinson's, other neurodegenerative disorders or movement disorders. Some are written by complementary practitioners who seek to treat people diagnosed with Parkinson's disease holistically in an effort to improve quality as well as quantity of life.

To my knowledge, there is no other book that explores the variety of aetiological pathways that may create Parkinson's disease symptom patterns and gives details of developed strategies to treat each pathway and combinations of pathways.

In my career as a naturopath I, at first, resisted the temptation to become a "specialist". But, as patient after patient came to me, I saw that the majority had been diagnosed with Parkinson's disease, had heard my story, and were looking to me for a pathway to recovery. Each patient had consulted Western allopathic medical practitioners (those using treatments that attack the symptoms of a disease) – often general practitioners, then one, two or three neurologists – looking for answers to their symptoms and feelings of illness, and ways to become well again.

They had all been offered similar advice:

1. You have Parkinson's disease
2. This disease is progressive, degenerative and irreversible
3. We don't know what causes it
4. There is nothing you can do for yourself to reverse the disease process
5. We can give you drugs to reduce the symptoms for a few years
6. Eventually you will need lots of drugs, perhaps deep brain stimulation
7. We're spending millions of dollars on research so, one day, we will find a cure. You can help by raising money for this research.

The next obvious move for my patients, and one I made myself when diagnosed, was to join a Parkinson's association looking for more detailed advice, support, news of research breakthroughs and companionship. What they, and I, heard from Parkinson's associations was:

1. You have Parkinson's disease
2. This disease is progressive, degenerative and irreversible
3. We don't know what causes it
4. There is nothing you can do for yourself to reverse the disease process
5. Doctors can give you drugs to reduce the symptoms for a few years
6. Eventually you will need lots of drugs, perhaps deep brain stimulation
7. We're spending millions of dollars on research so, one day, we will find a cure. You can help by raising money for this research.

I began to see that it was my responsibility, and a brand-new adventure, to try and discover why I had recovered when so many do not, whether others had also recovered, what the disease process really looked like, and how I could help more people reverse the process and become well.

This book is the result of the last twenty-five years of working to understand my own life, disease process and return to health;[4] how I and over 2000 of my patients diagnosed with Parkinson's disease became ill; how and why I became well after being so debilitated with Parkinson's disease symptoms; and what research (mainstream and obscure) is telling us about Parkinson's disease, its causes and hope for wellness.

The most distressing part of my story is the response of doctors and neurologists when faced with the unmistakable recovery of people who had been diagnosed with Parkinson's disease (often with a second and third opinion) and then presented with no symptoms after taking charge of their health. I naively expected their neurologists, especially, to be fascinated by their story of recovery. I thought they would ask their patients for details, take note of what each patient did that was different from the norm, confer with their colleagues to collect information on similar "aberrant" patients, and urge for research into these success stories.

What actually happened was that patients were ignored, dismissed or abused for daring to disagree with the "experts". Where a conversation took place, patients were told they had been "misdiagnosed" in the first place, but there was no explanation of their Parkinson's disease symptoms that had led to diagnosis.

Many patients called me, angry and puzzled, telling me that they had attended an appointment with their specialist, attempted to explain what they had done, how their symptoms had slowly subsided, that they were able to gradually reduce their reliance on medication and now lived without symptoms, only to be dismissed without any comment or attempt to engage with their story.

A few tried to tell their story to Parkinson's disease associations or support groups, but were roundly abused for daring to give "false hope" to those who had been condemned to lives of increasing misery by "experts". They were forbidden from discussing their experiences within that forum and asked to not return.

In 2001, I was invited to present my story of recovery at a major Parkinson's disease conference. I made no attempt to explain why I had recovered or to usurp the place of the experienced specialists in the audience. While I was speaking, at least ten doctors walked out. Following my presentation, there were three questions from people with Parkinson's but none from doctors. The following day, the person who had arranged my presentation was dismissed from their position on a national Parkinson's disease body because I was spreading "false hope" and should never have been allowed to speak.

Some years later, I was interviewed on a television show about food and Parkinson's disease. I told my story very briefly, expressed my views on the importance of food, and felt that there was a small chink in the armour of ignorance surrounding the treatment of Parkinson's disease in the Western world. A neurologist was interviewed about the "Mediterranean Diet" on the same show. The show was aired but, instead of being stored on the TV channel's website for a week as usual, was pulled within hours. I called to ask why and was told that the neurologist had demanded the show be taken down as it gave "false hope" to people with Parkinson's disease. The journalist who told me this then proceeded to abuse me for telling lies about my health, and (again) giving people "false hope". He told me that I had been misdiagnosed, that I was a charlatan and should be ashamed of myself for telling lies just to make money. This journalist had no knowledge of health matters, had never met me, read my medical or health history, and was totally ignorant of the process and treatment for Parkinson's disease. Yet, despite his enormous ignorance, he was arrogant enough to tell me about my own life.

Some of my patients have received similar abuse from doctors and other ignoramuses like that journalist – people without knowledge who have the temerity to preach to those with personal experience of recovery.

It is vital to tell the story of recovery. Not just case histories, but an understanding of how and why people diagnosed with Parkinson's disease reversed their symptoms and were able to live free from any sign of the disease.

Hope

What about "false hope"? Does it exist? In my view there is either hope or no hope. Hope is always real and helpful. Hope helps us to try harder, attempt new ideas, look in different places for ideas that may bear fruit.

"False hope" is an oxymoron. If hope is false, it is not hope but a delusion. Doctors often give patients hope without substance – "support this research and we will find a cure soon", "this treatment will shrink the tumour", "we are on the brink of a breakthrough". These are hopeful statements I often hear but are without substance. Does that mean they are harmful? Not necessarily. Hope is good, even if sometimes misdirected. We have seen in war times that those prisoners holding on to hope of escape or rescue were far more likely to survive the horror than those who lost hope. Patients diagnosed with serious cancer who are given hope of remission survive longer and have better quality of life than those told "there is no hope".[5]

Anomalies

Hope helps us look at anomalies. Those who come to me have read my story, or heard other stories of recovery, and see that this is a different dialogue than they have with their medical professionals. A few ask me to "cure" them and go away disappointed – there is no "cure" and probably never will be. But most ask, "What must I do to be well?" They have hope that they will have the determination and strength to follow a pathway to wellness.

There are many who seek to destroy hope for wellness – most Western allopathic medicine practitioners have been taught (and are expected to comply) that only Western allopathic medicine can provide hope for a "cure"; family members who see only symptoms sometimes pressure patients to accept their "fate" and comply with conservative medical processes only; many in the media are paid to preach the conservative gospel of "the only hope is 'cure' and only Western allopathic medicine can find a 'cure'".

Investigating anomalies and holding on to hope have brought us the greatest breakthroughs in health and wellness. The process usually involving strident opposition from those who are comfortable in conservatism and do not wish to be disturbed.

Dr Ignaz Philipp Semmelweis (1818–65) discovered the anomaly of hand washing before delivering babies. He found that washing hands saved lives; women and babies had a much greater chance of survival. He presented his findings to colleagues who, at first, ridiculed him, then incarcerated him in a mental asylum where he died of septicaemia. It was over thirty years before his principles of hygiene were adopted and, in the meantime, thousands of women and babies died unnecessarily.

Dr Louis Pasteur was ridiculed and ignored for over twenty years before his bacteria hypothesis was supported and investigated further to allow development of better treatment.

Dr Alexander Fleming, in 1928, accidentally noticed that bacteria in a petri dish with a particular mould were dead. Instead of ignoring this "accident" (anomaly), he investigated and the world was blessed with penicillin.

Barry Marshall and Robin Warren were ignored for twenty years after they discovered that Helicobacter pylori was implicated in the development of gastric ulcers. Their work was recognised eventually and gastric ulcers became more treatable but, again, conservatism kicked in and doctors now seek to "cure" an overgrowth of H. pylori without seeking to understand why it has proliferated. The anomalies of patients who reverse H. pylori overgrowth without antibiotics and proton pump inhibitors (PPI) are ignored.

Hope is never "false", always good, and anomalies are exciting.

By the time this is published, I am sure there will be more news, understanding and ways to create wellness; so this should be a starting point for your own adventure of discovery. Joyful wellness is our right and goal; never give up striving to reach that. When others tell you to "stop looking, believe the 'experts' and just settle down to the misery of a degenerative disease", remember the words of James Arthur Baldwin: "*Those who say it can't be done are usually interrupted by others doing it.*"

CHAPTER 2

WHAT IS PARKINSON'S DISEASE?

Is it a disease?

"Disease" is defined in a variety of ways by different bodies and organisations, depending on their culture, experience and commercial interests (or lack thereof).

In the past, disease has often been defined as an absence of wellness, leaving us with the problem of defining "wellness". The World Health Organisation's claim that health is "a state of complete physical, mental and social wellbeing, not merely the absence of disease or infirmity" (WHO, 1946)[1] has been praised for embracing an holistic viewpoint, and equally strongly condemned for being wildly utopian; the historian Robert Hughes remarked that it was "more realistic for a bovine than a human state of existence" (Hudson, 1993).[2]

Accepting the WHO definition of wellness, we must accept that Parkinson's disease is definitely a disease. However, in the context of twenty-first century Western allopathic medicine, the term disease is predicated on the notion that the disease being discussed or diagnosed is a singular matter of ill health (or absence of wellness) with a single cause that has been or will be defined, and a treatment process that can, or will be able to "cure" the disease (remove all the symptoms and restore the patient to a state of wellness).[3]

Another phenomenon I have noticed over the last twenty plus years is that diseases are defined ("created") when a profitable treatment becomes available. For instance, gastroesophageal reflux disease (GORD or GERD depending on how you choose to spell oesophagus or esophagus) only became a "disease" when drugs like proton pump inhibitors were seen to be profitable, if unsuccessful, treatments. Parkinson's disease will be defined as a "disease" while there are profits to be made from treating the symptoms.[4]

In my view, Parkinson's disease does not fit within this definition of a disease. It is, instead, a set of symptoms that vary from person to person, stemming from one or more of a wide range of aetiological pathways ("causes") that cannot be "cured", but *can be reversed*.

Try to forget that you have been diagnosed with a "disease". You simply have symptoms and, together, we will discover the causes of your symptoms, then develop strategies to reverse those causes. Once the causes have been removed, the symptoms will no longer exist and you can continue to work towards a state of wellness.

The Parkinson's process

We will be discussing, in some depth, the known causes of Parkinson's disease and strategies to reverse their effects, so this is probably a good time to look at what the journey to Parkinson's disease looks like.

Let's work backwards. Parkinson's disease symptoms may include: tremor at rest, paucity of movement or slowed movement (bradykinesia), loss of facial expression, rigid muscles, stooped posture, reduced sense of balance and gait problems (festination) or shuffling walk. Festination occurs when our steps become shorter while our centre of balance moves forward involuntarily, culminating in a complete loss of balance and falling forward. These can be considered dysregulations caused by relative deficiencies of dopamine, serotonin, anandamide and several other neurotransmitters. Other symptoms, not always associated with Parkinson's disease by medical professionals, but commonly experienced by patients, include loss of smell and taste senses, sleep dysregulation, dysuria and constipation. These symptoms, with "diseases" such as hypertension, gastroesophageal reflux disease and hypercholesterolemia are generally treated separately. Mild to moderate depression may also be present.

By the time Parkinson's disease is diagnosed, some symptoms have usually been present, often unnoticed, for several years. Many of my patients have been treated for hypertension for twenty years, depression for five to thirty years, GORD for ten to twenty years and hypercholesterolemia for many years also.

It seems likely that there can be direct influence on the brain that reduces production of those neurotransmitters required for optimal function (injury, toxins absorbed through scalp and skull, infections, electric and magnetic fields [EMF]) but also indirect influences, primarily via the gut.

Recent studies are showing that alpha-synuclein, a protein implicated in the processes we call various forms of dementia or Alzheimer's disease when misfolded, is also implicated in the expression of Parkinson's disease symptoms.[5] Extensive studies of gut bacteria are being funded to try to gain better understanding of the differences in the gut microbiome of those diagnosed with Parkinson's disease and "healthy" people, and whether changes in the gut microbiome causes mis-folding of alpha-synuclein. Dr Paul Clouston notes the finding of Lewy bodies (intraneuronal aggregates of a number of cellular proteins, the most prominent being a misshapen (misfolded) version of a normal neuronal protein called alpha-synuclein), normally expected in the upper brain stem (substantia nigra pars compacta), are also found in the lower brain stem, anterior olfactory nucleus, cerebral cortex, control centres for sleep physiology and vagus nerve function and, more significantly, in the walls of the bowel.[6] Dr Clouston goes on to say that this is "raising the intriguing possibility of the spread of Lewy body pathology into the central nervous system from the gastrointestinal tract via the vagus nerve".[7]

So our symptoms are caused by relative deficiencies in several neurotransmitters, which is caused by toxic assault to the brain or gut dysregulation and inefficient transport via the vagus nerve, which, in turn, are caused by inappropriate physical or emotional environments.

This is where we must start in our quest to find the real "causes" of Parkinson's disease and the means to create strategies for recovery.

One of the areas we will explore is more appropriate treatment of other chronic disorders such as hypertension, hypercholesterolemia, GORD, failing smell and taste sensations and mild depression which may reduce or eliminate the risk of developing Parkinson's disease in later years. Another question to be asked is why the average age for diagnosis of Parkinson's disease is falling. Once considered a disease of the ageing, people are now more commonly diagnosed with Parkinson's disease in their forties and fifties, but even as early as twelve years old![8] As we work through the known causes of neurodegeneration and chronicity, I think we will see answers to these questions.

Once we understand the aetiological pathways (basic processes) leading to a diagnosis of Parkinson's disease, we can take action to become healthy.

CHAPTER 3

A BRIEF HISTORY OF PARKINSON'S DISEASE AND ITS TREATMENT

It is difficult, if not impossible to know when Parkinson's disease was first noticed. Certainly there are descriptions of similar symptoms in ancient documents; Ayurvedic medicine and traditional Chinese medicine describe these symptom patterns and attribute them to various energy (Chi, Vata) dysregulations; Galen of Pergamon (also known as Aelius or Claudius Galen, 129 AD to circa 210 AD), wrote about the "shaking palsy" in 175 AD.[1]

The early descriptions and understanding of the "shaking palsy" are interesting in that each philosophy attempted to explain why the symptoms developed. The disciplines of anatomy and physiology were not sufficiently developed for physicians and researchers to explain the neurological mechanisms of the symptoms, with many medical philosophies based on a Hippocratic theory of four "humours".

Hippocrates of Ur (460-377 BC) is still considered the father of modern medicine, but much of his philosophy of medicine and healing has been forgotten in modern medical practice (to our detriment), including his continuing search for *why* disease symptoms develop rather than focusing only on *what* the symptoms are.

Galen extended our knowledge of anatomy based on animal dissection (and vivisection), so produced inaccuracies as he was not able to dissect human bodies. He was, undoubtedly, a most influential and important medical researcher who differentiated between tremor at rest and tremor with action, and described other cardinal signs now accepted to demonstrate Parkinson's disease.[2]

Medicine in the Western world (primarily Europe, England and America) moved away from "Why Medicine" to "What Medicine" during the nineteenth and early twentieth centuries. Wonderful progress in research techniques and medical devices allowed greater access to human anatomy and physiology, bringing ever-increasing knowledge of the minute, microscopic and even sub-microscopic activity that is part of the human existence.

This new knowledge was so exciting that many forgot the age-old question of WHY? We learnt about circulation, respiration, cells, organelles, bacteria, viruses, bone structure, hormones, enzymes and neurotransmitters among many thousands of other bits of knowledge about our marvellous bodies.

With this new, fantastic knowledge, it was tempting to believe that all answers about health and disease lay within the disciplines of anatomy, physiology and biology; that the answers to disease states could be gleaned through dissecting the tiny parts of the body to even tinier parts and watching them work or not work. We lost sight of the place of humanity in the world, and the influences for health and illness that are so powerful in our environment.

A further change occurred with the accidental discovery of penicillin in 1928 by Alexander Fleming. Howard Florey, Norman Heatley, and Ernst Chain (medical scientists) performed the first in-depth and focused studies on the drug and, in 1942, Anne Miller became the first civilian to receive successful treatment with penicillin, narrowly avoiding death following severe infection after a miscarriage.[3]

Penicillins and other antibiotics have saved countless lives from death and disablement from infection, but have created challenges with bacterial resistance (caused by overuse of these "wonder drugs") and an established medical view that, if we can identify a disease, we can find a drug or a surgical procedure that will "cure" it.

James Parkinson (1755-1824) sought a "cure" for Paralysis agitans (the shaking palsy), suggesting bloodletting and "emptying the bowels" could help, and urged others to work to this end. He did not suggest any environmental influences that may have caused the symptoms.[4]

Jean Martin Charcot (1825-93), a French neurologist, undertook significant research into the shaking palsy during the late nineteenth century, and named it Parkinson's disease in honour of James Parkinson.[5] However, it was not until the 1960s that low levels of dopamine in Parkinson's disease patients were observed and synthetic levodopa was first administered in 1961, but with uncertain results. In 1967, increasing doses of levodopa were tried with significant reduction of Parkinson's disease symptoms, but also increasing adverse effects.

It was not until the early 1970s that decarboxylase inhibitors were added to levodopa to reduce absorption of levodopa before entering the brain through the blood-brain-barrier, bringing much better results. The first commercially available "packaged" drug (levodopa packaged with carbidopa, a decarboxylase inhibitor) was introduced, and this has become the first-line treatment for people with Parkinson's. Many variations of the "dopamine theme" have been introduced – dopamine agonists (to stimulate dopamine receptors in the brain), COMT inhibitors (to reduce the activity of Catechol-O-Methyltransferase, an enzyme that breaks down dopamine in the brain), MAOB inhibitors (to reduce the activity of monoamine oxidase B, another enzyme that breaks down dopamine) – all with the aim of increasing the supply of dopamine in the brain. None have been as effective as levodopa replacement therapy although are still often prescribed.[6]

The view that the destruction of dopaminergic cells (cells that make dopamine) in the striatum nigra pars compacta (a tiny part of our mid brain rich in dopaminergic cells) is the sole or predominant cause of Parkinson's disease symptoms has persisted despite a lack of success in finding treatments and research describing a much wider view of aetiological pathways leading to Parkinson's disease symptoms.

Tim Lawrence, a former stuntman, was diagnosed with Parkinson's disease in 1994 and prescribed levodopa drugs but, by 1997, found his resultant dyskinesia (jerky, uncontrolled movements – an adverse effect of Parkinson's disease medication) almost unbearable. During a night out, he popped an ecstasy pill (MDMA) and found his dyskinesia symptoms almost disappeared for some hours.[7]

His case was studied at Hammersmith Hospital in London, where tests and scans showed that the ecstasy effect was not placebo and did not produce more dopamine. Rather, ecstasy stimulates production of serotonin (and also seems to increase hydration in the brain – more about that in later chapters).

Research with MDMA on mouse models followed and various hypothesis explored. However, the aim of all this research seemed to be finding new drugs to either offset the adverse effects of older drugs or stimulate dopamine production. Once again, there was/is an apparent lack of interest in environmental influences on our health status and/or strategies to create an overall state of health that will not allow Parkinson's disease symptoms to develop, or will reverse the external/endogenous influences that created the symptoms in the first place.

This is the reason for writing this book. Medical treatments for Parkinson's disease symptoms can be useful and helpful, but won't help you become well. Ninety-nine per cent or more of Parkinson's disease research money is spent on seeking new medications that may mitigate symptoms and will provide enormous profits to pharmaceutical manufacturers.

Diagnosis of Parkinson's disease must, ideally, include assessment of what has caused the symptoms in each individual. This will take much more time than the 20–30 minutes normally allowed for the first, diagnostic visit to a neurologist. Treatments must be aimed at not only mitigating symptoms (which is important, if possible without creating more "illness symptoms") but, primarily, at reversing the influences that created symptoms. Much of that will be self-help strategies.

There are, possibly, up to ten million people worldwide diagnosed with Parkinson's disease. A few have found ways to reverse the process and live without symptoms, yet these people are not studied or even interviewed by neurologists or scientists, and Parkinson's disease associations refuse to even consider the possibility of wellness.

We have the opportunity and knowledge to slow and even stop the epidemic of neurodegenerative disorders, including Parkinson's disease but, at the moment, we lack the will. Perhaps we can be the beginning of a healthy change.

CHAPTER 4

WESTERN ALLOPATHIC MEDICINE TREATMENT OF PARKINSON'S DISEASE

Diagnosis

One of the great challenges faced by those displaying symptoms that may be diagnosed as Parkinson's disease is the process of diagnosis; its efficacy and limitations.

The most common diagnostic pathway is a visit to a general practitioner (GP) or primary care physician (PCP) because some symptoms have begun to concern the patient, or someone close to them has noticed changes that are concerning. In a few cases, the GP/PCP will make a diagnosis of Parkinson's disease and prescribe medication (usually levodopa) without referring on to a specialist. More commonly, the patient will be referred to a neurologist/ movement disorder specialist who, ideally, will conduct a thorough physical examination and order a variety of scans and tests to rule out possible confounding or concomitant disorders such as tumour, stroke, multiple sclerosis or Wilson's disease.

The specialist may or may not conduct some specific tests to differentiate between Parkinson's disease, Multisystem Atrophy and Progressive Supranuclear Palsy if there is any suspicion of "atypical" symptoms (e.g. I was ultimately diagnosed with both Parkinson's disease and Multisystem Atrophy because of my complex pattern of symptoms).

In more recent years, a number of practitioners and patients have undertaken gene testing to see if they have a "Parkinson's gene". If the test indicates a mutation in one of the many genes now associated with Parkinson's disease and/or there is a family history of Parkinson's disease in close relatives, the diagnosis may be "familial" or "genetic" Parkinson's disease and the patient told that there is nothing to be done except mitigate symptoms.[1]

If there is no known genetic influence, and all tests for other possible disorders are negative, the diagnosis will be "idiopathic" Parkinson's disease – idiopathic meaning that the cause is unknown.

Once the pronouncement of "You have Parkinson's disease" is made, it is rarely questioned unless the patient seeks further examination from open-minded practitioners. In these rare cases, it is most likely that the aim of any further testing is to decide whether the patient has Multisystem Atrophy or Progressive Supranuclear Palsy (sometimes called "Parkinson's Plus" disorders) rather than idiopathic Parkinson's disease.

During the diagnosis process, there is no thought or examination of the possibility of nerve damage caused by heavy metals or other toxins such as glyphosate, the effects of early trauma (despite the findings of the Adverse Childhood Experience studies[2]) or underlying "stealth" infections. There has never been, to my knowledge, an examination of pharmaceutical drug consumption over ten or more years to understand the possibility of nerve damage as an adverse effect of a drug or polypharmacy rather an idiopathic process.

Western allopathic medicine specialists and researchers claim that around 20 per cent of people diagnosed with Parkinson's disease are, in fact, misdiagnosed. This means that up to two million people worldwide are being treated with potentially toxic therapies for an illness they do not have. As many Parkinson's disease treatments can create Parkinson's disease-like symptoms, these diagnoses become self-serving.[3,4,5]

Treatment

Parkinson's disease is known as a dopamine deficiency disorder, and Western allopathic medical treatment has focused on either replacing dopamine, reducing the uptake of dopamine, or preserving the effects of dopamine in the striatum nigra of affected people.

With the introduction of drugs containing levodopa packaged with decarboxylase inhibitors in the 1970s, quality of life for people with Parkinson's caused by dopamine deficiency was greatly enhanced, at least for several years.

Research into dopamine replacement/enhancing therapies continued apace. Pharmaceutical companies were well aware of the prevalence of Parkinson's disease estimated to now be between seven and ten million people worldwide (2019)[6] – and produced variations on the levodopa/decarboxylase inhibitor theme, dopamine agonists to stimulate dopamine receptors, COMT inhibitors to reduce the metabolic effects of catechol-O-methyltransferase which breaks down dopamine, and MAOB inhibitors to reduce the effects of monoamine oxidase which also breaks down dopamine. To overcome some of the long-term adverse effects of conservative pharmaceutical treatment of Parkinson's disease, doctors sometimes added back in some of the old anticholinergic drugs and even an old influenza drug that showed some promise in controlling tremor (albeit with some rather unpleasant adverse effects of its own).

There are many erudite and excellent texts on conservative treatments for people with Parkinson's, and most public libraries, and certainly any Parkinson's disease association, will be able to provide a number of books explaining in detail how and why Parkinson's disease is treated in the Western world. Reading some of these texts is a useful exercise in order to understand the entrenched view of this "mysterious, debilitating disease" we call Parkinson's disease.

Reading books by acknowledged "experts" in Parkinson's

disease and movement disorders will enhance our understanding of the Western allopathic medicine view of Parkinson's disease as a discrete, "stand-alone" disease with, potentially, a single cause and a single "cure". Western allopathic medicine research and publications can enhance our knowledge of the processes that degrade dopaminergic cells in and around the striatum nigra, and the focused approaches that are, and have been, used to preserve dopamine and attempt to slow or stop cell destruction.

This reading will also enhance our understanding of the limited view of Western allopathic medicine regarding possible causes and therapies. While there has been useful evolutionary research over many years, there has been no real revolutionary research into Parkinson's disease within the cloisters of Western allopathic medicine since levodopa experiments in the 1970s.

During the ten years following my recovery, I attempted to present information to Western allopathic medicine practitioners and organisations about the, then, hypothesised causes (or aetiological pathways) leading to a diagnosis of Parkinson's disease. My approaches were, for the most part, totally ignored while, in a few instances, I was accused of "quackery", "charlatanism", and anyone in these organisations who chose to listen to my presentations was demoted or fired.

It seemed, at that time, that Western allopathic medicine practitioners and organisations were only interested in maintaining and expanding the status quo of treatment – that is, a focus on dopamine – and complementary/alternative medicine ideas and hypotheses looking at other possible aetiological pathways and strategies for reducing symptoms were not worth even considering.

In the first part of the twenty first century, some symptom-reducing strategies have become more acceptable. Exercise, dancing, singing, meditation and some bodywork strategies are encouraged rather than dismissed as useless, and many patients benefit from this changing attitude.

Treatment of people with Parkinson's by Western allopathic medicine practitioners will almost invariably focus on replacing dopamine, preserving the life of dopamine in the striatum nigra and mitigating symptoms where possible. There may be some brief discussion of the "Mediterranean Diet" (a very poorly understood concept, usually translated to include grains and animal dairy – both damaging; but much better than the standard American/Australian diet), but little or no actual instruction.[7] Patients may be referred to a dietitian, especially if they are constipated, and often referred to a physiotherapist who may or may not be helpful. There may be a brief mention of exercise with no details.

Advantages of Western allopathic medicine treatment for Parkinson's disease include moderately rapid relief of symptoms if the patient is deficient in dopamine (not always the prime factor), a sense of security in having a definite diagnosis and prognosis (even if they are wrong), full or part payment of treatment costs by public health funds or private health insurance, access to full or partly funded allied health professionals such as physiotherapists, dietitians and psychologists, access to hospital treatment if necessary and the possibility of some respite accommodation.

Disadvantages include no acknowledgement of the possibility of the aetiological pathways discussed later, lack of knowledge in regard to health-giving food choices and other environmental impacts on the illness/health process, the possibility that Western allopathic medicine treatment of concomitant "illnesses" (hypertension, anxiety, depression, gastroesophageal reflux disease, migraine, etc.) may exacerbate Parkinson's disease symptoms and Parkinson's disease treatment may exacerbate these other "illnesses". In my experience, there is little coherent communication between medical specialists, and interactions between prescribed drugs is common.

Perhaps the two greatest disadvantages are "nocebo" and the

impact of treatment on those misdiagnosed. Almost all Western allopathic medicine practitioners will tell their patients that they cannot get well and there is little or nothing patients can do the help themselves. This attitude can and does often exacerbate symptoms by causing feelings of hopelessness and helplessness. Thoughts and feelings are chemical processes and negative thoughts/feelings reduce the supply of dopamine, serotonin and anandamide, all of which are critical for wellness.

Parkinson's disease drugs, by their very nature will, over time, exacerbate or create Parkinson's disease symptoms such as tremor, bradykinesia, "frozen face", anxiety, constipation and confusion, "proving" a diagnosis in the long-term.

In order to move towards wellness, patients must accept the support and knowledge of their Western allopathic medicine doctor and/or specialist but seek advice and support for health-giving strategies from open-minded allied health therapists or complementary/alternative medicine practitioners.

My dream is many holistic health centres dotted around the world where practitioners from many disciplines work harmoniously together to bring peace and health to patients and explore the enormous gaps in our knowledge of degenerative disorders. These centres would see Western allopathic medicine and complementary/alternative medicine practitioners working together, acknowledging the benefits and shortcomings of all therapies, being respectful and supportive to each other, and working together to benefit patients first.

This cannot happen while money dominates the discussion as now. It is time to remember three important principles laid down by Hippocrates of Ur, the "Father of Modern Medicine":

- First, do no harm
- Let food be thy medicine and medicine thy food;
and, in my view, the most important:
    The measure of love he gives to his patient counts above all.

CHAPTER 5

COMPLEMENTARY/ALTERNATIVE MEDICINE APPROACHES TO PARKINSON'S DISEASE – AN OVERVIEW

Complementary/alternative medicine practitioners are often unwilling to treat patients diagnosed with Parkinson's disease as there is little offered in the universities and colleges to encourage a view of assisting wellness.

The most common attitude from teachers is that we can only mitigate symptoms by offering alternatives to common Parkinson's disease drugs, albeit with less adverse effects than pharmaceutical drugs.

During the twenty years following my recovery in 1998, I approached several colleges in Australia and USA offering my research, experience and services to bring clearer and expanded knowledge to the discussion about Parkinson's disease and its treatment. My own college engaged me as a guest lecturer for final-year students where I was able to tell my story and explain the principles behind holistic treatment of Parkinson's disease, and I continued this work until the college closed. No other Australian college or university has evinced any interest in this work. Standard complementary medicine texts in Australia quote the Western allopathic medicine view of Parkinson's disease as a dopamine deficiency disorder, but they do emphasise the importance of gut health, nervous system support and mitochondrial health, which is a great advantage over Western allopathic medicine texts.[1]

My approaches to some of the largest and most respected colleges in USA were met with a total lack of interest. While those I spoke with were courteous, my follow-up correspondence was ignored. One of my challenges in approaching such institutions was/is lack of academic qualifications. It is unfortunate that, within the hallowed halls of complementary/alternative medicine education, a PhD in almost anything health-related carries much more weight than experience and results. I hope this will change in time.

There is some potentially useful research emanating from one of these colleges, but its impact is reduced by a limited aim and poor study design. Much, if not all the information to be gained from this study is already available from a variety of other studies and research projects, perhaps not as coherently, but still available, and the money spent on this Parkinson's disease study could well have been directed towards looking at one of the aetiological pathways and ways to reverse the illness results of that pathway.

However, even though I am critical of the limited view of complementary/alternative medicine academia, there is some excellent work done in supporting those diagnosed with Parkinson's disease and helping them achieve a higher quality of life.

Therapies supporting gut function, immune system and mitochondria are a general focus, while therapies mitigating drug adverse effects help many patients. Detox protocols (when not over-rigorous) are helpful to many, and can assist in reversing one of the major aetiological pathways.

Many complementary/alternative medicine practitioners are able to provide body work (Bowen therapy, massage, Feldenkrais and others), exercise direction (Pilates, yoga, boxing, high-intensity interval training, directed exercise regimens), emotional and psychological support, and may encourage self-help activities such as meditation, singing and dancing.

Advantages of complementary/alternative medicine include general lack of toxicity (assuming prescriptions comply with current research), a more holistic approach to health, a more common application of the Hippocrates principle of "first do no harm", repair of some body systems which improves overall health and so reduce the impact of Parkinson's disease symptoms, and a general willingness to engage with and listen to patients in clinic.

Disadvantages are a lack of willingness to focus on aetiological pathways, so reducing the helpful impact of therapies, extra costs for the patients as most public health funds and private health insurance pay little or nothing for complementary/alternative medicine treatments, and unwillingness on the part of most Western allopathic medicine practitioners to engage with or correspond with complementary/alternative medicine practitioners; this reduces the possibility of excellent outcomes through utilisation of combined therapies.

One rather unpleasant disadvantage is the plethora of "quacks" claiming to be complementary/alternative medicine therapists with answers. Now, there are certainly "quacks" in Western allopathic medicine, although we could consider these to be ignorant bigots rather than quacks perhaps. Complementary/alternative medicine quacks claim to have "cures" for many illness, including Parkinson's disease, offer expensive multi-level marketing "remedies", and/or sell their own brands of formulas and supplements without any evidence of efficacy or safety. These are despicable human beings who deserve condemnation. The same can be said about Western allopathic medicine practitioners who refuse to see the evidence of patients improving their health, close their eyes to Western medical research proving many complementary/alternative medicine principles, and continue to condemn patients to lives of misery.

We must weed out quacks and pretenders, and use "people power" to change the attitude of doctors to one of hope and helpfulness.

Parkinson's disease is a set of symptoms that may be "incurable", but the fact remains that we can reverse the illness process and become well.[2]

SECTION 2

WHAT CAUSES PARKINSON'S DISEASE?

CHAPTER 6

CAUSES AND DEVELOPMENT OF PARKINSON'S DISEASE

Conservative, considered, contentious

Millions of dollars are being spent to find a single cause for this set of symptoms we call Parkinson's disease. Most of this money is being used to study minute proteins, enzymes or cells that may, or may not, be involved in the development of Parkinson's symptoms.

At the same time, we can see some excellent research into the effects of lifestyle and food, childhood health and experiences, response to infections, exercise and social activities. Much of this research shows increased risk of neurodegenerative disorders in certain circumstances; not just Parkinson's disease, but including Parkinson's disease in the disorders more likely to develop, given specific life circumstances, food choices, environmental impacts or social structure.

Given that most of the "risk research" is conducted by medical experts and/or medical researchers, one could ask why someone in Parkinson's research has not joined the dots and instituted research to look much more deeply into these likely aetiological pathways and, from this, develop recovery strategies.

Many erudite books and papers have been presented on this subject and I do not consider it my place to explain the workings of research organisations. Suffice to say that most medical research is funded largely by commercial interests who want to see the prospect of profit at the end of the research period, and this is their right and responsibility to shareholders. Unfortunately, this funding model excludes research that may lead to development of self-help strategies and reduced reliance on pharmaceutical medication or medical intervention. Improving health and recovery is not profitable.

More concerning is the influence of Western allopathic medicine "experts" and the "single-cause-disease-single-cure" (SCDSC) view of disease in prominent Parkinson's organisations led by celebrities or business people who have been affected by a Parkinson's disease diagnosis. This view allows for development of one or a small group of pharmaceutical interventions that will "cure" a "disease". But this assumes that every case of Parkinson's disease is caused by the same thing or things, develops along the same pathway, and will respond identically to intervention. We know that this is simply not true. But the imposition of this SCDSC view on these organisations funnels many millions of dollars into studies of minutiae or trivial changes in microscopic particles that, while interesting or even fascinating, bring us no closer to understanding aetiological pathways or recovery strategies.

Another challenge is the entrenched belief that Parkinson's is a single, separate, discrete "disease", hence its name of Parkinson's "disease". There is an alternative view (which I share) that Parkinson's is, actually, a group of debilitating symptoms stemming from a number of aetiological pathways that may be identified as one of a wide range of "diseases" supported by numerous organisations seeking "cures" for their "disease", rather than combining their efforts to find ways to create wellness.

Studies are being or have been conducted to support the hypothetical aetiological pathways discussed in this book. Yes, they are, as yet, hypothetical simply because there is not sufficient financial support to conduct large-scale randomised studies to prove (or disprove) the hypotheses. But there is a large body of evidence that does support these hypotheses – not specific Parkinson's disease studies, but well-designed, large-scale population studies that show increased risk for Parkinson's disease given particular influences or circumstances. As most people diagnosed with Parkinson's disease have experienced more than one of these increased-risk circumstances, we can calculate that their risk increases exponentially with each extra increased-risk circumstance.

For instance, if person A experienced a high-stress childhood (perhaps they were abused in some way), chooses to eat inflammatory foods known to increase the likelihood of neurodegenerative disorders, and finds work in a factory using a lot of degreasers or petroleum-based products, their risk of developing a neurodegenerative disorder is very high, and that disorder may be Parkinson's disease, or it may be another form of neurodegenerative disorder such as dementia, amyotrophic lateral sclerosis (ALS), progressive supranuclear palsy (PSP), etc.

Person B may have a wonderful childhood and enter a career where toxic chemicals are rare, but still eat a typical Western diet high in inflammatory foods. While they have some risk of disease because, perhaps, their work is sedentary and their food choices unfortunate, they have a lower risk of developing a neurodegenerative disorder such as Parkinson's disease.

There are genetic influences that enhance our predisposition to develop certain disorders (or sets of symptoms), given appropriate gene triggers. Scientists have found several "Parkinson's genes" that may increase the risk of developing Parkinson's disease; but, remember, genes don't *cause* disease; genes express proteins and must be activated by some form of trigger before their activity becomes troublesome.[1,2]

The pathway to illness (any degenerative or chronic illness) is:

1. Circumstances that create an unhealthy environment around cells
2. Messages from the environment changing gene expression

3. Inappropriate production of proteins (such as misfolded alpha-synuclein)

4. Cell damage

5. Symptoms manifested

6. Disease diagnosis.

Current research indicates three major aetiological pathways that can lead to the ultimate diagnosis of a chronic degenerative disease:

1. Unresolved trauma or long-term stress early in life

2. Environmental toxins (including foods)

3. Chronic infections.

These are the pathways we will explore over the next few chapters, then look at ways to reverse the pathways and their physiological effects.

CHAPTER 7

WHAT CAUSES PARKINSON'S?

Aetiological pathways leading to diagnosis

Is it genetic?

Genes are groups of DNA which act as instructions for cells to produce protein molecules.

Some genes are very firmly established during conception and gestation (pregnancy) and are unlikely to change ("switch on or off") without significant external intervention. Others tend to switch on or off (change their gene expression) according to stimuli provided from around the cell.

With the rapid increase of relatively inexpensive tests to determine our genome and genetic predispositions, many people are becoming afraid of genetic inheritances which may never cause any problems.

For instance, we may inherit the gene for cancer, so undertake rigorous treatment to prevent cancer that may not develop if we eliminate all triggers for the expressions of that gene. A tragic case in point are women who undergo bilateral mastectomies because they have the "gene for breast cancer", yet continue to live a stressful and carcinogenic lifestyle. Many go on to develop cancer elsewhere caused by lifestyle, not genes. On the other hand, many others with the breast cancer gene live a healthy, wellness-creating lifestyle, retain their breasts, and never have a hint of developing cancer.

We can switch genes on and off depending on how we choose to live. Professor Bruce Lipton explains this wonderfully in his book *The Biology of Belief*,[1] while there is a very clear explanation of epigenetics on page 4 of *The Dark Side of Wheat*.[2] It is often fairly easy to estimate our genetic inheritance by looking at our family history without going to the expense of undergoing gene testing. For instance, I can tell that I have genetic predispositions to Parkinson's disease, heart disease, stroke, cancer and dementia simply by observing the health and illness of my ancestors and immediate family.

It is estimated that we all carry around 1000 single nucleotide polymorphisms (SNPs), the so-called gene mutations that have gained the reputation of causing disease.[3,4] If we don't have our genome mapped, we will never know what SNPs we carry and, for most of us, it will never matter. Genetic SNPs will only affect us if we choose to live lives that will trigger unhealthy expression of proteins controlled by those genes that are lying dormant until lifestyle choices or involuntary exposure to disease triggers cause mutation.

Population studies tell us that between 5 and 15 per cent of diagnosed Parkinson's disease cases occur in family clusters, leaving up to 95 per cent thought to be non-genetic in origin.[5]

A word of caution: some of my patients have done genetic testing and been told that they have the gene for Parkinson's disease, with the implication that there is nothing they can do about it.

Here's the truth of the matter: there are many "Parkinson's genes", including LRRK2, PARK1, PINK1, PRKN and SNCA,[6] that are of no concern unless switched on by other triggers; if we live well, they will not be activated. Even if they are, we can reverse the process that triggered the expression of the genes, therefore eliminating their influence.

Other aetiological pathways (causes)

There seem to be three major groups of triggers that begin the process of degeneration, ultimately creating groups of symptoms diagnosed as Parkinson's disease. We will discuss each one and suggest strategies to reverse their influence in later chapters, but here are details of each pathway.

CHAPTER 8

THE TRAUMA PATHWAY

Trauma, Oxford Dictionary:[1]
> A deeply distressing or disturbing experience
> Emotional shock following a stressful event or physical
> injury, which may lead to long term neurosis
> Physical injury
> Origin: Late 17th Century: from Greek; literally "wound".

Esther Giller, president of the Sidran Institute, writes, "But the key to understanding traumatic events is that it refers to extreme stress that overwhelms a person's ability to cope. There are no clear divisions between stress, trauma, and adaptation." She goes on to say, "What I want to emphasise is that it is an individual's *subjective experience* that determines whether an event is or is not traumatic."[2]

Stress:
> A physical, chemical, or emotional factor that causes
> bodily or mental tension and may be a factor in disease
> causation.[3]

The experience of stress or trauma is different for each person. Circumstances that create little disturbance in the physical and emotional equilibrium of one person may cause ongoing mental and emotional challenges in another, with the possibility of physical challenges or "disease" in the long-term.

Undoubtedly, repeated traumas, or ongoing stress, have higher risk of long-term damage than one incident, no matter how horrible. Ongoing stress may seem minor or unimportant, even to the person experiencing that stress, but it can create emotional, mental or physical challenges over many years.

Stress is a word (with its derivatives) bandied around by us all, sometimes correctly (working permanent night shift on a North Sea oil rig is stressful), sometimes over-emphasising the importance of a circumstance with little impact (*"I was stressed out because I couldn't find my mascara"*). The word "stress" has lost much of its true meaning, and the real impact of long-term stress has become discounted by many, including health professionals.

The discovery of Helicobacter pylori as a cause of peptic ulcers led to many public figures (including a previous Australian Prime Minister) stating that stress had no part to play in the development of peptic ulcers. This position ignored the questions of why do some people, but not all, develop overgrowth of Helicobacter pylori? Why do some people develop peptic ulcers without the presence of H. pylori? What is the long-term effect of antibiotics on the gut microbiome and overall health? How well is food digested when gastric acid secretion is inhibited as required in standard treatment of peptic ulcers?

Victoroff,[4] McEwen[5] and others have elegantly described the detrimental effects of long-term stress on gut function and our ability to digest food. Reduced gut function also increases the risk of infection, increasing the possibility of H. pylori overgrowth and other infectious diseases of the gastrointestinal tract.

Studies in 2015–17 showed that a protein associated with the onset of Parkinson's disease, alpha-synuclein (aS) is formed in the gastrointestinal tract as a protective mechanism when infections occur.[6] Repeated or ongoing infections may cause the production of aS to overwhelm the aS clearance system, allowing aS to migrate to the brain and cause cell damage there.[7]

Medical logic would then indicate that suppressing gastrointestinal tract infections with antibiotics may prevent the overgrowth of aS and reduce the risk of Parkinson's. But overuse of antibiotics creates antibiotic-resistant bacteria which can then cause infections we cannot treat conventionally, creating more aS as our body struggles to cope with infectious overwhelm, leading to further brain damage.

We need to remember that a prominent underlying cause of suppressed gut function and propensity to disease is long-term stress. A pathway to Parkinson's disease might be (and this is yet to be proven) many years of unremitting stress, gut infection, overproduction of aS, migration of aS to the brain via the vagus nerve, cell damage and the appearance of physical symptoms diagnosed as Parkinson's disease or dementia, or some other "disease".

But unremitting stress has far more insidious adverse effects than a propensity to increased gut infection. The long-term effects may directly lead to neuro-dysregulation, which may then be diagnosed as Parkinson's disease or similar.

Since 1998, I have examined and worked with over 2000 people from many countries diagnosed with Parkinson's disease. In each case, I have taken the most thorough life and health history possible, examining all aspects of childhood, growth and adult experiences.

One factor stands out as a common denominator among 98 per cent of these patients. Each person has experienced high stress or trauma at some stage during their first fifteen years. Some traumas began in utero; for others, in early childhood; for a few, in early teens. Many of the traumas are obvious – abuse of various types, loss of a parent or sibling, life-threatening disease or accident. Some are not so obvious and we must look closely at our patient's life history to find circumstances that may result in unremitting stress or perceived trauma. In 2 per cent of cases, we have been unable to find a direct link to early-life trauma. Only 2 per cent!

For some patients, trauma/stress is a primary pathway to Parkinson's. For many, it is one of two or more aetiological pathways that, together, have created a degenerative state of being. We cannot ignore the influence that long-term stress and trauma has on all human physiological processes.

Stress can be good for us as it motivates us to activity and provides the physiological resources for that activity. Without some level of stress, we would not get out of bed in the morning. Our alarm device wakes us as planned, hunger drives us from bed, our need or desire for income sends us to our work, the needs of our children extend from early morning to late evening.

These stresses are a normal part of life and, if they bring rewards of satiety, income or love, are beneficial stresses with few, if any, disadvantages. However, if we allow the circumstances causing stress to become onerous or dominant, they may then cause health challenges.

For instance, I have seen many young business people who were fatigued, struggling to accomplish their tasks each day, and displaying depressed mood because of their tiredness and struggle to perform. But some simple changes to eating habits, a couple of basic nutritional supplements and hygienic sleep habits transformed their energy and mood. Their various stresses then became incentives to complete rewarding tasks each day or care for children who responded with love.

But many people experience stress that is onerous yet difficult to change, either in perception or in fact. We may feel locked into work where we experience bullying or unfair expectations, and be unable to see a way to leave or alter our circumstances because we have family responsibilities and really need the income. Or we may be in an unsatisfactory or even emotionally abusive relationship and feel unable to leave because of financial dependence, responsibility for children, or because we are under threat.

Long-term night shift creates physical and emotional stresses that are often unrecognised. Sleep patterns are disturbed, especially as rest days are experienced in "normal time", then night shift recommences; relationships with friends and lovers may be difficult because free times are different. Chronic fatigue is common among night shift workers, as are feelings of isolation and disorientation during rest days.

Rotating shift patterns can also create difficulties as workers struggle to adapt to constantly changing sleep and meal patterns, attempt to maintain relationships with those on normal time and seek to maintain energy.

Trauma need not be physically damaging if it is treated and resolved healthily and holistically. But there are traumas that are not or cannot be treated and healed for a variety of reasons – traumatic abuse is often hidden for many years and its effects may become embedded physically as well as emotionally; social trauma (war, invasion, natural disasters, oppressive government) may take years to escape and the physiological effects remain unrecognised; post-traumatic stress disorder (PTSD) is still usually treated as an emotional/mental disorder rather than physical or physiological.

Prolonged stress and unresolved trauma trigger our body into continuous stress reactions that, over a long time, become damaging.

The initial physiological reaction to any type of significant stress or trauma is the "flight, fight, freeze" response. Simply put, the process is this:

- Our adrenal glands, situated on top of our kidneys, have two major sections, the medulla and cortex;
- Excretion of adrenal medullary hormones is directly triggered by stress and trauma;
- Stress and trauma stimulate the hypothalamus to release Corticotropin-releasing hormone (CRH);
- CRH stimulates the release of Adrenocorticotropic Hormone (ACTH) from the pituitary gland;
- ACTH regulates excretions from the adrenal cortex.

Hormones released by the adrenals are:

Medulla (adrenaline and noradrenaline)

(US: epinephrine and norepinehrine) – derived from the amino acid Tyrosine (with co-factor tetrahydrobiopterin). As levodopa (precursor to dopamine) is also derived from tyrosine (in the biopterin cycle), increased production of adrenaline/noradrenaline "competes" with the production of dopamine.

Cortex (steroids)

- mineralocorticoids (aldosterone)
- glucocorticoids (cortisol)
- adrenal androgens (testosterone)

Effects of adrenal hormones

Adrenaline

- Increases blood glucose by activating cyclic AMP.
- Increases glycogen breakdown (decreases reserves of glucose)
- Increases intracellular metabolism of glucose in skeletal muscles (for action)
- Increases breakdown of fats in adipose tissue
- Increases heart rate
- Increases force of heart contraction
- Constricts blood vessels in skin, kidneys, gastrointestinal tract (GIT) and other organs not needed for fight/flight
- Dilates blood vessels in skeletal and cardiac muscle.

Prolonged expression of adrenaline at stress levels may create exhaustion, elevated blood sugar, hypertension and heart stress.

Aldosterone

- Increases rate of sodium (Na) reabsorption in kidneys
  * Increased plasma Na
  * Increased water reabsorption (may lead to oedema?)

* Increased blood volume (may lead to hypertension?)
- Increases potassium (K) excretion (lower plasma K)
- Increases hydrogen (H) ion excretion (acidic urine, increased metabolic pH – alkalosis)
- Changes in Na/K balance can affect cellular hydration which, in turn, can affect cell efficiency.

Chronic expression of aldosterone may be implicated in changes to tissue pH (causing loss of efficiency and/or pain).

Cortisol

- Increases catabolism of fats
- Decreases glucose and amino acid uptake in skeletal muscles
- Increases glucose synthesis from amino acids in the liver, leading to increased blood glucose
- Increases protein degradation (causing muscle weakness/atrophy, osteoporosis)
- Decreases inflammatory response by decreasing number of white cells and the expression of inflammatory chemicals (causing depressed immune system).

Over-expression of cortisol is implicated in reduced immune function, fatigue and weakness, making patients more vulnerable to seasonal or opportunistic infections.

Testosterone (indirect and mainly in women)

- Increases pubic and axillary hair
- Increases sexual drive (but may reduce potency).

Short-term stress is a normal part of life. We need it for motivation, and we need the physiological responses to stress in order to survive. Our forebears faced immediate dangers and stimuli every day in living – for instance, they needed to chase down prey, or run away from predators, or fight enemies to protect their territory or families.

In all these cases, the stress was resolved quite quickly – they won or lost, caught the prey or waited until the next day, got away or got eaten.

We have negative feedback systems to adjust levels of adrenal hormones so they do not become damaging. However, *long-term stress can override these negative feedback systems* so that we go on hyper-producing stress chemicals. All animals have developed a fight/flight/freeze response to enhance survival prospects in dangerous environments. For most animals in their natural habitat, safety and danger are easily recognisable conditions. We do see, however, chronic stress behaviours and illnesses manifesting in animals kept in captivity, for instance, or deprived of their ability to roam over their normal territories. Humans are now constantly deprived of natural environments suitable for healthy living. We confine ourselves in immovable houses, restrict our activities to regulated programs to earn income or support families, operate under artificial light for much of the day, subject ourselves to noise, toxins, EMF and poor-quality foods.

Professor Bruce McEwen has estimated that constant stress for only six weeks can lock our body into permanent fight/flight/freeze response unless specific action is taken to break the cycle.[8] As the effects of six weeks plus of stress are rarely, if ever, recognised by primary care practitioners, restorative action is not taken.

Many stresses in this society are not resolved, and many traumas go unrecognised. We live surrounded by noise, pollution, busy-ness and poisons. Child abuse is the world's best kept secret (even though there is much more acknowledgement of this scourge now than in previous decades); family breakdown is seen as traumatic for the partners, but not necessarily for the children; the loss of a sibling or grandparent or friend is often borne in silence by the young in our society.

Prolonged and unresolved stress or trauma can result in:

- Increased plasma sodium
- Decreased plasma potassium
- Cellular dehydration
- Reprogramming of the hypothalamus
- Chronic heart stress and eventual failure
- Alkalosis (often treated with antacids when the primary symptom is reflux!)
- Hypertension
- Weak skeletal muscles
- Acidic urine
- Hyperglycemia leading to diabetes mellitus
- Deficient immune system
- Muscle atrophy
- General weakness and debility
- Osteoporosis
- Weak capillaries
- Thin skin that bruises easily
- Impaired wound healing
- Inappropriate fat distribution (face, neck, abdomen)
- Mood swings (euphoria and depression).

In women

- Hirsutism
- Increased sex drive
- Diminished breast size
- Menstrual irregularities.

People facing prolonged, unresolved stress or trauma will respond in different ways, possibly dictated by their genetic inheritance and/or environment. Some will develop heart disease, cancer, arthritis, diabetes, skin disorders, depression or other psychological disorders, gastric ulcers (with an overgrowth of H. pylori) or inappropriate behaviours such as substance addictions, addictive gambling or violent behaviour.

Some will develop neurological and/or autoimmune disorders. The reprogramming of the hypothalamus and cellular dehydration, as well as many of the other effects shown above, increase production and distribution of misfolded alpha-synuclein, allow some brain cells to become damaged or inactive, or even die, over many years, ultimately resulting in the expression of neurological disorder symptoms.

Many patients who come to my clinic do not recognise any high stress or trauma in their past, primarily because their childhood circumstances were "normal" to them. For instance, a child growing up with a father who was often drunk after work, became abusive and violent when intoxicated, but only abused their mother rather than the children, may not consider that traumatic, as the abuse was not directed at them personally. However, the circumstance of seeing their mother abused by someone who was supposed to care for them creates fear, uncertainty, perhaps frustration with themselves for being incapable of protecting their mother, and conflicts of love and hate for their father.

A patient reported that they had experienced a "pretty good" childhood. On questioning, however, we found that their mother had died when they were very young so they relied on their father for some years. Father remarried when my patient was five and, while my patient reported that "she was a pretty good stepmother", there was a difference in the way children and step-children were treated, causing a sense of loss for their birth mother.

Traumas between conception and birth are not uncommon. Perhaps the circumstances that are most obvious are social traumas during pregnancy – war, imprisonment (concentration camps, refugee detention, for instance), or natural disasters such as fire and flood. The overwhelming fear experienced by the mother creates hormone imbalances in the womb. The baby is provided with inappropriate amounts of testosterone and cortisol, affecting growth patterns of their nervous system. In fact, the baby may be born already locked into fight/flight/freeze response.

Other circumstances during pregnancy may have similar effects. The mother, losing their parent or sibling, becomes locked in grief, fear and uncertainty; or may be involved in family squabbling over inheritance creating moderate to long-term fight/flight/freeze response. Disruptive or abusive relationships during pregnancy can have devastating effects of baby's progress.

> **Patient A:** *Mum was living in London while pregnant during World War II. When the first air raid warning siren sounded, Mum ran towards the nearest shelter, slipped on the wet road, fell heavily and lost the baby. A little over a year later, she gave birth to a healthy child, despite air raids continuing. Eighteen months or so after the birth, Mum was pregnant again, running towards a shelter with her toddler, fell and lost her baby again. My patient grew up in a household heavy with grief and anger, feeling inadequate to fulfil the needs and wants of her parents.*

> **Patient B:** *During pregnancy, the father became discontented with the constraints of parenthood, began drinking heavily and was emotionally and physically abusive to his pregnant wife. The mother escaped the household before giving birth, but circumstances were difficult, with little money or support. The child was born in fear and uncertainty, without a father's care.*

Trauma or high stress during childhood is easier to trace if we spend time to fully explore our patient's early life. Sometimes stories have not been told before we ask the questions; perhaps patients have told only therapists who do not see a connection between emotional disruption and physical illness symptoms; perhaps children have been told to "buckle up and get on with it", so have suppressed their feelings of fear, anger, frustration or worthlessness and "got on with it" until the chronic fight/flight/freeze response they were sublimating created physical symptoms.

Patient C: *He was seventy-eight when he came to see me and had been a fit, hardworking farmer all his life. He left school early and loved working on the land. Being diagnosed with Parkinson's disease was a great shock and the prognosis left him devastated. His written history showed no sign of trauma in his childhood but, during a conversation about school, he mentioned a distrust of priests. Talking about this feeling became more and more difficult until he began to cry (for the first time in memory) and revealed that he had been sexually abused by a priest at his school. He felt unable to tell his parents as they were staunch church members and respected that priest. My patient had suppressed that horror, anger and grief for seventy years, not even telling his wife, until physical illness opened a way to reveal his past.*

Patient D: *As an only child in a conservative home, my patient was sometimes lonely so, when an uncle offered a picnic by the river, she was very happy. Rather than a picnic, the uncle raped her repeatedly until she lost consciousness, then threw her into the river to drown. My patient managed to escape and found her way home, but felt unable to speak about her horror to her parents. The uncle had reported an "accident" and joined the joyful celebrations when she was found "safe and well". She was in her sixties before finding her voice and revealing that childhood experience. By then illness symptoms had become obvious.*

Patient E: *A lovely baby girl was adopted by wonderful parents at nine months of age. She was nurtured and cared for by her adoptive parents and loved them dearly. However, the first nine months of her life had been spent in the care of her birth mother who loved her despairingly (she knew she could not keep her child long-term), breast fed, bathed and changed her child with enormous love. The* *trauma of being taken from her birth mother, even into a loving family, was not recognised until, in her thirties, illness symptoms began to develop. Sometimes love is not enough.*

Adverse Childhood Experiences (ACE) Study

This remarkable study, the result of cooperation between the Centers for Disease Control and Prevention USA (CDC) and Kaiser Permanente (an American integrated managed care consortium, based in Oakland, California USA), followed the health outcomes of over 17,000 Health Maintenance Organisation members from Southern California receiving physical exams who completed confidential surveys regarding their childhood experiences and current health status and behaviours. Data was collected in two waves between 1995 and 1997.[9]

The CDC says: *"Childhood experiences, both positive and negative, have a tremendous impact on future violence, victimisation and perpetration, and lifelong health and opportunity. As such, early experiences are an important public health issue. Much of the foundational research in this area has been referred to as Adverse Childhood Experiences (ACEs)."*[10]

This study was, and probably still is, the largest and most wide-ranging of its kind, and has yielded important information for healthcare and welfare agencies, allowing better distribution of scarce resources and improved management of chronic illness.

As with any large study, there are limitations on the experiences classified as ACEs, and health outcomes are generalised rather than nominating specific "diseases" which, in my view, is a sensible approach.

ACEs, in this study, were classified into three sections: Abuse; Household Challenges; Neglect.[11] There was no data collected on social trauma (war, rebellion, oppression), traumatic events (flood, fire, injury), "inherited trauma" (e.g. children and grandchildren of Holocaust victims or survivors; children of refugees) or dramatic changes in circumstances such as moving from country to city, frequently changing addresses or striving to fit within a blended family. However, the results are valuable as they show a marked propensity to physical and mental dysregulation following even one adverse childhood event. The impact on physical and mental health increases with the number of adverse events and the length of time the event lasted.[12]

All ACE questions refer to the respondent's first eighteen years of life.

ACE definitions in this study[13] were:

Abuse

- **Emotional abuse:** A parent, stepparent, or adult living in your home swore at you, insulted you, put you down, or acted in a way that made you afraid that you might be physically hurt.
- **Physical abuse:** A parent, stepparent, or adult living in your home pushed, grabbed, slapped, threw something at you, or hit you so hard that you had marks or were injured.
- **Sexual abuse:** An adult, relative, family friend, or stranger who was at least five years older than you ever touched or fondled your body in a sexual way, made you touch his/her body in a sexual way, attempted to have any type of sexual intercourse with you.

Household challenges

- **Mother treated violently:** Your mother or stepmother was pushed, grabbed, slapped, had something thrown at her, kicked, bitten, hit with a fist, hit with something hard, repeatedly hit for over at least a few minutes, or ever threatened or hurt by a knife or gun by your father (or stepfather) or mother's boyfriend.
- **Household substance abuse:** A household member was a problem drinker or alcoholic or a household member used street drugs.

- **Mental illness in household:** A household member was depressed or mentally ill or a household member attempted suicide.

- **Parental separation or divorce:** Your parents were ever separated or divorced.

- **Criminal household member:** A household member went to prison.

Neglect*

- **Emotional neglect:** Someone in your family helped you feel important or special, you felt loved, people in your family looked out for each other and felt close to each other, and your family was a source of strength and support.†

- **Physical neglect:** There was someone to take care of you, protect you, and take you to the doctor if you

---

* Collected during Wave 2 only.

† Items were reverse-scored to reflect the framing of the question.

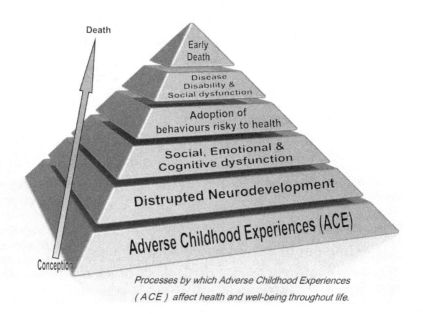

Processes by which Adverse Childhood Experiences
(A C E) affect health and well-being throughout life.

needed it,‡ you didn't have enough to eat, your parents were too drunk or too high to take care of you, and you had to wear dirty clothes.

The prevalence of ACEs in this study was estimated at nearly 64 per cent. That is, more than six out of ten children experienced one or more adverse events from the above list. Data from other government agencies in USA, Australia and Europe indicates that this may be a low estimate, particularly if other ACEs are included.

Nothing in this study suggested that Adverse Childhood Experiences *cause* Parkinson's disease. However, there is a very distinct move towards ill-health, unhealthy lifestyles and risky behaviour. There is certainly an increase in autoimmune disease and other chronic disorders.

The ACE Pyramid represents the conceptual framework for the ACE Study. The ACE Study has uncovered how ACEs are strongly related to development of risk factors for disease, and wellbeing throughout the life course.[14]

This study supports my clinical findings that childhood experiences are a major influence on adult health and this must be considered when working with an ACE survivor to help them recover from Parkinson's disease.

Adverse childhood experiences, plus trauma and/or continuing stressful circumstances during growth and adulthood are factors to be investigated and treated when assisting a people with Parkinson's towards recovery.

---

‡ Items were reverse-scored to reflect the framing of the question.

CHAPTER 9

THE ENVIRONMENTAL TOXIN PATHWAY

A variety of toxic substances have been studied and shown to increase the risk of Parkinson's disease, or to exacerbate the development of symptoms. Generally, these studies have been on chemicals that we are subjected to with little or no choice, or have been exposed to without knowing the dangers.

Agricultural chemicals have been the subject of more studies than most, although the results showing health dangers are generally ignored. A few domestic gardening chemicals have been shown to be damaging but, again, these findings are often ignored and suppressed where possible.

While it is important to be aware of these very dangerous chemicals, and to explore ways of reducing exposure, there are toxins in our immediate environment that we *can* control and avoid once we know about them. Many of these toxic substances lie hidden in our refrigerators, pantries, kitchen cupboards, bathrooms, toilets and cleaning cupboards. Yes, I am talking about food, drink and common household products.

Food choices (including drink)

Parkinson's disease is a world-wide phenomenon and does not discriminate between first and third worlds (or "developed" and "developing"), race or gender, but does tend to affect older people, although that is changing as many people under forty, and even in their twenties, are diagnosed with Parkinson's disease. What we do see, however, is that neurodegenerative disorders are on the increase in the developed world with few, if any, answers coming from "experts".

There are no significant studies on food and Parkinson's disease for very good reason. Food does not *cause* Parkinson's disease and food will not *cure* Parkinson's disease. However, food does have the power to improve or diminish our health.

Our food provides our sole source of energy, growth and functional chemicals, no matter how we ingest it. We can eat and drink orally, intravenously, insert a percutaneous endoscopic gastrostomy (PEG) or even use a nasogastric tube (gavage feeding). We need food and fluids to keep us alive and functioning.

Intravenous, PEG and gavage food administration are effectively used to save lives and rehabilitate after trauma or surgery. Without these interventions, many more would die unnecessarily. We have little or no choice about what is administered through these interventions and, while some improvements could be made, they are not the subject of this book. However, this type of food delivery affects only a tiny percentage of the population and, generally, for only a short time.

We can, and do, choose what we eat and drink in most circumstances. Whether we are at our home, work or eating out, we have the opportunity to choose food that will enhance rather than inhibit our health. In the developed world, we have a vast array of foods available from which we can choose. We have access to huge supermarkets filled with products, some of which can, rightly, claim to be food and some that are called food but have little or no nutritional value.

Even our acknowledged "experts" seem confused about what constitutes a healthy food selection and what will create a pathway to illness. And this is the crux of the matter. Our unhealthy food choices, for the most part, will not *cause* Parkinson's disease but may create levels of dysregulation in our body and, combined with other toxic influences and aetiological pathways, lead to a set of symptoms diagnosed as Parkinson's disease.

Let's talk about *diet*. I don't like that word as it implies a regimented, restricted way of eating that limits choices. We have the Mediterranean diet, Paleo diet, Vegetarian diet, Vegan diet, Keto diet, and numerous other diets aimed at achieving weight loss, muscle enhancement, performance or better skin.

A most significant diet is the Standard American/Australian Diet or SAD. This is significant because more people eat some variation of this in the developed world that any other diet.

The SAD food pyramid looks something like this:

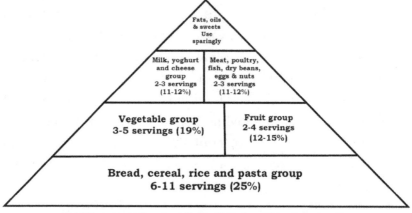

Food choices recommended by government health authorities in most western developed countries.
Often referred to as the Standard American Diet or Standard Australian Diet (SAD)

These are the food choices encouraged by healthcare "experts" in the developed world who claim that this will provide suitable nutrition and the basis for good health. Let's see if this is true.

Grains: The basis of the diet is grains (bread, cereal, rice and pasta group). The experts recommend six to eleven servings per day. That's at least one-third of our food intake. The experts certainly recommend wholegrain products, believing that this will offset disadvantages of grain consumption.

Humans have consumed grains as a major part of their dietary intake for only roughly 10,000 years. While there is some evidence of wild grain consumption up to 105,000 years ago, the definition of "grains" during this era by archaeologists seems rather vague and broad-ranging, including African false banana, pigeon peas, wild oranges, African wine palm and African potato, so the actual percentage of grain-based foods consumed is uncertain.[1] Storage and significant consumption of lectin-dense grain foods appears to have commenced around 10,000 years ago as reliance on hunter-gatherer type food use diminished over the preceding 30,000 years.[2] This is not nearly enough time to develop the enzymes required to fully utilise the substances in grains, nor mechanisms to defend against toxins. All true grains contain over 30 lectins (of which gluten is one) that are there to protect the plant against predators. Lectins cause inflammation in the human gastrointestinal tract (GIT), irritate the gut wall causing tight junctions between cells to open wider allowing large proteins to enter the interstitium, but block absorption of other, helpful nutrients. The inflammatory response extracts calcium and magnesium to buffer that, so reducing stores of those minerals for useful purposes. Coeliac disease (not really a disease, but a set of symptoms) is end-stage gut damage from an inappropriate dietary intake of many foods (plus, often, a stress response and reaction to other contaminants). While there is a genetic marker for Coeliac disease, the gene must be triggered before the proteins it produces affect us.[3] There are many healthy alternatives to grains that we will explore in the strategies section.

Animal dairy products: The myth promoted by dietitians, doctors, nurse practitioners and the industry is that animal dairy products such as milk, cheese, cream and yoghurt provide calcium, protein and a number of other nutrients. It is true that there are quite large amounts of helpful nutrients in these products; the challenge is that we can't absorb or utilise them. The milk molecule is so large that, in a healthy gut, it will not fit through the tight junctions to enter the bloodstream. Like grains, dairy molecules irritate the gut wall, causing tight junctions to open, allowing large molecules to inappropriately enter the interstitial space and bloodstream, causing more irritation and inflammation. Organic, grass-fed butter and ghee are exceptions to this (see food choices in the strategies section). The result of feeding our children the milk and milk products from other animals, and continuing this bizarre habit into adulthood, is a higher risk of osteopenia/osteoporosis, irritable bowel syndrome, Crohn's disease, Parkinson's disease,[4] anxiety, dementia, breast cancer, prostate cancer and bowel cancer.[5,6,7]

Sugar is now a dirty word, at last. Many foods contain sugars (fruits and many vegetables, for instance) but we humans, as we developed a taste for sweet foods, have found ways to refine sugar from plants and add it to already sweet foods. An excess of sugar in our food creates inflammation, increased production of insulin and, eventually, insulin resistance. We are made very aware of the dangers of diabetes with long-term heart disease, blindness and peripheral neuropathy as a consequence of poorly controlled, or even well-treated diabetes. However, in addition to adding refined sugar to food, we consume refined grains/carbohydrates that turn to sugar in our gut and have the same effect.

Artificial sweeteners: In a bid to avoid refined sugar, many have changed to artificial sweeteners which claim to reduce our sugar and calorie intake. Well, both these claims are true; but what manufacturers, food companies and supporters do not tell us is that most artificial sweeteners are highly toxic to humans. One in particular, aspartame (which is labelled under a variety of names), is directly linked to a number of autoimmune and degenerative disorders such as multiple sclerosis, Ankylosing Spondylitis, dementia and Parkinson's disease. If it is artificial (created in a laboratory), don't add it to your food or drink, or consume food or drink containing these sweeteners.[8,9,10,11]

Extracted sugars and syrups: Many are fooled by the "natural sounding" names of some sweeteners offered on the alternative foods market. Agave, palm sugar, coconut sugar, rice syrup, and a number of fruit syrups are all touted to be "natural" and therefore good for us. Don't be persuaded by good-sounding words. These "natural" sweeteners are extracted and refined and, therefore, far from natural; and they are, in practice, no better than refined cane sugar. Remember too that "natural" is not necessarily good. Cow droppings are natural, but not good food.

Coffee, tea and other caffeinated drinks: Don't be fooled by the hype. Coffee will not prevent, slow or reverse Parkinson's disease! Coffee contains antioxidants and is reputed to be one of the most antioxidant active drinks. This is not so; just hype by those who have not looked beyond the public claims and raw, unfiltered statistics, and those with vested interest. If we read the "breakthrough" stories, we will be told that six or eight cups of coffee daily will prevent or reduce the risk of just about every chronic disease, including some cancers! If only it were so.

There is no doubt that freshly ground coffee contains active antioxidants that can mop up Reactive Oxygen Species (ROS – which are the "oxidants" that antioxidants target) plus, for those of us fond of coffee, it has a vibrant aroma and tastes so fine. However, caffeinated coffee also causes an artificial activity boost to our adrenal glands, forcing them to produce additional adrenaline and cortisol, as if we were under severe stress – a fight/flight/freeze response. This is why coffee is habit-forming. We like the lift and extra burst of energy. So, when that fades, we grab another cup of coffee to lift us again; and again; and again.

Another fatal flaw in the argument for coffee is oxidation of the coffee itself. The "good-for-you-data" is based on freshly-ground, freshly-brewed coffee that has not had time to oxidise. As soon as coffee beans are roasted and ground, carbon dioxide begins to dissipate and the coffee oxidises, leaving us with the possibility of increased ROS to deal with.

Decaffeinated coffee should be healthier, but most is chemically decaffeinated, leaving residues of those chemicals, most is presented as ground coffee so is oxidising rapidly and, other than some attractive aroma and flavour, has no benefits (and may be even more detrimental).

Other caffeinated drinks – black tea, green tea, white tea, sports and energy drinks – produce the same caffeine lift as coffee, although usually to a lesser extent.

Apart from overworking our adrenals, caffeine, tannins and some other compounds in coffee, tea and caffeinated drinks, cause inflammation which can affect our nervous system.[12]

An interesting, but not "scientific" fact is that over 90 per cent of my 2000-odd patients diagnosed with Parkinson's disease drank coffee for many years (including me, by the way), while the rest drank tea.

A further thought on green tea, which is touted as a super healthy drink: the polyphenols in green tea can block the biopterin cycle (part of our methylation detoxification process) and, in the process, reduce the production of dopamine.

In the strategies section, we will look at warm drinks that will enhance our health without these challenges.

Nutrition-free food: The SAD (standard American/Australian diet) which is similar to the standard food habits in many other Westernised countries, is low in nutrients essential to health. Many meals are composed of refined carbohydrates with some overcooked vegetables and fatty protein. Add challenges of caffeinated drinks, sugary soft drinks or alcohol accompanying the meal, it is no wonder that many people in the Western world are suffering from sub-clinical malnutrition and scurvy.

To be well and combat all the toxic challenges we face in today's society, we need the best possible nutrition. When we choose foods that are devoid of nutrition, inflammatory and, in some cases, have a direct link to degenerative disorders, we are simply asking for illness.

Case history: *I was conducting a recovery workshop in 2004, expounding my views on food choices, meditation and other self-help activities that could help reverse the symptoms of Parkinson's disease. The participants included a doctor with stage 3 Parkinson's disease who accepted most of my teachings, loved the food, but drank one litre of diet cola each day. He was addicted. When I called him on it, he became angry and left the program. His addiction to aspartame was more important to him than wellness.*

Household toxins

We have become fanatical about cleanliness and a "germ-free" environment. To aid us in our quest, scientists have developed strong cleaners and anti-bacterial compounds which we spray, drip, spread, bathe and slosh around our homes. Our intention is to achieve no grime and no germs.

I believe in cleanliness, don't get me wrong, but not at all costs. Using powerful chemicals to do the job that hot water, bicarbonate of soda, some white vinegar and elbow grease will do is counterproductive.

Many household chemicals are either neurotoxic, carcinogenic, or both. Many people are sensitive to the chemicals. (Western medicine places a very narrow definition on allergic, so sensitive is a more acceptable term here.) Often these sensitivities go unnoted unless the person sees an holistic practitioner who can identify their sensitivities among the background noise of daily stress, busy-ness, poor food choices and other lifestyle challenges.

Many washing and dishwashing detergents can damage cell membranes on contact, strong-smelling cleaners can affect the brain directly via the olfactory nerve (especially ammonia, but there are others), oven cleaners are particularly nasty while antibacterial sprays, wipes and hand cleaners destroy our skin microbiome, which is a vital part of our immune system.

It is not hard to keep our homes clean without destroying our health in the process.

Personal care products

Body odour became an anathema in polite society and we at first attempted to combat its inevitability with bathing, powders and perfumes until scientists developed antiperspirant deodorants. We retained our love affair with perfumes and make-up, and applied the new, aluminium-based deodorants with enthusiasm.

We now know that there were/are two major problems with antiperspirant deodorants based on aluminium – firstly, perspiring is a natural detoxification pathway for us to help eliminate inflammatory and infectious toxins, so stopping perspiration can lock them into our body to cause long-term health challenges; secondly, aluminium is implicated in many serious disorders including Alzheimer's disease, dementia, chronic fatigue syndrome, chronic infections and Parkinson's disease.[13,14]

Shampoos, conditioners and shower gels may also contain chemicals that are either neurotoxic, carcinogenic or both.

Make-up, except in very rare cases, is highly toxic. It contains poisonous colours, coal tar, and a variety of chemicals to make it flow and/or stick on our skin. Many make-up contents are carcinogenic and some are neurotoxic.

Avoiding household and personal care products

If we wish to be well, we must be vigilant about what we become intimate with (and there is nothing more intimate than what we apply to our body, or wash in often). These chemicals, commonly used in both household and personal care products, must be avoided at all costs. Most of these are derived from petrochemicals, but some are otherwise synthesised in the laboratory. Avoid polyethylene glycol (PEG), sulfates and sulfides, laurel sulfates and ammonium sulfates, ethoxylates, parabens, propylene glycol, silicones, phthalates, mineral oils, artificial colours, flavours and sweeteners. This list is not exhaustive as new chemicals are introduced each year. We don't know what most of them are, their names or composition, as manufacturing companies only need approval from a government department. They don't have to tell us what they are or what they do. In most countries, manufacturers do have to list contents on the pack of each product (the thoroughness of this varies widely between countries). However, often the chemicals are listed by number rather than name. In this case, my policy is *if you can't spell it, pronounce it, understand it, or know what the number means, don't buy the product without further investigation.*

Common environmental toxins

There are at least 500,000 neurotoxic chemicals in our environment that we did not know about before they were released, we are not told about, we are not warned about, and are almost impossible to avoid.

In the strategies section, we will look at ways to protect ourselves against the toxic influence of our society but, in the meantime, here are some highly toxic areas we may be able to avoid at least some of the time.

Supermarkets use powerful cleaners, air-conditioning, deodoriser sprays and strong lighting, all of which are assaults on our senses. The off-gassing in their household and personal care aisles is very powerful. Smaller shops are sometimes safer.

Workplaces may be toxic, depending on our industry, position and employer. Most commercial properties employ cleaning firms that use chemical cleaning compounds (often ammonia-based), air-conditioning and deodorisers. Some industries, of necessity, use strong, neurotoxic chemicals in their processes. It is smart to examine your workplace, ask your employer about chemicals used or in the environment, then consider whether you need to be there.

Traffic can be toxic on a number of levels. If we live on a busy street, or in a high-trafficked suburb, we are constantly assaulted with noise and fumes from burnt fuel. If we commute by motor vehicle, the stress of driving in busy traffic increases our fight/flight/freeze response, exacerbating inflammation and reducing dopamine production.

Public transport is often a better way to commute as there is less stress involved. However, we are once again assaulted with powerful cleaning compounds, noise and crowded facilities.

Public spaces like parks and playgrounds are wonderful additions to our cities, providing open air recreation for many. However, most management bodies take the easy way out when caring for these spaces and use neurotoxic weed control (often glyphosate or Roundup) and somewhat less toxic, but still dangerous fertilisers. A few have taken their responsibilities to heart and are managing recreational spaces organically. Check out your area and encourage organic management.

Roadside: Just driving in the country and enjoying the peaceful scenery can be toxic. Most road managers use glyphosate to control weeds and often even more toxic chemicals for specific weeds like blackberries in Australia. If you see any signs of spraying when out driving, consider going somewhere else.

Gardens: While it is important to restrain weed invasions in our gardens, some chemical herbicides and pesticides are extremely toxic. Glyphosate (part of Roundup) is among the most neurotoxic chemicals currently in the environment,[15,16] and there are others used for specific weed and pest species. There are non-toxic alternatives that are effective and inexpensive. Always read the label; if the product contains chemicals or numbers you do not understand, do not purchase or use without much more investigation. Remember, too, that chemicals used in your neighbourhood (even several streets away) may drift into your environment and cause damage.

Agrochemicals: Farming is big business. Farmers work hard over long days to produce foods we need, or think we need, on slim margins of profit. To do this, most utilise chemicals to restrain weeds and pests and/or to encourage growth. Broadacre farming requires efficient means to distribute those chemicals, so long-arm spray units and spraying from aircraft are common. This means spray drift, even in very light breezes. Chemical drift may migrate up to 50 km (31 miles) from the source as spray deposits in road dust is thrown into the air by passing traffic, then further distributed by breezes or wind. Run-off during rainfall may contaminate creeks, rivers and lakes.[17,18]

Cattle and sheep dips also utilise very neurotoxic chemicals. While arsenic and DDT are no longer used, there are still residues of these chemicals contaminating many dip sites and they may affect animals and humans in those areas. The newer dip chemicals are still neurotoxic. The effects are primarily apparent in farming communities where farms and farm workers are in contact with the chemicals several times each year, although the long half-life of some means that ancillary industries (abattoirs, butchers, food packers, etc.) may also be affected to some degree.

In my practice, I have seen a number of clusters of neurodegenerative disorders in farming communities, including Parkinson's disease, depression, motor neurone disease (ALS), dementia and suicide.

Pharmaceutical medications: There is no doubt that pharmaceutical drugs, prescribed appropriately by qualified medical practitioners, play a valuable role in controlling illness symptoms in our community. Prescribed drugs are, apparently, tightly controlled in the Western world. However, there are some gaps in those controls and public knowledge of long-term effects of some drugs. While each drug is more or less well tested and trialled before release (although some trials fail to meet the "gold standard" set by Western medicine), there are no trials for off-label prescriptions (drugs approved for one use, but prescribed for another), concomitant use of drugs for different diagnoses (e.g. hypertension, plus anxiety, plus asthma, plus arthritis, plus insomnia), known as polypharmacy, or very long-term use of drugs recommended for short-term use (antihypertensive drugs and antidepressants, for instance).

Many of these drugs may cause adverse effects mimicking one or more symptoms of Parkinson's disease. These adverse effects may accumulate over time and with the number of different drugs with similar adverse effects. This may lead to a diagnosis of Parkinson's disease when the symptoms are, in fact, the result of long-term use of a number of drugs. (*MIMS ANNUAL Drug Guide 2018*)

Alice

Alice was diagnosed with Parkinson's disease at sixty-three years old, and prescribed levodopa drugs which made her feel nauseous, depressed and weak. She had been taking antihypertensives for over thirty years, an antidepressant for twenty-two years and an anticonvulsant drugs for insomnia since her husband died eight years ago. Her family history also included many years in farming communities. As we dealt with toxic contamination and lifestyle issues, we were able to, very slowly, wean her off drugs one by one until, four years later, she was free from symptoms and feeling really well.

Over-the-counter (OTC) drugs pose a more immediate problem in that they are rarely understood by the user (self-prescriber) and often misused or overused. While generally having less severe adverse effects than prescribed drugs, all pharmaceutical drugs do have adverse effects (not "side effects" – the adverse effects are always there), and these may accumulate significantly over time. No OTC drugs are thought to create Parkinson's disease-type symptoms, but a number of OTC analgesics and anti-inflammatory drugs do have neurological effects that may, over time, create mimicking symptoms. Some proton pump inhibitors are now available OTC (for reflux and heartburn) and these may cause significant damage to our digestive systems by raising the pH in the stomach, thus reducing our ability to digest proteins and other solid foods required for health and healing.[19,20]

Recreational drugs: Many recreational drugs are known to cause neurological and psychological damage. These are well studied by expert practitioners and there is excellent literature available. However, we tend to ignore the damage caused by "soft" drugs that are more socially acceptable. Alcohol and cannabis are two quite dangerous drugs – not because of the immediate effect (unless grossly over-used), but because the long-term damage is often irreversible.

Alcohol is a very social drug, and there is no doubt that the effects of modest consumption can be pleasant – relaxation, encouragement of conversation, pleasant flavour. However, even low consumption on a regular basis can exacerbate dehydration (unless significant repair is activated – more than just drinking water) and this may combine with other degenerative influences to adversely affect our health. Views on what constitutes modest consumption varies a great deal but, in my opinion, one small drink no more than three times per week is the limit if we want to be well.

The "cannabis conundrum" is a very different and more difficult challenge to unravel. Marijuana has been used for many, many years as pain relief for those at the end stage of dreadful diseases. I see no problem with that use, in the same way that I sadly accepted the need for "Brompton's Cocktail" (pethidine, morphine, cocaine) during the last few days of my son's life. These circumstances are appropriate for use of the strongest pain relief available.

However, we now see cannabis and medical marijuana promoted as a wonder drug capable of preventing, reversing or "curing" a wide range of disorders, including seizures, neuro-degenerative disorders, autoimmune disorders, stealth infections and cancers. These claims are made with very little, if any, real evidence.

Anecdotes, often consisting of heart-wrenching stories about children or beautiful young people, illustrate "miraculous" recoveries – seizures stop, patients walk again, symptoms are relieved – yet there is no long-term evidence of safety or efficacy. We do not know if the apparent recoveries can be sustained or what the long-term adverse effects will be. Remember thalido-mide? A wonder drug for pregnant women suffering insomnia or intractable nausea (morning sickness). Ten thousand babies later, we know the tragedy of using a drug without appropriate stringent testing. Remember Tolcapone (Tasmar), a COMT inhibitor for Parkinson's patients? At least three people died before the drug was suspended and we do not know how many more suffered liver damage.

Some serious research projects on cannabis are underway now (2019) but we are a long way from answers. We *do* know that recreational use of marijuana can cause psychological and neurological damage, fracture relationships, harm career paths, and exacerbate the progression of some cancers.

CBD (cannabidiol) oil, from cannabis or hemp, is thought to be a "safe" alternative to cannabis as it contains only very small amounts of tetrahydrocannabinol (THC), the psychoactive can-nabinoid. However, there is some, as yet anecdotal, evidence that CBD may block one or more of our methylation pathway cycles and reduce production of dopamine endogenously. In my practice, I have found that those few patients who used CBD oil against my advice, became dependent on it quite quickly, rein-forcing the thought that it reduces the production of dopamine (a "reward" neurotransmitter).

Research into other cannabinoids as therapeutic options is in very early stages, and we may see useful results in two or three years.

Vaccine adjuvants: This is not a discussion on whether to vaccinate or not. I support rational, effective, evidence-based and non-toxic vaccine programs. However, all current vaccines contain adjuvants that may be neurotoxic. Adjuvants in vaccines from childhood to old age include mercury (Thimerosal – reduced and no longer declared in most vaccines but still present), aluminium, animal cells/DNA, monosodium glutamate (MSG), formaldehyde, squalene, peanut oil, aspartame, formalin, ammonium sulphate and many others. It is up to each individual to choose whether they want to have these substances injected into their body (or injected into their children) and it is each person's responsibility to thoroughly investigate each vaccine offered. Ask your vaccine provider, or pharmacist, for *complete details* of all contents in each vaccine, together with any trials of combined vaccinations where offered (e.g. MMR, DTP).

Electromagnetic fields: We are constantly surrounded by ever-increasing electromagnetic fields (EMF). While we do not yet know how much is safe for each person, there is no doubt that our society has benefited from many of the mechanisms that create EMF, but research is emerging about damage caused by long-term exposure.

I was born towards the end of World War II when there were very few EMF. We had a small electric cooktop for emergencies (most cooking was on a wood-fired stove), a radio we listened to for one hour each evening and one incandescent electric light in each room. We sometimes passed high-tension wires when travelling by train to the city.

Fast forward seventy years, and we have multiple lights in many rooms, bedside electric clocks and radios, televisions, computers, mobile/cell phones, cordless phones, video games, smart meters, high-tension wires by or over many busy roads, television and cell towers repeating signals, and wi-fi present in most locations. Many non-aligned researchers are warning that frequent and long-term exposure to EMF may damage our nervous system.

While there is no evidence, as yet, that EMF cause neurodegenerative disorders, wisdom dictates that we should avoid them as much as we can and utilise protective measures when we can't.

"Polytoxicity"

I have seen very few cases of people with Parkinson's where we can say with certainty that contact with a specific chemical at a specific time caused their Parkinson's disease symptoms. However, we often see patients who have experienced frequent or ongoing contact with neurotoxic chemicals that have damaged cells and cell function. Many of the toxins we encounter are man-made and our body does not have mechanisms capable of eliminating them. The toxins become locked into cells, causing damage over may years.

As the toxic load increases day by day, we begin to feel their effects – fatigue or headaches at first, slowly escalating to irritability, loss of short-term memory, suppressed immunity and symptoms of chronic disease.

Environmental toxins must be investigated as a possible aetiological pathway for anyone expressing symptoms of a chronic disorder, including Parkinson's disease.

CHAPTER 10

THE INFECTION PATHWAY

Stealth infections and their association with chronic diseases is one of the most controversial health topics today. Stealth infections, "popularised" as Lyme disease or Lyme-like illness, have been understood by only a few doctors brave enough to diagnose and treat them. Many other hitherto neglected infections have become associated with the Lyme disease controversy.

The greatest amount of angst and argument centres around the question of whether ongoing symptoms remaining or reappearing after Lyme disease has been treated with seven to thirty days of antibiotics constitute "chronic Lyme disease", some sort of disease syndrome unrelated to the infection, or is completely psychosomatic.

At least fifty-two strains of Borrelia have been identified since 1992, of which at least ten can infect humans.[1] Only one strain, Borrelia burgdorferi sensu stricto, is specific to "Lyme disease"[2] (named after the township of Lyme, Connecticut, USA, where it was first identified), while others are associated with different symptom pictures. Some cause "Lyme-like" illness, others cause relapsing fever, others create milder forms of febrile illness, while some create significant neurological symptoms.

Infectious Borrelia species are often collectively known as Borrelia burgdorferi sensu lato,[3] creating confusion with Borrelia burgdorferi sensu stricto (actual Lyme disease). This is one of the major distractions in the discussion about chronic infectious syndromes caused by these bacteria. Medical authorities argue that Borrelia infections are of limited duration and can be successfully treated (even "cured") with antibiotic administration. More radical medical practitioners claim that Borrelia infections may be of very long duration and become chronic, especially if not treated shortly after the initial infection, and so need long-term administration of antibiotics, often over years rather than weeks or months.[4]

Other infectious pathogens (sometimes called co-infections), may be transmitted to humans by the same vectors as Borrelia and coexist, causing a confusing overlap of symptoms. Bartonella, Babesia and Mycoplasma (several species of each) are commonly found in patients diagnosed with Borrelia infections. There are also opportunistic infections that may be latent within patients and become active as Borrelia and co-infections suppress immune function. Epstein-Barr virus, other herpes viruses and, sometimes, more serious diseases such as Guillain-Barré syndrome may become challenging and need assertive treatment.[5]

Once identified, antibiotics, anti-inflammatory drugs, anti-protozoa drugs or steroids may be employed to combat the diagnosed infection.

Less destructive treatments (lifestyle, herbs and frequencies among them) are discussed more fully in the chapter on treating infections, but the important point to ponder here is whether the symptoms of chronic infections can mimic symptoms of Parkinson's disease and cause misdiagnosis.

There is strong evidence showing that many cases of chronic disease are caused by, or exacerbated by infections. Common diagnoses later found to involve chronic infections include fibromyalgia, chronic fatigue syndrome, rheumatoid arthritis, multiple sclerosis, motor neurone disease and Parkinson's disease.[6,7,8]

In my clinical practice, up to 30 per cent of patients presenting with firm diagnoses of Parkinson's disease, often confirmed by two or more neurologists, are found to be carrying a chronic infection – usually Borrelia or Bartonella. The infections are only diagnosed after persistent discussion with my patients and involve either serology, PCR or challenge tests.

Healthcare professionals treating those presenting with Parkinson's disease or Parkinson's-like symptoms will do well to familiarise themselves with the history of the Lyme disease controversy, and the symptom pictures of Borrelia species and common co-infections. Laboratory tests are notoriously inaccurate for these infections and positive identification may take months and many tests, and leave our patients in limbo, or being treated inadequately for all that time.

Recognising the likelihood of a stealth infection early is critical to effective treatment. This requires excellent history taking and inclusion of questions likely to elicit information about lifetime risks of infection, familial symptom pictures and symptoms experienced by your patients that seem unrelated to their presenting disorder.[9]

Dr Richard Horowitz, in his book *Why Can't I Get Better?: Solving the Mystery of Lyme and Chronic Disease*, includes a questionnaire for self-assessment and gives permission for its general use.[10] I have incorporated this questionnaire (without the self-scoring section) into my pre-consult questionnaire for all patients. This gives me clues about their risk of infection before we meet, and can alert me to symptoms that may warrant further investigation.

Dr Hororwitz's book is an excellent resource for those wishing to understand the deeper ramification of stealth infections, and some of the complexities of treatment. In terms of Parkinson's disease diagnosis and treatment, understanding stealth infection vectors, symptom patterns, acute and chronic manifestations, testing options and neurological challenges will enhance the effectiveness of your clinical practice.

However, diagnoses of an infectious process is not always welcomed by patients already thoroughly embedded in the process of treating a known "incurable" disorder like Parkinson's disease. Many patients are simply looking for a way to reduce their reliance on Parkinson's disease drugs or improve their quality of life, without making any radical changes or challenging the medical authorities who made the diagnosis of Parkinson's disease.

A number of patients, diagnosed with Parkinson's disease (or multiple sclerosis or motor neurone disease) have left my care precipitously after I broached the subject of stealth infections. This was too complex for them to contemplate; especially as they were usually not significantly debilitated and did not want to accept the complexities of treating more than one "disease" or aetiological pathway.

Diagnosis with a stealth infection does not necessarily mean that our patient does not have Parkinson's disease, but rather that we have identified another aetiological pathway leading to the symptoms diagnosed as Parkinson's disease. Patients often want a "simple" diagnosis (a disease name and straightforward treatment process), rather than discussion of a number of aetiological pathways and how these may be reversed.

Anna

Anna came to see me after being treated for multiple sclerosis for nearly two years. At our first consult, I suspected a stealth infection was one of her challenges, but she needed to make changes to her lifestyle, food choices and supplements to enhance her general health, so focused on that.

Anna returned after six weeks, and I broached the subject of a possible Bartonella infection. She became quite angry and refused to discuss the matter. At her third visit, I again broached the subject of Bartonella and persuaded her to undertake a challenge test. Within a week, the test showed positive for the presence of Bartonella, but Anna claimed that she was under a lot of stress and so the test was possibly inaccurate. We decide on a wash-out period and to re-test.

The second test quickly proved positive also but, again, Anna found excuses for the result and became quite angry in discussion with me. When a third test also proved positive, Anna returned the test formula with a note saying that I was "not a practitioner I want to be associated with" and "talking about Bartonella is causing me too much stress".

Anna preferred to be ineffectively treated for an "incurable" disease rather than reverse a major aetiological pathway leading to her diagnosis.

Susan

Susan was diagnosed with Parkinson's disease three years before seeing me. Her clear intention was to reduce her symptoms (especially her tremor) so she could function professionally without having to reveal or discuss her "illness". Discussion of possible aetiological pathways fell on deaf ears as she just wanted symptom reduction.

We had an uneasy relationship for several years until her symptoms increased to the extent that they could not be hidden, no matter how much medication she took. I suspected a Borrelia infection and, this time, Susan agreed to blood and urine PCR tests which were positive.

I naively thought that such positive tests would persuade Susan to focus on treating the infection as well as developing lifestyle habits to enhance her health. This was not the case. Susan continued to focus on suppressing symptoms rather than making changes to enhance her health. The Borrelia infection was an "inconvenience" and she was not able to make serious inroads into the ravages if was causing.

Susan continues to deteriorate in health, focus on symptom suppression, and make half-hearted attempts at following my advice on lifestyle and food choices. She is not treating the diagnosed Borrelia infection.

Another serious influence on health that may be mistaken for neurodegeneration (or a factor causing neurodegeneration) is moulds. Over the past fifteen years or so, the profound damage caused by moulds, often invisible in our immediate environment, has been recognised and studied in depth.[11] Dr Ritchie Shoemaker is a prime mover in this field and has trained many practitioners in his knowledge and strategies. Patients at my clinic are closely questioned about the possibility of mould infection, current and past, and encouraged to examine their homes and work environment. If necessary, we guide them to building biologists to assist in finding and remediating mould damage.[12]

MSIDS Questionnaire

From *Why Can't I Get Better? Solving The Mystery Of Lyme And Chronic Disease* © 2018 by Dr. Richard Horowitz, MD. Reprinted by permission of St. Martin's Press. All Rights Reserved.

Answer the following questions as honestly as possible. Think about how you have been feeling over the past month and how often you have been bothered by any of the following problems. Score the occurrence of each symptom on the following scale:
0 = none, 1 = mild, 2 = moderate, 3 = severe

SECTION 1: Symptom Frequency

0 None   1 Mild   2 Moderate   3 Severe

1. ____ Unexplained fevers, sweats, chills or flushing.

2. ____ Unexplained weight change; loss or gain.

3. ____ **Fatigue, tiredness.*

4. ____ Unexplained hair loss.

5. ____ Swollen glands.

6. ____ Sore throat.

7. ____ Testicular or pelvic pain.

8. ____ Unexplained menstrual irregularity.

9. ____ Unexplained breast milk production; breast pain.

10. ____ Irritable bladder or bladder dysfunction.

---

* See how to score starred points on p. 81

11. _____ Sexual dysfunction or loss of libido.

12. _____ Upset stomach.

13. _____ Change in bowel function (constipation or diarrhoea).

14. _____ Chest pain or rib soreness.

15. _____ Shortness of breath or cough.

16. _____ Heart palpitations, pulse skips, heart block.

17. _____ History of a heart murmur or valve prolapse.

18. _____ **Joint pain or swelling.

19. _____ Stiff neck or back.

20. _____ Muscle pain or cramps.

21. _____ Twitching face or other muscles.

22. _____ Headaches.

23. _____ Neck cracks or neck stiffness.

24. _____ **Tingling, numbness, burning, or stabbing sensations.

25. _____ Facial paralysis (Bell's palsy).

26. _____ Eyes/vision; double, blurry.

27. _____ Ears/hearing; buzzing, ringing, ear pain.

28. _____ Increased motion sickness, vertigo. _____

29. _____ Light-headedness, poor balance, difficulty walking.

30. _____ Tremors.

31. _____ Confusion, difficulty thinking.

32. _____ Difficulty with concentration or reading.

33. _____ **Forgetfulness, poor short-term memory.

34. _____ Disorientation; getting lost; going to wrong places.

35. _____ Difficulty with speech or writing.

36. _____ Mood swings, irritability, depression.

37. _____ **Disturbed sleep; too much, too little, early awaking.

38. _____ Exaggerated symptoms or worse hangover from alcohol.

SECTION 2: Incidence Questions

Please place a tick below for the incidences applicable to you.

1.____ You have had a tick bite with no rash or flulike symptoms.

2.____ You have had a tick bite, an erythema migrans (bull-seye rash), or an undefined rash followed by flulike symptoms.

3.____ You live in what is considered a tick-borne infection-endemic area.

4.____ You have a family member who has been diagnosed with tick-borne infection and/or other tick-borne infections.

5.____ You experience migratory muscle pain.

6.____ You experience migratory joint pain.

7.____ You experience tingling/burning/numbness that migrates and/or comes and goes.

8.____ You have received a prior diagnosis of chronic fatigue syndrome or fibromyalgia.

9.____ You have received a prior diagnosis of a specific auto-immune disorder (lupus, MS, rheumatoid arthritis), or of a non-specific autoimmune disorder.

10.___ You have had a positive Lyme test (IFA, ELISA, Western blot, PCR, and/or Borrelia culture).

SECTION 3: Overall Health

1. Thinking about your overall physical health, for how many of the past thirty (30) days was your physical health <u>not</u> good? _____ days

2. Thinking about your overall mental health, for how many days during the past thirty (30) days was your mental health <u>not</u> good? _____ days

---

ADDING SCORES (see instructions in boxes below)

Section 1: _____

Section 2: _____

Section 3: _____

Section 4: _____

Final: _____

MSIDS QUESTIONNAIRE SCORES

SECTION 1	SECTION 3	SECTION 4
Add scores as given	**1 Physical**	Add 5 if each starred point in section 1 scored 3.
	0-5 = 1	
SECTION 2	6-12 = 2	
1 = 3	13-20 = 3	
2 = 5	21-30 = 4	**OVERALL**
3 = 2	**2 Mental**	46+ highly probable
4 = 1	0-5 = 1	21-45 possible, worth investigating further
5 = 4	6-12 = 2	
6 = 4	13-20 = 3	Less than 21, look elsewhere.
7 = 4	21-30 = 4	
8 = 3		
9 = 3		
10 = 5		

This questionnaire should be completed honestly by every person diagnosed with any chronic disorder. Think long and hard about how you feel before answering each question.

If possible, have someone close to you also complete the questionnaire about you without any reference to your answers. Sometimes those around us see us differently and their observations can be very helpful.

If there is a great divergence in scores (e.g. you score 38 and your independent assessor scores 60), discuss the differences and reach an agreement on the most accurate assessment.

Once you have agreed on a final score, consider the following strategies:

If less than 21, spend time reassessing your exposure to toxic substances and review your actions in both avoiding further exposure and removing those accumulated toxins that are adversely affecting your health. Also review any possible past trauma/stress influences on your health and make sure you are fully engaged in anti-stress strategies like self-love, laughter, meditation, singing and dancing.

21-45: Seek advice from a health practitioner who has awareness and experience in diagnosing and treating stealth infections. This may be a medical doctor, naturopath, herbalist or homeopath with relevant experience. Avoid kinesiologists/biofeedback practitioners, live-blood analysis practitioners and similar who claim quick diagnosis and "cures". You may need to seek help from a remote practitioner with whom you communicate via Skype. While not ideal, this is better than being misled by an inexperienced or misguided practitioner.

Your need, at this score, is further assessment and discussion on what stealth infection is the most likely to be affecting you. Once this is established, you can move ahead with treatment – preferably while maintaining contact with your experienced practitioner but also following the strategies detailed in later chapters.

If your score is **46 or higher**, you are very likely (almost certainly) affected by one or more stealth infections, and it is critical that you move ahead with diagnosis and treatment. See Chapter 21 for my suggestions to find a practitioner to help you.

If you have any suspicion of a stealth infection (MSIDS), I highly recommend that you read *Why Can't I Get Better? – Solving the Mystery of Lyme and Chronic Disease* by Richard I. Horowitz, MD.[13]

CHAPTER 11

FINDING THE AETIOLOGICAL PATHWAY

Patients usually reach my clinic after being diagnosed with Parkinson's disease by at least one, and generally two or more Western medical practitioners. There is often a tentative diagnosis by a general practitioner (GP), followed by a referral to a neurologist specialising in movement disorders or Parkinson's disease, sometimes followed by a visit to a second neurologist for another opinion.

Rarely, a patient will consult with me because they have realised that they are displaying health challenges that may involve the nervous system. In these cases, I ask them to also consult their GP and/or a neurologist so we can obtain all possible information and a number of independent assessments.

No patient consulting with me has been questioned, by their doctors/specialists, about their lifestyle, health history beyond five years prior to diagnosis, or engaged in exploration of possible aetiological pathways. They are generally (although not always) sent for an MRI to rule out stroke, tumours and other scannable events, then told they have idiopathic (of no known cause/origin) Parkinson's disease.

Whichever route patients take to see me, they all complete a very thorough questionnaire, then attend a two-hour (or longer) initial consultation to explore and assess all possible aetiological pathways before we begin any treatment.

Questionnaires and the patient's history can tell us much about the possible aetiological pathways leading to illness. Questions to be answered and details investigated include the items below. There may be more details needed for some individuals.

Place of birth? Checking the birth environment can be very telling. A rural area? Check for the possibility of agrochemicals (especially organophosphates/glyphosate, arsenic and DDT). Mining areas? Check for heavy metals. Areas of heavy traffic or EMF? Be certain they will need detoxing and protection against EMF damage. Countries of social conflict? Check for family trauma.

Did they move during childhood? Some patients move from relatively "safe" areas to more toxic districts while in their formative years. Again, check for agrochemicals, heavy metals, smog, EMF and social conflict. Immigrant families face enormous challenges and, while they move seeking a better life, learning a new language, fitting into a new culture, finding work (often at a much lower status/pay than in their home country) and facing frequent discrimination can be the basis of long-term hidden trauma. Refugees are treated horribly in many Western countries (including Australia and USA), and the trauma from these experiences may tip their nervous system "over the edge" into neurodegeneration.

Family history: The health history of parents, grandparents and siblings may provide clues about genetic predispositions in the family and/or lifestyle choices not apparent from other questioning. Traumatic events experienced by our grandparents can be a factor in our genetic predispositions to neurodegenerative stress responses. For instance, I have treated the grandchildren of Holocaust survivors who displayed hyper-alertness and hyper-sensitivities possibly first triggered during the horrors their grandparents experienced, exacerbated by attitudes expressed by parents and grandparents, openly and/or implicitly, as they dealt with normal challenges.

Significant research early in the twenty-first century is indicating that we can and do inherit "cellular memory" of ancestral experiences. Cellular memory will not *cause* Parkinson's disease (or any disease), but may make us vulnerable to moderate stresses, or very resilient to major stress, depending on what our ancestors experienced and how they responded.

On a more immediate note, it is, of course, significant if grandparents or parents developed Parkinson's disease, Multiple System Atrophy, Progressive Supranuclear Palsy, Alzheimer's, dementia, multiple sclerosis, or any other neuro- or autoimmune disorder. Information of symptom development, treatment received and lifestyle, while often difficult to obtain with any accuracy, can be useful, when available, in assessing the current patient's likely responses.

My father and paternal grandmother both developed Parkinson's disease. My grandmother died before I was born, but I have a couple of photos of her in a wheelchair, obviously unable to function without assistance, but always smiling. I have been told that she was a gracious and resilient woman who did not allow the disease to rob her of humanity. Treatment in those days was largely anticholinergic drugs and palliation. On the other hand, my father displayed mild symptoms for over twenty years and took only levodopa drugs plus some intermittent medication for angina. He died at ninety-three after a short exacerbation of heart disease. My father worked hard through to his mid-eighties then, in retirement, continued his church involvement, gardening and taking train travel holidays on his own (my parents did not like each other much). Like his mother, he chose to resist the debility of Parkinson's disease.

Sibling health may also give clues to family predispositions in expressing stress responses. Siblings with chronic disorders may alert us to family factors affecting the health of the whole family.

Relationships within the family may point to significant trauma or help discount that pathway. Comments like "Mum was always busy", or "Dad was an alcoholic" can provide the basis for further probing to discover how much influence those relationships had. On the other hand, a quick chat about the family, school and friends may serve to discount trauma as a significant part of the illness pathway and allow more time for exploring other pathways.

If there was little support from parents or siblings, discussing other support networks can give insights into possible toxic exposure or trauma.

Where they **work and past employment** history may provide clues regarding exposure to toxic chemicals (production line, mechanic, farming, mining, hospitals and many other places of work).

Parental employment may also give indications of toxic exposure. For instance, a patient reported that their father owned a scrapyard and, as children, my patient would play with rusty metal, grease, old batteries and tanks containing the remnants of unknown chemicals. Another patient's mother worked at a fertiliser factory and had residual chemicals on her clothing after work. One father was a plumber in the days of lead pipes, "red lead", soldering fluxes and other toxins which clung to his clothing when he came home. Another patient said that, while his father was a farmer, the family lived in town, so he was not there when crops were sprayed with pesticide. However, Dad did not use protective clothing, so organophosphate residue was often on his clothing.

In all these examples, exposure to toxic chemicals was slight, but persistent, and occurred at times of growth when children are most vulnerable to toxic effects. All these toxins persist in the body for many years and can affect cell function.

The patient's **medical/health history** can provide many clues. Have they been treated for hypertension, anxiety/depression, hypercholesterolemia, reflux or other gut dysfunction, frequent infections or an inflammatory condition like arthritis? These histories may indicate early signs of neurodegenerative disorders or the treatments provided may have created the symptoms now manifesting as Parkinson's disease.

Accident/injury history may be important, especially if those accidents were traumatic or involved head injury. We do not think, at this stage, that head injury necessarily *causes* Parkinson's disease, but dysregulation between parts of the brain/nervous system may exacerbate symptoms. For instance, injury causing poor communication between the vestibular and ocular systems may exacerbate poor balance, velocity storage or dizziness. Injuries may cause "mis-communication" between many parts/lobes of the brain, creating or exacerbating symptoms otherwise blamed on the disease process.

Workplace injuries can be particularly devastating unless the employer is very supportive and understanding. Patients may be fearful about losing income, being unable to return to work, or having to change career paths and these stresses, in conjunction with other factors, can play a role in escalating degenerative symptoms.

It is important to note *pharmaceutical drugs* taken up to five years before symptoms became noticeable. *Polypharmacy* is especially important as it has been shown that, while one drug with (say) an adverse effect of tremor is unlikely to be a problem, several drugs taken together, all with tremor as an adverse effect, are much more likely to cause tremor. Length of time taken is also important to note. Antidepressants, for instance, are recommended for short-term use only. However, many patients take these drugs for months or years, vastly increasing the likelihood of experiencing adverse effects. As noted above, drugs such as antidepressants, statins, antihypertensives, proton pump inhibitors and recreational drugs can all create symptoms that may be mistakenly diagnosed as Parkinson's disease.

Complementary medicine is important to note. While complementary medicine is inherently much safer that Western allopathic medicine, there is strong evidence of interactions between some pharmaceutical drugs and specific herbs and a few supplements, and some complementary medicine prescriptions blocking or reducing the effect of some drugs. Lists of these interaction and contraindications are readily available and constantly updated by the TGA, FDA, similar bodies in other countries, professional bodies relating to Western allopathic medicine and complementary medicine practitioners and pharmacists, and many drug/herb guides.

There is, moreover, knowledge of toxic doses of most herbs and supplements. Again, most are inherently safe at well above sensible doses, but some (e.g. Phytolacca, black cohosh and others) may be dangerous at high doses or in certain circumstances. Herbs and supplements should always be prescribed and supervised by a well-qualified complementary medicine practitioner who is a member of a recognised accreditation body.

Because complementary medicine lacks coherent regulation in many countries (despite very strong campaigns by complementary medicine practitioners to create a useful regulation model), inexperienced, poorly qualified or negligent practitioners may prescribe complementary medicine treatments that are contraindicated for patients already having treatment from Western allopathic medicine practitioners. As most Western allopathic medicine practitioners choose to remain ignorant (and scornful) of complementary medicine, they, too, may prescribe drugs or treatments that are contraindicated for patients already taking complementary medicine prescriptions.

Studying each patient's intake of pharmaceutical medicine, complementary medicine and other (sometimes self-prescribed) OTC substances may trigger warnings about interactions and contraindications. Resolving these may mitigate symptoms and clarify the aetiological pathway that has led to a diagnosis of Parkinson's disease.

Onset of symptoms may provide clues regarding the accuracy of the diagnosis. I see many people told they have Parkinson's disease with "atypical onset", or "atypical Parkinson's disease", or "Parkinsonism" because the symptoms fit the accepted picture of Parkinson's disease but have manifested more quickly than usual, or been noticed after significant life changes, or just seem "not quite normal". "Atypical" should trigger more investigation to find out what has caused the onset of symptoms.

Extreme diets, current or from the past, should also be noted as they may have compromised the immune system or damaged the nervous system. The reasons for undertaking the extreme diet may also indicate past trauma or poor self-image causing constant fight/flight/freeze response.

Current food choices are, of course, critical to understanding what may be causing symptoms. Inflammatory foods may be exacerbating illness symptoms, nutrition-free foods increasing fatigue, grains and dairy inhibiting digestive activity and production of neurotransmitters in the gut for transport to the brain, and caffeine increasing the fight/flight/freeze response. The manner of eating is also important as many people eat on the run, which greatly inhibits digestive ability. A salad eaten while rushing between appointments and under stress is just a nutrition-free as poor-quality breakfast cereal eaten at rest.

Stealth infections: Every patient I see completes Dr Richard Horowitz's **MSIDS questionnaire** without being aware of the object of these questions. Dr Horowitz, in his wonderful book *Why Can't I get Better?*[1] includes this questionnaire as a self-assessment tool together with a scoring key. I ask each patient to complete this as part of my general clinic questionnaire, with no scoring key. I can then score the answers and gain a good idea of whether stealth infection may be one of the pathways leading to symptoms. This questionnaire is readily available from Dr Horowitz's book and can be used separately (I have, at times, used it this way) or as part of a more comprehensive questionnaire for new patients as in my practice. The answers and scores in this questionnaire will not tell us what infection is the challenge, but can indicate that infection is unlikely, possible, very likely or almost certainly there as one of the pathways to illness.

If infection is possible, likely or very likely, then we need clinical skills to ascertain what infection. A few are traceable via readily available blood tests. However, real stealth infections like Borrelia, Bartonella, Babesia and some others are highly unlikely to show up on standard blood tests. There are only a handful of specialist pathology laboratories worldwide that are capable of reasonable accuracy in detecting these debilitating stealth infections via serology or PCR investigation. However, even these laboratories can claim only 50-70 per cent accuracy, depending on factors such as time since the first infection, symptom picture, time of day and month the blood is drawn, medication taken at the time of the test and concomitant morbidities. All ethical laboratories include a statement with the test results to the effect that diagnosis of Borrelia, Bartonella and Babesia is primarily by clinical examination and pathology tests may be used only as confirmation of clinical findings.

It is, therefore, very important for patients to seek out practitioners skilled in diagnosing and treating stealth infections and for practitioners who do not have these skills to network with appropriate colleagues.

Diagnosis of a stealth infection does not mean the patient does not have Parkinson's disease, but does mean that the infection is one of the prominent aetiological pathways creating Parkinson's disease symptoms.

Tests: Many patients have a number of tests and scans to eliminate other possible causes of their symptoms diagnosed as Parkinson's disease. Some will provide useful information for tracing or eliminating probable aetiological pathways.

Full blood examination (FBE) is always useful for indicating general function status. Haemoglobin, inflammatory markers, liver enzyme levels, white cell levels, cholesterol, vitamin D can all give information about the patient. Additional useful information is thyroid hormones – free T3, free T4, TSH, reverse T3 and thyroid antibodies may indicate thyroid dysfunction caused by stress or infection.

Online Visual Contrast Sensitivity (VCS) Aptitude Test:
https://www.survivingmold.com/store1/online-screening-test
If moulds/biotoxins are suspected as a symptom trigger or aggravation, this free online test from Dr Ritchie Shoemaker is a useful assessment. There are instructions on the site for taking the test. This is not a diagnostic test, but will give an indication of an individual reaction to mould/biotoxin infestation. If the test is positive, the patient's environment must be examined for moulds (by a building biologist if possible) and careful remediation undertaken. It is best for the patient to be absent during remediation and for some days following (again, if possible) as some remediation processes, especially for severe mould infestations, are quite toxic and may exacerbate the illness process. However, mould must be removed if the patient is to recover wellness. The patient will need to seek help from a naturopath or doctor experienced and skilled in treating mould/biotoxin infections.

Hair mineral analysis: Heavy metals and other toxins may be a significant influence on the health/illness processes within individuals. Blood tests for minerals and heavy metals are, in general, quite inaccurate so we need to look elsewhere for this information.

Twenty-four-hour urine analysis can be quite accurate but may need significant "flushing" of minerals before taking urine samples over twenty-four hours. This process can cause physical and emotional stress and, if the patient is already debilitated or anxious about their diagnosis, the extra stress may exacerbate symptoms.

Hair mineral analysis is available worldwide through many reputable laboratories. The test involves supplying a small quantity of clean, uncontaminated hair (no "products" or colours) to the chosen laboratory which will provide mineral levels within six weeks or so. Hair grows at roughly 1.25 centimetres (1/2 inch) per month, so the test results are "historical" – that is, they will show mineral levels two to three months ago. But, as symptoms in most patients have taken many years to develop, this is still very useful information, and the process is not stressful nor invasive. For those lacking head hair, pubic hair may be used. I have found hair tests to be very useful in showing critical mineral levels (e.g. calcium, magnesium, zinc), toxic levels (e.g. lead, mercury, arsenic, aluminium), and mineral ratios that may need correction.

Tests for infections: As discussed above, some infections may not be easily revealed using standard blood tests. However, blood tests from reputable laboratories can be useful for many infections that could be aggravating illness symptoms and need treatment. Herpes, Epstein-Barr virus, significant staphylococcus infections and many species of Rickettsia may show on blood tests. The decision then is whether to treat each infection separately or consider them as an aggravating factor, or else treat the underlying causative infection and allow the immune system to take care of the rest. This requires much discussion and skilful assessment by an holistic healthcare practitioner and may need cooperative treatment between complementary/alternative medicine and Western allopathic medicine practitioners.

Many of my patients, obviously symptomatic for Borrelia or Bartonella, have been referred for standard blood tests by their doctors which have shown negative for infection. Given that standard blood tests for these infections are only 10–15 per cent accurate, this is to be expected, especially if the patient was infected many years previous to the tests.

There are currently (2019) four laboratories worldwide that I can recommend for stealth infections testing: Igenex (California, USA), Infectolab and Armin Labs in Germany, and Aust Bio in Sydney, Australia. These laboratories have the most sensitive tests available at this time (I am sure there will be more in due course) but even these tests are 50–70 per cent accurate, not 100 per cent. Some strategies can ensure the highest degree of accuracy possible – drawing blood at the full moon (when the bacteria are likely to be the most active in replicating, so may appear in the blood), having a massage and/or undertaking some aerobic exercise before the blood draw. However, blood test results must always be considered in conjunction with clinical assessments and symptom pictures.

Challenge tests for stealth infections can be up to 98 per cent accurate. In this process, the patient is given an antimicrobial (herbal or pharmaceutical) aimed at the specific pathogen suspected. Killing the pathogen will cause it to dump toxic products into the patient's system and may overwhelm elimination pathways causing a "herx" (Jarisch-Herxheimer reaction). This reaction tells us that the pathogen is present. Strategies are then applied to stop the reaction, detox and treat correctly.

While challenge tests are very accurate, some patients are too debilitated or anxious to undertake a process that will, essentially, make them feel worse for some time, so we must rely on skilled clinical assessment. The key here is to make sure that the practitioner involved *is* skilled and experienced in detecting and treating stealth infections, and is open to the presence of *chronic* stealth infections.

Be wary of biofeedback testing (via muscle testing or machine) that indicates a plethora of infections, or rapid onset/resolution of stealth infections. Biofeedback can be useful and valuable in many illness and wellness settings, but can only reveal factors apparent to our body but below the level of our conscious awareness.

Stealth infections, by their nature, are not apparent to our body. Many stealth infections are able to disguise themselves (by changing the antigens on the outer membrane) so fooling the immune system into seeing the pathogen as normal. In these circumstances, biofeedback will be highly inaccurate and should not be relied on for diagnosis or disease tracking.

Where there are indications of more than one stealth infection, the practitioner must make decisions about priorities of treatment as, by treating the dominant infection(s), other co-infections/comorbidities may well be resolved by improved immune function.

Finding the aetiological pathways for each patient: This is the first and most important responsibility for each practitioner in conjunction with each patient and their support network. Until we ascertain what *caused* the symptoms diagnosed as Parkinson's disease, we are unable to reverse the illness process and assist in a return to wellness.

As patients, we must be thoughtful and honest about our symptoms, the onset of illness symptoms, our lifestyle, food choices, hobbies, recreation and history. We must also find out as much as possible about our family history.

As a practitioner, we must *look, listen and learn*.

Look at each patient as an individual person with characteristics unique to them. Look at how they walk, sit, move, stay calm or become agitated, changes in expression (or lack of), colours and style of clothing, hair style/colour/treatment, make-up and/or nail treatments. Each feature will tell a story about how the patient cares for themselves and possible toxins. Look at any companions present to see how supportive they might be.

Listen to what each patient says, how they say it, the real meaning behind the words, the sounds of fidgeting or foot tapping. If the patient is accompanied by a spouse, partner, family member or friend, listen to what they have to say, or sounds of agreement/disagreement with what the patient says.

Learn from what we see, what we hear and what we read in our questionnaire and any test results. The more we learn, the more likely we can accurately assess the aetiological pathways affecting this patient.

Most patients will be affected by two or more aetiological pathways. Most will have some level of toxicity which is almost inevitable in current Western society. We are surrounded by over 500,000 neurotoxic chemicals that have been released over the past fifty years with, or without, our knowledge. Some we have welcomed as making life more convenient, while others have been introduced to aid production of consumables or increase profit margins. Therefore, toxic load is always high on the list of factors affecting health for each patient.

Looking and listening for evidence of unresolved trauma, and looking for signs of infection take time but, once established or eliminated, facilitate our treatment plan and pathway to wellness.

The process of finding the aetiological pathways must be a cooperative effort between the patient and practitioner(s), and may involve family, partner or friends, pathology laboratories and other practitioners to make sure that all possible information is accessed and accurate.

SECTION 3

REVERSING THE ILLNESS PROCESSES

CHAPTER 12

LIVING WELL

This is for everyone

When diagnosed with any disease or disorder, our aim is to find the cause or causes, then work to reverse their effects on our health. In later chapters, I will give details of strategies to reverse the effects of specific aetiological pathways leading to a diagnosis of Parkinson's disease.

However, if we want to be well we must live well. And that means using strategies to live healthily in our current environment, no matter what aetiological pathway led to our diagnosis.

For a moment, let us indulge in a simplistic and fairly inaccurate analogy: let's compare our body with a computer (a modern, sophisticated, high-power super computer, but still much simpler than our body). Here are some what-ifs to consider:

1. What if we allow the operating system to become outdated and corrupt? The computer will stop working properly and provide inaccurate information.

2. What if we load cheap, non-compatible or corrupt programs? The programs won't work correctly and may corrupt our whole system.

3. What if we enter incorrect information into a program? We will receive incorrect information or results out of the program.

4. What if we never update a program or refresh it? It will stop working.

5. What if we never shut down the computer; just keep it running day in and day out for months or years? It will become sluggish and worn, and may stop working.

6. What if we allow dirt, liquid or other pollutants to enter the computer workings, or even the keyboard? The computer will no longer work correctly.

I think you get the picture. We must provide the environment, input and care that will allow our body (our "computer") to work efficiently over our lifespan. To do this, we all need to be involved in strategies that will maintain our "operating system", load up-to-date "programs" and update them periodically, and avoid pollutants.

Our operating system includes our brain, nervous system, blood and lymph circulation, immune system, fascia, skin, bones, muscles, ligaments and tendons. That's a complex collection of systems and parts that all need to be cared for and maintained. That means we must provide ourselves with a healthy environment as well as healthy inputs.

Our programs consist of our thoughts, our intellectual inputs (reading, study, discussion, debate) plus the nutrients to support those thought processes (food, drink, supplements), and the emotional complexities surrounding our thoughts and nutrients.

Creating a healthy environment means much more than removing obvious toxins from our home, although that is very important. I have included lists of potentially toxic products in the Environmental Toxins Pathway sections, and it is vital that we avoid all possible neurotoxins at all times.

However, much of our environment is emotional and/or spiritual, if the focus of our thoughts is stressful, negative or demeaning, then our endogenous chemical environment will be imbalanced and potentially neurotoxic. If our focus is peaceful, fulfilling, joyful and content, our endogenous chemical production will reflect that.

Case history: *I met Arthur in 2002. He was only forty-six years old and had been diagnosed with Parkinson's disease about six months earlier. His symptoms were mild – right hand tremor, some loss of mobility. He was a businessman and focused on business "success"; that seemed to mean making more profit than he had the year before.*

It quickly became obvious that Arthur's business was a major stressor, and his vision of success created unhealthy expectations for his own performance. When I suggested meditation, he didn't have time. Taking time off was not an option as he had not achieved his financial goals. Changing part of his current exercise program (weights plus intense cycling over 150 kilometres twice weekly) to Pilates and yoga was not considered, as it seemed to him that this would be a backward step.

Arthur could not see that his focus on driving his body hard and driving his business harder was maintaining a constant fight/flight/freeze response in his body. He wanted to achieve business and exercise goals that were unreasonable for his level of physical health.

To allow him to function more to his level of satisfaction in his business, Arthur started increasing his Parkinson's disease medication much more quickly than I considered wise. In less than twelve months, his medication input was creating adverse effects that inhibited his ability to function to a greater degree than his earlier symptoms. He stopped seeing me (not surprisingly, as he had refused to do most of what I had advised) and became involved in promoting fundraising to find a "cure" for Parkinson's disease. It was only a couple of years later that he chose deep brain stimulation which alleviated some of his medication-induced symptoms for a while, but he later had to cease involvement in business altogether.

This was a sad, but not unusual, story. Arthur was unable to see that he had chosen to create a neurotoxic environment that exacerbated the disease process when he had the option to create a calmer, more healing environment that could have supported all the physical changes he made and improved his health.

When I met Ronald, the story was very different. He was a little older than Arthur, at fifty-two, but had similar goals of success. However, within just a few months, Ronald had made significant changes to his environment by reducing his working hours (even though this had financial implications), revised his exercise program to include clinical Pilates as well as walking and medium weights, meditated daily and shifted his focus to being well joyfully. His reward was a steady improvement in physical health.

If our immediate environment is relatively free from toxic impact (there are many more details in the section on treating the toxic pathway), we need to consider our physical inputs.

CHAPTER 13

FOOD, HELPFUL AND HARMFUL

It does not matter what aetiological pathway led to diagnosis with Parkinson's disease, we must consume only food that will provide the nutrients we need to function healthily, feel energetic and motivated, and remain free from illness symptoms.

While many circumstances in our lives are largely beyond our control (although that is no excuse to give up), food is one we *can* control in almost every circumstance. This may require some negotiation with partners, spouses, live-in friends, meals-on-wheels providers or other food providers. But control can be and must be applied to ensure the best environment for healing.

Food and drink consumption is the only means (other than nutritional supplements) of providing our body with the nutrients we require for function, growth, thought, repair and healing. We can choose foods that help us or foods that harm us. There are no neutral foods. They either help or harm.

We must avoid all foods that create inflammation, reduce our immune integrity or our capacity to function healthily, or adversely affect our mood.

Far from being restrictive, our appropriate food choices will include all fresh, seasonal foods that are naturally suitable for human consumption, which includes a vast array of vegetables, fruits, eggs, fish, organic meat and chicken, nuts and seeds and, perhaps, some nutrient-dense supplements such as super green powders or protein powders (but not dairy or soy based).

We may prefer raw or cooked foods, and that is often a reflection of our body's needs. While our early ancestors ate most food raw, our digestive system may be unused to raw, fibrous foods at first, and we may need to introduce them slowly. For a few of us, raw foods are difficult because of past illnesses or surgery, so cooked foods may be a better choice. This is a matter for individual discussion between practitioner and patient.

We looked at the SAD food pyramid in the Toxic Pathway section and saw how this consumption pattern, promoted by "experts", is exacerbating illness pathways. A far healthier approach is this food pyramid which is closer to our need for seasonal, unpolluted food as nourishment and fuel.

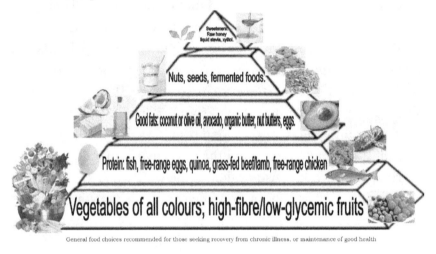

Sweeteners:
Raw honey
liquid stevia, xylitol.

Nuts, seeds, fermented foods.

Good fats: coconut or olive oil, avocado, organic butter, nut butters, eggs.

Protein: fish, free-range eggs, quinoa, grass-fed beef/lamb, free-range chicken

Vegetables of all colours; high-fibre/low-glycemic fruits

General food choices recommended for those seeking recovery from chronic illness, or maintenance of good health

Developing our food intake in line with this pyramid will assist in alkalising our body (while improving acid production in our stomach), improve nutrient uptake, reduce food sensitivities and allergies, and increase energy production.

Where possible, certified organic food is always the preferred choice. However, this may not be possible for many of us, either because of cost, or because organic food is just not available locally. However, some foods are more laden with agro-toxins than others. The so-called "Dirty Dozen" are foods most likely to be polluted (see below), so we should buy certified organic forms of these foods whenever we can.

- strawberries
- spinach
- nectarines
- apples
- peaches
- pears
- cherries
- grapes
- celery
- tomatoes
- sweet bell peppers/capsicum
- potatoes.

All these foods have the potential to be good for us in providing many nutrients that will help heal and maintain our computer. However, current growing processes include high rates of pesticide sprays that are often toxic to humans, so buy organic wherever possible. Where organic produce is not available, wash thoroughly, or peel, or avoid.

Despite some television advertising and patient concerns, being healthy does not mean that our food has to be restrictive, bland, unappetising, boring or weird. Examining the pyramid above will show that most naturally-occurring food and some carefully prepared foods will help us.

We have a vast array of vegetables available in most centres these days. Green, yellow, orange, red, white and even purple vegetables offer different flavours, textures, colours and nutrients to our meals. Vegetables may be eaten raw, steamed, baked or roasted, depending on the vegetable and your requirements.

A lovely combination for a family meal (especially when there are a variety of ages, backgrounds and needs together) is roasted vegetables, including potato, sweet potato, pumpkin, parsnip, beetroot, carrots and garlic; plus a selection of crunchy and colourful salad vegetables – lettuce, capsicum/bell pepper, celery, roquette, tomato, etc., with a lemon, lime and olive oil dressing; plus some steamed green beans and broccoli florets dressed with Himalayan sea salt, butter and nutritional yeast flakes; plus your choice of protein foods – fish, chicken, red meat or eggs. There are many more choices for this combination depending on location and season.

Buying local food wherever possible is good for our health, our community and our carbon footprint. In many cities and towns there are community gardens where you can be involved with growing your own food, or you can purchase food from local growers. Farmers markets are a great place for buying local, organic foods at reasonable prices. Some people are working with neighbours, growing different varieties of vegetables and fruit, and swapping excess production with each other.

Protein is important for our recovery and continued health. Eggs are brilliant food (free-range-organic of course), providing excellent protein, good fats and a wide variety of nutrients that our body easily absorbs. A few people are allergic to eggs, and this is unfortunate but not disastrous, as there are other proteins available. Eggs have received a bad reputation over many years because the yolk contains cholesterol. The cholesterol myth is a matter for discussion elsewhere. However, the important matter here is that research since 2014 has shown that egg consumption (up to three eggs per day) has no negative effect on serum cholesterol and, in some excellent studies, a positive effect on serum cholesterol. These recent studies have shown that, even when there is a small increase in serum LDL concentrations, the size of the LDL molecule increases which is, in fact, healthy for us, as large LDL molecules are less likely to be incorporated into arterial plaque.[1,2,3]

Wild-caught oily fish, such as salmon, trevally, mackerel, sardines, trout and herring are also excellent sources of protein and provide the benefits of anti-inflammatory oils as well. There is a legitimate concern about mercury pollution in some fish, and a much greater concern about the treatment of farmed fish. Realistically, there is probably not one unpolluted fish on earth today. In fact, I doubt there is any unpolluted food available. Our job, as patients and practitioners, is to find the sources of the least polluted foods, and strengthen our innate immune and elimination systems to cope with unavoidable toxins. If we purchase with care, we can find good quality oily fish with minimal pollution that will be of benefit to our health.

Organically farmed chicken is a pleasant change of flavour and texture, while organic red meat (especially young meat like lamb and veal) provides protein, iron and a number of other nutrients.

When cooking protein foods, especially fish, chicken and red meat, we must avoid the Western society habit of barbequed "burnt sacrifice". Charred or burnt meat and oxidised fats are *bad*. They exacerbate inflammation and carcinogenic processes (causing cancer). Cook gently on a hot plate, in a pan, or roast, bake or stew. Eggs can be fried in olive or coconut oil at low to medium heat, poached, boiled, scrambled or made into omelettes. I have learned to "froach" my eggs – break the eggs into a pan over low heat with a tiny amount of oil, add a teaspoon of water, pop on a lid and let the eggs fry/steam lightly. With this method, I produce "fried" eggs with cooked but soft whites and lovely runny yolks.

A very useful and nutritious protein for vegetarians, vegans or anyone wanting a change is quinoa (*Chenopodium quinoa*). This wonderful seed is often misnamed an ancient grain or a gluten-free grain. But it is *not* a grain at all. It is a seed originating from South America and grown domestically for over 3000 years. Quinoa is high in protein (higher than grains or most vegetables, but not as high as animal products), plus B vitamins, calcium, magnesium and other minerals. Quinoa may be used in most circumstances otherwise calling for rice, noodles or grains. It is available as seed, flakes or flour. There are many recipes for quinoa on the internet and in good cookbooks. Suffice to say that quinoa may be cooked in water (a bland but useful meal reinforcement), stock, bone broth or coconut cream/milk to bring a variety of flavours, textures and nutrient values to your meals.

Fermented foods such as sauerkraut, pickles and kimchi are good for supporting beneficial bacteria in our gut. There is a great deal of information online about fermented foods and how good they are for us. However, we need to be careful about the basic foods used for fermentation as not all are healthy.

Yoghurt is a healthy food if it is made from coconut milk and not pasteurised. It is not healthy if it is made from animal milk (inflammatory) and/or pasteurised (which kills the beneficial bacteria).

Kefir is healthy if made from coconut milk, nut milk, vegetables or plain water. It is not healthy if made from animal milk.

Including healthy fermented foods in your diet will assist your gut to digest other foods better.

There are groups of foods and pseudo-foods that must be avoided at all costs. Some may surprise you as they are foods commonly promoted as "good", "nutritious" and "necessary".

Grains (wheat, barley, rye, oats, rice, corn, spelt, millet and sorghum are common) in their current form are quite recent introductions into the human diet. It is difficult to know exactly when the first grains were added to our intake, but wild grains may have been introduced over 100,000 years ago. Domestication of grains (cultivation) probably started between 8,000 and 10,000 years ago, using seed from wild grains.

With the evolution of agriculture and the gathering of families into groups or villages that remained in place rather than staying nomadic, our choices of foods became restricted to those capable of farmed reproduction, supplemented with hunting in some areas, and thus selective breeding began.

Grains, which are seeds from grass, are fortified with lectins (proteins) that assist in warding off predators. There are many lectins of which gluten, the most infamous, is best known.

Many foods contain lectins, including vegetables, legumes and some fruits. However, the amount and type of lectin per gram of food is an important factor. A few lectins may be of benefit in the human body by assisting beneficial bacteria in the gut to replicate. Most, however, cause damage to the gut wall, may increase gut permeability, increase inflammation and, in many cases, create intolerance symptoms. The lectins in grains are inflammatory and, over time, will cause gut dysregulation with consequences of constipation, diarrhoea, IBS, autoimmune disorders, brain dysregulation and emotional lability.[4]

Coeliac disease is really end-stage lectin intolerance. Ninety-nine per cent of those diagnosed with coeliac disease show the presence of one or more variants of the HLA-DQA1 and HLA-DQB1 genes, so coeliac disease is classed as genetic. However, most people with these variants do not develop coeliac disease, so we can accept that lifestyle and environment are much more important influences on gut health than these gene variants.

Alternatives to grains are quinoa (*Chenopodium quinoa*), buckwheat (*Fagopyrum esculentum*) and amaranth (*Amaranthus species*). Flours made from nuts, coconut and seeds can be used for baking, and many recipes are available.

Animal dairy foods are touted as being high in protein, high in calcium and other minerals, and "good for us". The science supports the claims of contents but contradicts the latter (good for us). Population studies show that those consuming animal dairy products (milk, cream, cheese, yoghurt) regularly have a higher to much higher risk of Parkinson's disease, osteopenia, osteoporosis, IBS, cancers of the bowel, breast and prostate, memory challenges and dementia.[5,6,7,8]

There is no doubt that animal milk contains useful nutrients, including the calcium so often promoted. However, the human gut is not constructed to process these products appropriately. Milk molecules (A1 or A2) irritate the gut wall, causing inflammation. The irritation may also cause tight junctions between cells to open, thus allowing large proteins to enter the interstitial space. These actions create an acidic, inflammatory environment that our body must buffer to become more alkaline. To do that, the body extracts calcium from bones, nerves and lymph, so beginning the process of osteoporosis.[9]

Teenagers (especially girls) who have consumed animal dairy have a significantly higher incidence of bone fracture than non-dairy consumers. Importantly for this document, women who have consumed animal dairy habitually show up to 60 per cent higher risk of Parkinson's disease while male dairy consumers show a dose-related increase of risk.[10,11]

Exceptions to damaging dairy are organic, grass-fed butter and ghee. These may be used moderately for flavour or cooking.

Do we need milk? Not really. We use it mostly to eat with grain cereals that we will no longer be eating (see above), so a major use of milk is gone. Cheese? This is certainly an indulgent and tasty addition to many meals, but simply is bad for us. We can use coconut cheese as an alternative, or add nutritional yeast flakes to foods where we would normally use cheese for flavour and texture.

There are useful alternatives to animal dairy, some of which have positive benefits. Nut milks such as almond milk (unsweetened) and hemp milk are useful as fluids where needed. Coconut milk and cream are tasty, easy to use and contain some useful fats. As mentioned above, we can now obtain coconut cheese which is a great alternative for foods like pizza (with a non-grain crust), pasta (from pulses, buckwheat or seaweed), omelettes, etc. Coconut cream solids may be whipped to replace whipped animal cream in desserts.

Processed and "cured" foods are ubiquitous in our supermarkets and stores today. Three-quarters of supermarket shelves are loaded down with packets of pseudo foods that have little to no nutritional value. The packages are strategically placed and brightly coloured to attract buyers already prepared by constant visual and aural advertising. Reading the details on each packet will reveal that many have little of the claimed "food" in them and, what there is, has been steamed, sterilised, cleaned, refined, bleached, coloured, flavoured, added to, modified, emulsified and rendered unrecognisable from the original. Many packets show, in very small print, added cane sugar or similar, salt, artificial flavours and colours, preservatives that may be toxic to humans, palm oil and canola oil.

Casual observation at supermarket checkouts will often see trolleys loaded with packaged foods, sugary drinks, frozen sweets and not a fresh vegetable to be seen. These goods are seductive and addictive. They are also convenient to buy and prepare quickly (throw them in the microwave) but yield no benefit to our health.

"Cured" foods, such as bacon, ham, pressed chicken, etc., pose different challenges. Processing changes the constituents and develops carcinogenic chemicals. As people with Parkinson's, we are already very sensitive to chemical pollution, so it seems sensible to reduce our risk of developing cancer by not consuming carcinogenic foods.

Artificial sweeteners: Refined cane sugar has, correctly, been condemned as something to avoid (see below). Many alternatives have been researched and promoted as lacking calories and being many times sweeter than sugar. Many of these statements are true in that the substance has almost zero calories and is very sweet (sometimes hundreds of times sweeter than sugar). However, there are dangers lurking in omissions from these statements.

Many artificial sweeteners cause damage to our nervous system either directly or by increasing inflammation. When added to drinks (such as soda) the damage can be increased dramatically.

Claims that replacing cane sugar with artificial sweeteners will assist in reducing weight are simply untrue. Most people using this strategy gain weight. Another omission from promotors is that many artificial sweeteners are addictive, so total consumption of calories can actually increase.

Regular consumption of artificially sweetened soda may be a prime cause of inflammatory disorders, especially if the person also consumes inflammatory foods.[12]

> **Case history:** *Rachel was diagnosed with ankylosing spondylitis at seventeen years of age and treated conservatively with analgesics and steroids. By the time I saw her thirteen years later, she was almost crippled, in constant pain despite swallowing over thirty pain pills each day, and very despondent. Scans of her spine showed almost complete fusion from C3 to L5. Her foods of choice were meat pies, some cooked vegetables and three litres of diet soda per day.*
>
> *We began introducing better foods, added some homeopathic treatment and gentle bodywork, and I asked her to slowly reduce her diet soda ingestion over six weeks to zero. She did everything I asked, except decided to go "cold turkey" in stopping her diet soda. She suffered bad withdrawal symptoms (headache, depression, anxiety, shaking, diarrhoea) for about a week, then settled down into her new routine.*
>
> *Within three months, Rachel was free from pain, her spine had unfused and her mood was hopeful, happy and, sometimes, joyful.*

Cane sugar is almost ubiquitous in packaged foods today. Sugar is a huge industry using every marketing ploy possible to persuade the public, governments and health authorities that the consumption of cane sugar is "normal" and "healthy".

Fortunately, after many years of pressure from complementary/alternative medicine practitioners and holistic nutritionists, Western allopathic medicine researchers and practitioners began to see the damage caused by this white poison and began the process of getting governments onside. Response has been weak, as there is enormous dollar pressure from the sugar industry to maintain its "healthy" status and, there is no doubt, it is a source of employment for thousands of workers.

There has been a satisfying reduction in sugar promotion and some moves towards legislating for clearer labelling of foods, and reduction of sugar content in drinks.

One of the unfortunate offshoots of this sugar-reduction campaign has been the growth of the artificial sweetener industry (see above), but any reduction in refined sugar consumption is a good thing.

Refined sugar, that is, sugar not naturally occurring in foods we consume, creates challenges for our digestive system that spread throughout our body. Briefly, we produce large amounts of insulin to deal with the extra sugar, convey it into cells and use it to produce energy. Over time, this can lead to insulin resistance – that is, insulin receptors become jaded and unable to accept and utilise the increased amounts insulin produced. This can then lead to a reduction in insulin production, raising the level of sugar in our blood.

The symptoms of diabetes are well known but there are more subtle and less well recognised adverse effects of refined sugar consumption. Diabetes Australia (www.diabetesaustralia.com.au) notes the following as complications of diabetes:

- People with diabetes are up to four times more likely to suffer heart attacks and strokes
- Diabetes is the leading cause of preventable blindness in Australia
- Kidney failure is three times more common in people with diabetes
- Amputations are fifteen times more common in people with diabetes
- More than 30 per cent of people with diabetes experience depression, anxiety and distress.

These nasty effects begin long before diabetes is diagnosed or treatment commenced.

Furthermore, consumption of refined sugar increases inflammation. People with Parkinson's are in a state of chronic inflammation, and we need to reduce or eliminate any food or activity that exacerbates that state.

There are a number of naturally occurring sweeteners that we can use where necessary (fruit or raw organic honey, for instance) and it is a really good idea to get used to less-sweet foods. In fact, our digestive system will work better if we consume some bitter foods to generate hydrochloric acid in our stomach and digestive enzymes in our intestine.

Caffeine is being promoted these days as beneficial in quite large quantities. Drinking coffee at the rate of between four and eight cups daily is, according to some medical researchers, supposed to prevent diseases like cancer, dementia, Parkinson's disease and many other chronic disorders. For those already ill, there are claimed benefits from drinking coffee also.

We need to be very careful about this "research" (which is being supported by many coffee-drinking doctors) as there is much that is not revealed.

As an aside, the hype about coffee and Parkinson's disease reminds me of research I looked at many years ago which stated that smoking cigarettes would prevent or delay the onset of Parkinson's disease! We have since discovered the terrible toll smoking wreaks on our health (directly and indirectly) and the smoking/Parkinson's disease research has been largely filed under "interesting but …"[13,14] However, I am still occasionally asked by people with Parkinson's if they should start smoking after diagnosis with Parkinson's disease and noted that, in a 2018 medical story on Parkinson's disease, smoking was mentioned as a factor reducing risk!

The coffee research is much better presented and, with the

growth of the internet in social media, has gained a lot of traction with gullible people and those who are addicted to coffee.

Caffeine stimulates adrenal activity and promotes an artificial fight/flight/freeze response. This, in turn, exacerbates inflammation, anxiety, tremor and insomnia. It may also exacerbate other chronic disorders such as diabetes, arthritis and osteoporosis.

The adrenal stimulation can become addictive as, for a short time, it makes us feel better. We feel we have more energy, we may even feel sharper in thought, and it can stimulate bowel function. The disadvantage of this is, of course, that we must continue drinking coffee to sustain these apparent benefits.

We must also recognise that the research was conducted using good quality coffee, not the instant rubbish consumed by many coffee drinkers. The extra chemicals and lack of quality contained in instant coffees make them beverages to be avoided at all costs. However, even the best quality coffee will offer more disadvantages that advantages.

My clinical experience and patient notes reveal that over 90 per cent of my patients diagnosed with Parkinson's disease were coffee drinkers (including me), and all those who have recovered, stopped drinking coffee (again, including me).

You will find more comprehensive lists of foods to eat and avoid a little later. However, how we eat is also important. Our digestive system requires energy to process and absorb nutrients from food. Therefore it is best for our health to give our body time and attention so we gain the utmost benefit from the food we consume.

Eat calmly: Eating on the job while fending phone calls or rushing to meetings is detrimental to our digestive process and can create problems later diagnosed as chronic disorders such as gastroesophageal reflux disease (GORD), irritable bowel syndrome (IBS), Arthritis, Diabetes Mellitus, and many others. Eating without attention (mindfulness) is another way to throw our body into fight/flight/freeze response, with all the health consequences described in the section on the trauma pathway. Many years of stressful work and bad eating habits have resulted in many successful people in these positions suffering from mal-nutrition, even though they are surrounded by opportunities to eat well and are, ostensibly, consuming moderately healthy food. Their digestive system simply lacks the energy to process food properly because they are constantly diverting energy to phone calls, meeting, plans or projects.

Taking time out to enjoy food, look at it, smell it, note the flavours and feel it supporting our body brings great benefit. There are many enjoyable ways to do this. We can eat alone, just concentrating on the food and process of eating. We can use meal times as functioning meditations: focus on the food, be grateful for the colours, aromas and flavours, visualise the benefits it brings to us. We can listen to music (calming or uplifting), read relaxing books or magazines, or enjoy conversation with family and friends.

Mealtimes are not appropriate for business plans, arguments, or solving problems. They are times for laughter, intimacy, gentleness and love.

The number of meals we eat each day is not as important as the quality of the food and the time given for enjoying food. Each person needs to decide, possibly in conjunction with their healthcare practitioner, how many meals they require each day, and the best times to enjoy those meals.

Many of us were brought up on the principle of three square meals per day. This was generally interpreted as cereal for breakfast (non-food), sandwiches for lunch (inadequate and inflammatory), then meat and three vegetables for dinner with, possibly, a sweet or cake to follow. This is a very unhealthy principle.

There is an old adage stating we should breakfast like a king/queen, lunch like a prince/princess, and dine like a pauper. If we wish to stay with three meals per day, this is the best way to do it: a big, hearty, high-protein breakfast, substantial lunch with protein and vegetables and a light evening meal when we are likely to be less active.

However, there is no reason that we must have three meals each day. Two meals or even one meal per day may suit many of you. I have established a very satisfactory routine of two meals daily, which enhances my work process and suits my body. This will not suit everybody but has helped me significantly. The routine is rising reasonably early, some aerobic and weight exercises, then one to one and a half hours writing or work, a substantial breakfast later in the morning, work through the day, then an early dinner consisting of protein and vegetables but smaller in size than breakfast. I may have a piece of fruit or a cup of Rooibos tea during the day. I also take a short, five-minute break each two hours or so for meditation – more about that later.

Some people find one meal per day enough. A substantial meal during late morning or early afternoon may provide sufficient nutrition to be active, happy and well. Obviously, the meal will consist of quality protein, a variety of vegetables and, possibly, some fruit.

There are a few people with challenged digestive system who need to graze in order to sustain their nutrition levels. They may need to eat small amounts six or seven times daily to gain nutrition and avoid digestive discomfort. This is usually a temporary state that corrects over time with appropriate guidance and changes.

If you are a person with Parkinson's, it is important to find a member of your healthcare team who has been well trained in food, nutrition and health recovery. This may not be a doctor or dietician as many do not receive holistic training in food and eating. Holistic nutritionists, naturopaths or herbalists with additional nutrition training and/or long experience in treating people with chronic disorders may be the best choice. It is also very important for each person to pay attention to how food affects them, the number of meals that suit them best, and meal timing that is right for them.

Remember that what is *in* food is not as important as what our body can extract from that food and how we can use it.

Intermittent fasting may be helpful for many, providing we eat appropriate meals before and after the fast. The length of intermittent fasts may range from twelve hours to two days but, for those diagnosed with Parkinson's disease, twelve to sixteen hours seems to be the most useful.

This is not arduous as it simply means that we finish our evening meal at, say, 7 pm, then refrain from eating until after 7 am the next day. That's twelve hours. Sixteen hours is from 7 pm to 11 am, or 6 pm to 10 am. Really not difficult at all.

The benefits of intermittent fasting can include improved cell repair and removal of toxic waste, reduction of oxidative stress and inflammation, reduced risk of insulin resistance, reduced heart stress, improved cognitive function, reduced oxidised and serum cholesterol levels, and improvements in general wellbeing.

Foods

The lists of foods below are not complete as there are many foods unique to different countries and localities. However, the lists will give guidance when choosing foods. Choose wisely to create health and shun all foods that will harm you.

Best foods

80 per cent or more of your daily consumption

The following foods will supply you with all the nutrients required so that your body can produce the amino acids and glycoproteins necessary for its healing. Try to include as many of these as possible as your staple and snack foods (aim for at least 80 per cent of your food intake from this list).

All vegetables: (At least 70 per cent of each main meal recommended):

Best: raw and steamed

Okay: stir-fried and baked

Vegetables will provide vitamins, minerals, protein, fibre and hydration. Choose the widest possible range in your locality. Choose green, yellow, orange, red, white and purple if possible. Eat three to eight different vegetables with your main meal for the day (see notes on breakfast below). Include bitter, mild and sweet vegetables as well as pickled or fermented.

Fruits that are high in fibre and lower in sugar such as avocado (good protein and anti-inflammatory), lemons, limes, tomatoes, cranberries, fresh figs, fresh apricots, kiwi fruit, pears, Granny Smith apples, peaches, cherries. Avocado gives excellent protein, omega 3 and 9 fatty acids, and is anti-inflammatory. It is excellent for reproductive health as well as gaining wellness. Eat one per day if possible. Buy organic fruit whenever possible or wash the fruit thoroughly to remove pesticides and wax (used to make the skin shiny in shop displays).

Fruit is best eaten as snacks rather than as a main meal (other than avocado and tomatoes that fit well into main meals). However, lemon juice or fresh lemon before each meal can improve digestion.

Fish: (especially deep sea and oily fish):

Best: steamed or poached

Okay: baked, grilled, or fried gently in coconut or grape-seed oil or extra virgin olive oil.

Buy fresh fish if you trust your fishmonger and know where the fish is sourced. Most fishmongers are honest people eager to help customers; however, there have been cases of fish imported from other countries, caught in highly polluted waters, renamed and sold as good quality fish. So take time to befriend your fish merchant, get to know where the fish is sourced and make sure it is exactly what it is advertised to be.

There is a great deal of legitimate concern over heavy metal contamination of fish from coastal waters. We humans have done a great job of polluting our world with poisons that can kill us, so it is wise to be wary. There is probably not one gram of unpolluted food on the planet, so we need to seek out the least polluted and most local foods we can find.

Deep-sea fish are generally less polluted than surface feeders, while the larger predator fish tend to be more polluted – that is, large fish like sharks eat smaller fish that are polluted so tend to accumulate larger amounts of pollutants.

Good fish to look for are wild Atlantic salmon, blue-fin tuna, mackerel, Norwegian sardines, fresh water trout (especially from mountain areas), and other deep-sea fish.

If fresh fish is not available locally (as in my town), we have two options. We can travel intermittently to a quality fish market, buy in bulk and freeze for later use, or else purchase the best quality frozen fish available. Both options work well. If buying from a fish market to freeze, make sure you carry the fish home with ice in some sort of insulated or refrigerated container to prevent contamination. If purchasing ready frozen fish, read the packets to make sure it is genuine, from sustainable sources and, if farmed, farmed organically without polluted feed.

Frozen fish should be thawed in the refrigerator and cooked once thawed. Fresh or properly thawed fish should not smell unpleasantly "fishy", but carry an aroma of freshness. Yes, it will smell like fish, but pleasantly so.

Good quality canned salmon, tuna and sardines are useful as part of lighter meals. Again, read and research so you know where the fish is sourced.

Eggs: Free-range (organic if possible), boiled, poached, scrambled, or fried in a little coconut or olive oil. Omelettes are terrific too. Eggs may also be added to protein shakes.

It is true that egg yolks contain cholesterol. This is one of the valuable attributes of organic eggs. Not only is the egg cholesterol easily absorbed; eating organic eggs may help us reduce our serum cholesterol and improve our HDL/LDL ratio.

Large population studies have concluded that eating organic, free-range (pasture-fed) eggs in significant quantities has no bearing on serum cholesterol. The quality of eggs, however, is very important, as eggs from caged hens do not have nearly the same nutritional values as organic free-range eggs.[15]

Another important fact is that we need cholesterol to form cell membranes and hormones. We make most of our cholesterol internally, and cholesterol in food is a minor matter as far as quantity goes. If we reduce our cholesterol production, we reduce our ability to form new cells and hormones, leading to many adverse effects like confusion, anxiety, pain, fatigue and others.

Arterial plaque, the material that blocks cardiac arteries and causes heart attacks, is composed of calcium, fat, cholesterol (approximately 15 per cent), cellular waste, fibrin, foam cells and macrophages. Plaque forms when inflammation or oxidative damage causes the artery wall to become rough or damaged. The plaque forms to stop further damage but, as we rarely change our lifestyle when this happens, damage spreads, and so does plaque.

Oxidised cholesterol is damaging, but that comprises just a tiny percentage of cholesterol in our body. Lifestyle choices that reduce inflammation, improve activity and reduce stress may stop or even reverse the formation of arterial plaque. Eggs can be part of that lifestyle.

A few people are allergic to eggs and that is unfortunate, but not disastrous as there are other excellent protein foods available.

Quinoa (*keenwa*): A great source of complete protein, calcium, fibre and other minerals. Can replace all other grains as it is a seed rather than a grain; buckwheat is also good.

When we eat refined carbohydrates (e.g. refined flour, white rice), the food becomes sugar and requires insulin and other sugar processes. Refined carbohydrates can increase insulin resistance and exacerbate diabetes. A cup of cooked white rice equals about ten cubes of sugar!

Quinoa is more complex and contains significant dietary fibre, so creates much less sugar. After cooking, which is the typical preparation for eating, quinoa is 72 per cent water, 21 per cent carbohydrates, 4 per cent protein and 2 per cent fat. In a 100 g (3.5 oz) serving, cooked quinoa provides 120 calories and is an excellent source of manganese and phosphorus, and a moderate source of dietary fibre, folate, iron, zinc and magnesium.

The nutritional quality and appeal of quinoa can be enhanced by cooking in bone broth, stock or coconut cream.

Fresh whole nuts and seeds: Almonds, brazils, pecans, walnuts, pine nuts, macadamia and others (*not peanuts or cashews*) plus seeds such as pumpkin seeds, sesame seeds, sunflower seeds, flax seeds, etc. Nuts and seeds provide protein, fibre and minerals and are excellent as snacks or for adding to salads or other food dishes.

Peanuts and cashews are not nuts, but legumes. Many peanut crops are infested with aflatoxins (moulds) that are very toxic to humans, so are best avoided. Some cashew crops are also infested. European government testing has revealed that only a few cashew crops are infested, so choosing genuine organic cashews is a wise move. However, any recipe calling for cashews can be made using macadamia nuts, so we can do without cashews.

Fresh juices (especially vegetable juices) are packed with enzymes and provide easily assimilated nutrients to the body from an organic source. Fruit juices should be diluted with water by 30-50 per cent to prevent sugar hits from pure juice.

Remember that when we extract juice from a vegetable or

fruit, we lose fibre and many minerals, so have reduced the value of that vegetable or fruit. Juices are pleasant and a good snack drink, but cannot replace whole fresh vegetables or fruit.

Herbs: Culinary herbs: Use as many as palatable added to the vegetables and other foods.

Teas such as Rooibos, dandelion, peppermint, rosehip etc.

Medicines, as prescribed by a qualified herbalist or naturopath.

Breakfast

This is the most important meal of the day, and often the most neglected. We *must* eat a high protein breakfast to maintain our energy throughout the day and assist the healing process.

Breakfast timing may vary, of course, especially if we are choosing a routine of intermittent fasting. Breakfast time may range from 5 am for those leaving early for work to 11 am for those on a more relaxed schedule.

It is important, however, to fuel our body before we expect serious energy expenditure. We may choose moderate exercise before eating, followed by a refuelling meal but, if we are about to embark on a day of work, energetic entertainment or a marathon, we must give our body the fuel to produce the energy required.

Athletes make sure they feed their bodies before embarking on sporting events. As people with Parkinson's, we are undertaking a continuous marathon requiring all the energy we can muster, so we must fuel our body at the start of our daily journey.

Best breakfasts include: eggs (two to four) plus avocado, and add (as you wish) fish, vegetables, mushrooms, tomato, spinach, etc. You may, like me, enjoy the same breakfast each morning, or vary the combination sometimes for interest. As long as we give ourselves good protein plus some fibre and flavour, we will do well.

Alternative breakfasts: Quinoa porridge plus sunflower seeds, fresh fruit and almond milk (plus a little raw honey for sweetening if desired); or salmon/sardines/tuna and avocado, spinach and other vegetables.

Mediocre foods

Up to 20 per cent of your daily consumption

The following are foods that will not adversely affect your health and will provide some energy value and nutritional value. These are fine in smaller quantities or as snack foods, when the better-quality foods are not available.

Fruits higher in fructose (especially dried fruit) – small quantities only as snacks. Avoid these if you have, or suspect you have diabetes or a fungal/yeast problem such as candida. Check with your healthcare practitioner.

Lean young **meat** such as lamb, veal or game (e.g. kangaroo, deer and rabbit), or lean free-range chicken breast can be eaten two or three times weekly. Organic is always better.

Milk substitutes: Almond, coconut or hemp milk are the best alternatives to animal milk. Always buy the unsweetened organic varieties. Or make nut milk by soaking almonds in water overnight, then blending in the morning. Coconut cream is excellent to replace dairy cream or give a rich smooth texture to your food. Coconut cheese and yoghurt (unsweetened) are excellent substitutes for the animal sourced products.

Eliminate all grains: Quinoa *and* **buckwheat** are seeds rather than grains and may be used as substitutes for wheat, other grains, rice and noodles in most instances. Quinoa particularly is a good source of protein and calcium, and can replace rice and couscous in all dishes. **Wheat and other grains must be eliminated** and replaced with quinoa and/or buckwheat (pasta, flour, etc.). Gluten-free products may be used very sparingly.

Legumes such as lentils, beans and peas (e.g. chickpeas) may be eaten in moderate quantities to add nutrition, variety, fibre, protein and carbohydrates. Legumes may be difficult to digest for those from white Caucasian backgrounds and may cause flatulence as a result, but most people can get used to them over a fairly short time.

Raw, organic honey and **pure maple syrup** in very small quantities are useful sweetening substitutes in food preparation. Pure liquid **stevia** (not powdered stevia as this is often contaminated with other material) and powdered **xylitol** from *birch* (not from corn) are also useful.

Oils: Use **coconut oil** for cooking with high heat, and/or **extra virgin olive oil** for low to moderate heat (less than 180°C) and/ or for dressings.

Rooibos tea: Better than all green, white or black teas and coffee for antioxidant activity and free from caffeine and tannins. Most are organic, but check before you buy. Available in supermarkets.

Rooibos tea is a robust-flavoured herbal tea (sometimes known as Red Bush tea) which may be consumed without any additions (i.e. "black" – it is, in fact, a deep red colour), with almond or coconut milk ("white"), with or without a little honey for sweetening. Rooibos tea is naturally mildly sweet so is most enjoyable on its own.

Worst foods

The following foods give very little nutritional value, and are generally toxic to humans, especially fragile humans with symptoms of a chronic disorder. Their toxicity counteracts any energy and nutritional value that they may offer. Eliminate these from your diet as either staple meals or snacks. Consuming any of these foods may exacerbate your illness process.

All animal dairy products (i.e. milk, cheese, cream, yogurt) that come from cows, goats or sheep inhibit gut absorption, reduce calcium uptake, and may aggravate gut and lymph imbalances. **Organic butter and ghee** in small quantities are useful. Population studies indicate that those habitually consuming animal milk, cream, cheese and yoghurt have greatly increased risks of osteoporosis, Parkinson's disease, a variety of emotional challenges, gut disorders and some cancers.

Processed foods such as margarine, and processed meats such as bacon, ham, salami and others ("cured foods"), tinned and packaged foods should be generally avoided. Many of these foods contain trans fatty acids (artificial fats) that may be carcinogenic, artificial additives that may create illness symptoms, and other illness-creating properties caused by the processing.

Food with additives (such as chemical preservatives, colours and flavours including artificial sweetener). *NB: never consume any artificial sweetener – they are neurotoxic, suppress immune function, and may be carcinogenic.*

Coffee and other caffeinated beverages including **black, white and green teas** (Rooibos tea is a very good substitute). Recent research has shown that polyphenols from green tea can block the conversion of tyrosine to dopamine. This conversion of amino acids to neurotransmitters occurs during the biopterin cycle (part of our methylation detox pathway) and is vital to ongoing health, especially if we display symptoms of Parkinson's disease. While there is no research on the actions of polyphenols from other forms of tea (black and white) or coffee, there is the possibility that these also block production of dopamine.

Grains (especially wheat, but *all* grains) and refined grain products, such as breads, pasta, biscuits, etc. Lectins and gluten in grains inhibit gut absorption and interfere with gut permeability, and therefore aggravate digestive and bowel dysfunctions. Most foods contain lectins, so it is the type of lectin that is important. Lectins in grains are intended to ward off or kill predators by adversely affecting their gut and nervous systems. We are grain predators (we eat them) and, although we are much bigger than insects, repeated consumption of grains will create lectin-caused inflammatory illness.

Saturated fats from most animal sources, including dairy products (see above), fatty red meats, especially if fat is caramelised (burnt), lard, etc. The backyard barbeque can be very unhealthy, even while offering wonderful social support and interaction. Cooking/charring meat fats on the open grill creates carcinogenic properties. Look for lean meat and chicken, and cook on the solid hotplate or in a pan. I use a griddle pan that offers excellent fat drainage without exposure to naked flame. *Saturated fats from coconut, avocado, eggs and similar are healthy.* Butter and ghee from organic, grass-fed cattle are also safe to use in moderate quantities.

Peanuts and cashews can cause a reaction in certain people and cause bowel and digestive disruptions because of the moulds within the "nuts" (they are actually legumes) that have a toxic effect once eaten. Peanut crops suffer widespread infestation by aflatoxins and, while cashew crops are much less affected, only consume cashews if you are certain that they are organically produced and free from aflatoxins.

Old or sick animals and vegetables. This is logical. Fresh produce that is stored for too long may be infected with bacteria that can cause mild to fatal disease in humans.

Refined foods including refined sugar. Refined carbohydrates (especially grain flours, cereal, etc.) simply become sugar when consumed. Food that is refined and processed has much less nutritional value (if any) than fresh whole food.

Highly spiced foods such as the hotter curries, because they can inhibit gut function by reducing the action of villi and peristalsis. Mildly spiced foods may be used for flavour and variety.

CHAPTER 14

DETOXING

We are surrounded by toxic substances that may be detrimental to our health. We know that there are at least 500,000 neurotoxic chemicals in our general environment that are difficult to avoid. Many of these chemicals have been produced and permitted for limited usage but, through unwise practices, have spread into areas never intended.

Agrochemicals are a case in point. Many herbicides and pesticides are produced for limited use on particular crops and not recommended for release in populated areas. However, the areas under crop (often many hectares) mean that aerial spraying and long-arm spraying are now common. Even in the lightest breeze, spray particles can drift many kilometres. There is some evidence suggesting chemical drift of fifty kilometres from the spray site.[1,2]

Residual chemicals no longer used (e.g. lead in petroleum/gas) are still found in dust many kilometres from the area of original use. Old animal dipping chemicals (arsenic, DDT) remain in the soil surrounding dipping areas and may be in ground water.

Modern town/city/suburban life brings contact with many toxic chemicals from traffic pollution, cleaning chemicals in public places (shops, public buildings, parks, toilets) and construction chemicals (paints, coatings, adhesives) as well as the drift from gardens, roadside verges and flight paths.

While we can choose to create a toxic-chemical-free home for ourselves, we cannot avoid contact with carcinogenic and neurotoxic chemicals unless we seal ourselves in a bubble. Our best strategy then is to avoid toxic chemicals when we can, use detoxification techniques to remove chemicals from our body as much as we can, and protect ourselves against their effects.

In Chapter 6, we examined many common products that contain potentially neurotoxic chemicals. Our first obvious strategy, then, is to eliminate any of these products from our homes and, if possible, work environment. Many can be replaced with simple, inexpensive alternatives while other replacements, even though costing a little more than standard products, will protect your health.

Cleaning chemicals can be replaced with white vinegar, sodium bicarbonate, eucalyptus oil, lemon juice and, so often forgotten, hot water and "elbow grease". For instance, we clean our stainless steel stove top with hot water 95 per cent of the time with occasional use of bicarb. We have found organic, non-toxic dishwashing liquid, laundry liquid and dishwasher powder. Toilet cleaner can be made using white vinegar, psyllium husk (a tiny amount) a couple of drops of organic dishwashing liquid and eucalyptus oil. The toilet shines white and smells fresh. If this is too much trouble, there are organic toilet cleaners based on tea tree oil that work really well.

When we purchase body care products, we *must* read the small print on the labels. Products can be labelled "natural" or "organic" with very little natural or organic constituents. The permitted amount varies from place to place, but can be as low as 10 per cent! This means that some "natural organic" body care products may be 90 per cent toxic. Always read the labels and stick to the principle of "if you can't spell it, pronounce it, understand it, or know what the number means, don't buy it".

Once we have cleaned up our homes, we need to detox and protect ourselves. Protection is mostly based around boosting our immune system and enhancing elimination pathways. In the next section, I describe a number of nutritional supplements that will help boost our immune system integrity and performance. In general, nutritional supplements should be prescribed by a qualified and experienced healthcare practitioner. Most complementary/alternative medicine (CAM) practitioners are well trained in this while, unfortunately, most Western allopathic medicine (WAM) practitioners have no training in nutrition or nutritional supplements, but there are a few that can be helpful for almost everyone. Check them out when you finish setting up your detox strategies.

Simple and potent detox activities include:

- Drinking at least 1.5 litres (3 pints) of clean water each day (*not* alkaline water – the pH should be between 6.8 and 7.2)
- Including Rooibos tea, or other non-caffeinated herbal teas, in your daily routine
- Dry skin brushing daily (see Appendix 1)
- Strong lemon juice in warm water before each meal (enhances digestion, plus liver and gall bladder activity)
- Epsom salts (magnesium sulfate) baths or foot baths (see Appendix 1)
- Including vitamin C and magnesium in your supplement list (see next section)
- Drinking green smoothies (see Appendix 1).

Where toxins have been a long-term challenge (which means most of us over fifteen years of age), your healthcare provider may wish to prescribe certain detox formulas or remedies to assist. This is particularly important where industrial or agricultural chemicals are involved as these are very difficult to move out of cells without causing distress. Most agricultural and industrial chemicals are petroleum based or fat soluble, that is, they are absorbed into fatty tissue and stored in cells. While our normal elimination pathways may be efficient (bowels, bladder, sweat and respiration), these fat-soluble toxins remain in cells causing inflammation and, often, direct damage to our nervous system.

There are efficient methods to move the toxins out of cells, into the bloodstream where they can be processed and eliminated, But, if we do this too quickly, the dump of toxins into the bloodstream can cause illness and distress. So the process is best supervised by a healthcare professional who is experienced in treating fragile people (particularly people with Parkinson's) for toxic overload. These will be discussed in detail later.

CHAPTER 15

BASIC NUTRITIONAL SUPPLEMENTS

We are told by "health authorities" that we can obtain all the nutrients we need from a healthy diet. However, as we discussed in Chapter 7, most do not consume a healthy diet and, even if they do, according to health authorities, the food consumption is loaded with grains (sugar and inflammation), animal dairy (inflammation, calcium loss, etc.) and processed foods. I see many in my clinic who have been eating the Standard Australian/American Diet for most of their lives (thinking it is healthy) and show distinct signs of malnutrition.

We face another challenge in Western society. Most of our food is mass produced, harvested early, stored for a significant period of time, transported long distances and processed with a variety of preservation and appearance strategies to give it a longer shelf life and make it more attractive for sale. Foods may be harvested early and ripened in an artificial environment to give protection from weather and predators. This seems sensible, except that some of the nutritional value occurs during the last few weeks of maturation. Some foods are waxed to make them look nice and shiny on the shelves to encourage buyers. There are many other techniques used to encourage buyers to choose the high-profit, easier-to-produce foods over the organic, more nutritious foods that are, generally, more expensive anyway.

The upshot of all this is a lack of appropriate nutrients even in a carefully constructed and varied food intake. Add to that the stress of manifesting illness symptoms plus the challenges that created those symptoms, and there is no doubt that sensible nutritional supplementation will enhance our pathway to health.

It is always wise to talk to your healthcare practitioner about any supplementation you wish to commence. However, it is important to choose the people you talk to with care. Most Western allopathic medicine practitioners have little to no training in food or nutrition and certainly none in supplementation. Some complementary/alternative medicine practitioners are aligned to particular companies so will recommend one brand of supplement without necessarily considering your individual needs.

Try to find a practitioner with extensive training in nutrition and supplementation (most naturopathy degrees include many hours of lectures, research and assignments on this), and who recommends a range of brands based on efficacy rather than profit.

The suggestions below are to assist in maintenance of good health and may assist during the recovery pathway. The advice is general in nature, so may not apply to you as an individual. We should always choose the best quality food as our first line of nutrient supply, then the best quality supplements. These are **supplements**, not food, and must be considered in that light. All nutritional supplements should be taken with food unless otherwise advised by the manufacturer or your healthcare practitioner.

Vitamin C (everyone needs vitamin C supplementation – no exceptions)

Take from 4000 mg per day to bowel tolerance (the level that may cause your stools to become soft or loose) each day (divided doses throughout the day if possible). Powder with mixed ascorbates plus bioflavonoids. **Do not** use chewable tablets. Liposomal/ Lypo-Spheric forms of Vitamin C may be suggested in specific circumstances.

There are good quality powders available in practitioner-only lines, but there is great variation in quality even amongst these brands.

Vitamin C is ascorbic acid, and it is tempting to believe that, if we take high-dose ascorbic acid, we are taking the best. However, taking an acidic powder may cause irritation, burning or even ulceration of the oesophagus, exacerbating our woes. Manufacturers overcome this by buffering the acid with a mineral which is alkaline. Most manufacturers then show, on their labels, that we *gain* the benefit of that buffering mineral, so that the vitamin C supplement is also a mineral supplement. This is not correct.

One of the great pioneers of vitamin C supplementation for many disease states was Dr Frederick Klenner (1907–84) from North Carolina in USA. Dr Klenner treated many thousands of seriously ill patients, adults and children, using mega-doses of vitamins, including vitamin C. Dr Klenner used high-dose oral and injectable sodium ascorbate, even though many of his papers speak of ascorbic acid. His wife, Annie (née Hill Sharp) has stated that Klenner did, indeed, use primarily sodium ascorbate, but his papers describe the active therapeutic substance which is ascorbic acid.[1],[2]

I was desperate for information on vitamin C therapy in 1980 when my son was diagnosed with leukemia, and I was lucky enough to speak for over an hour with Dr Klenner via telephone. Dr Klenner was most helpful, gave me a great deal of information about how best to use vitamin C for my son, and rejected any idea of payment. One rather surprising piece of information was his warning about using high-dose mineral ascorbates and their effect on mineral balance. Klenner's experiments had showed that, when sodium ascorbate is absorbed by the body, it splits into ascorbic acid (which is what we want) plus an ion of sodium which is unstable, links to another sodium molecule, and is eliminated. He found that, when using very high doses of sodium ascorbate, his patients *lost* sodium, sometimes to a worrying level, and needed sodium supplementation. He later found similar effects when using calcium ascorbate orally.

During the early 1980s, I could only purchase ascorbic acid power, sodium ascorbate power or calcium ascorbate power, plus sodium ascorbate for intravenous delivery, so we focused on sodium ascorbate and observed my son's sodium levels.[3]

These days, it is possible to purchase excellent vitamin C supplements containing four or more mineral ascorbates, so helping to maintain a better mineral profile. At the dosages suggested above, your mineral levels will not be adversely affected if the right supplement is used. Most really good vitamin C supplements also include bioflavonoids.

Bioflavonoids are substances that occur naturally in many plant foods and help give those foods their colour and flavour. As part of our food, bioflavonoids can act as powerful antioxidants and anti-inflammatory substances, and assist cellular absorption of vitamin C. The inclusion of bioflavonoids in vitamin C supplements brings the supplement closer to a natural food formulation, so assisting in absorption and utilisation.

In order to obtain the most benefit from vitamin C supplementation, it is wise to explore all options available and purchase supplements with the highest number of mineral ascorbates, plus a range of bioflavonoids.

All vitamin C powders can have a laxative effect at high doses, which is often useful for those diagnosed with Parkinson's disease, as many report suffering from constipation for many years.

Liposomal (also known as Lypo-Spheric) vitamin C supplements can be useful in specific circumstances. Sometimes gut dysfunction is such that even a tiny amount of vitamin C powder will cause diarrhoea. For others, gut surgery or inflammation may render the use of powders difficult. In these cases, liposomal vitamin C is very useful as it is more easily absorbed with little to no effect on gut function.

There are two disadvantages in using liposomal vitamin C. These supplements are generally more expensive than powders gram for gram and, while it is claimed that we need less because of enhanced absorption, my clinical experience is that the difference is small so the overall cost is still higher than powders. The other disadvantage is that they do not contain mixed ascorbates or bioflavonoids, so we lose these benefits as well.

Vitamin C is required for ground substance integrity, immune function, nutrient absorption and metabolism. It is a strong antioxidant (the brain chooses vitamin C as an antioxidant over all others) and is required for brain and nervous system function, as well as for retinal health. It is stored in the liver, lymph, brain tissue and retina. Vitamin C "spill" through the bladder and bowel helps prevent infection and cancer; that spill remains relatively constant, no matter how much we supplement – this is not wasted vitamin C in excess of our needs, but a necessary part of health. Vitamin C can help us utilise other supplements and foods better and may enhance production of glutathione and CoQ10. Vitamin C intake may be increased greatly to assist in combating constipation, infection, abscesses or ulcers.

Folinic acid (5-formyltetrahydrofolate) or folate (5-methyltetrahydrofolate)

800 mcg (micrograms) to 1000 mcg per day are required for nerve health and function, to protects nerve cells and mop up homocysteine. Taking folinic acid or folate is critical if you are taking levodopa drugs (Madopar, Sinemet, Kinson or Stalevo in Australia). It is synergistic with vitamin C in this task. Folinic acid and folate are active forms of folic acid that do not require methylenetetrahydrofolate reductase (MTHFR) to be utilised by our body. This means we get more bang for our buck, our

body uses less energy to absorb and utilise the folate, and those challenged with MTHFR SNPs (genetic mutations) that inhibit this conversion can still gain the benefits of folate.

The metabolism of dopamine creates over forty metabolites, one of which is homocysteine. While we are healthy, this homocysteine is mopped up, converted to methionine which is then used in a variety of sulfation and, indirectly, methylation processes – part of our detoxification and immune function. This prevents an excess of homocysteine which may be cardiotoxic and neurotoxic.

When taking a dopamine supplement (i.e. levodopa drug), our body is not nearly as efficient at mopping up homocysteine, thus creating a risk of hyperhomocysteinemia (an excess of homocysteine). Taking additional folinic acid or folate will greatly reduce this risk.

Vitamin B complex or a multi vitamin/mineral complex with high-dose B vitamins

It is best to find a supplement including the active forms of the B vitamins. Most members of this group of nutrients require energy to convert to active, usable forms, unless we take the active form directly.

Vitamin B1:   thiamin diphosphate

Vitamin B2:   flavin mononucleotide or flavin adenine mononucleotide

Vitamin B3:   nicotinmide adenine dinucleotide

Vitamin B5:   pantothenic acid converted to coenzyme A

Vitamin B6:   pyridoxal 5'-phosphate

Vitamin B9:   5-methyltetrahydrofolate

Vitamin B12: methylcobalamin, cyanocobalamin, hydroxocobalamin

– may assist in handling stress, maintenance of energy levels and metabolic function.

Magnesium

Take up to 5 grams daily in powder form. Magnesium citrate is the best researched and, as shown in that research, the best utilised of all the forms of magnesium available. However, magnesium citrate supplements can be expensive and are not always readily available; I have found, in clinical practice, that mixed forms of magnesium can be helpful for most patients. Many powdered supplements contain mixtures of several types including citrate, malate, orotate, and glycinate. Magnesium powder supplementation can also help improve bowel function.

More recent research (2018–19) is indicating that magnesium threonate may be more efficient at crossing the blood/brain barrier and so be useful in treating neurodegenerative disorders.[4]

Magnesium in sufficient quantity reduces spasm and cramping, is required for brain health and many other body functions, may assist with rigidity and promotes a better response from bodywork. While it is best to obtain our required magnesium from foods, this is not always possible as our needs increase vastly with inflammation, stress, illness and some medications.

Mag Phos tissue salts (magnesium phosphate prepared as homeopathic dilutions but without potentisation) is also helpful in specific circumstances, especially as a first aid therapy for cramping, stiffness and some pain.

While soaking in Epsom salts (magnesium sulphate) or magnesium chloride baths is excellent for detoxification, and rubbing with magnesium oil may help relieve muscle pain, transdermal absorption of magnesium is very poor. An Israeli study comparing no supplementation, oral supplementation and transdermal application by measuring serum magnesium levels showed no increase in serum magnesium when applied transdermally, while a literature and data review found no good evidence for claims made for transdermal magnesium absorption.[5]

Vitamin D3

Many of us are deficient in vitamin D now that we are so frightened of sunlight. Campaigns such as "Slip, Slop, Slap" in Australia, and the apparent war against sunlight exposure waged by cancer authorities and organisations around the world has reduced sun exposure below healthy levels for many people. It seems ridiculous that, in a sunny country like Australia, we have an epidemic of vitamin D deficiency with its associated health challenges of autoimmune and inflammatory disorders, some cancers, mood changes, neurodegeneration and bone disorders.

It is sensible to avoid sunburn or other skin damage from over-exposure to hot sun so, in hot climates, limiting time of skin exposure and covering up at other times is a sensible strategy. However, many sunscreens contain carcinogenic chemicals so are best avoided.

It has been shown that we need early morning sun exposure over about 90 per cent of our body for ten to fifteen minutes daily to create sufficient vitamin D for health. This is critical when we are otherwise unwell.[6]

Sensible sun exposure can have a profound effect on our mood and willingness to participate in healthy life activities. A disorder called SAD (seasonal affective disorder) occurs most often in the northern hemisphere in countries where sunlight is scarce during winter months. Treatments include light therapy and vitamin D supplementation. I see some patients in Australia with signs of SAD because they avoid sunlight as much as possible.

It is often useful to supplement with vitamin D3 (cholecalciferol) and monitor your blood levels annually, aiming for the very high end of the standard/normal range. Take 1000iu (4000mcg/4mg) daily or 5000iu (10,000mcg/10mg) three times per week, or as advised by your healthcare practitioner.

Zinc

This is a mineral often deficient in most Western diets. It is particularly so in Australia where zinc has been leached from our soil over many millions of years. Zinc is required for thousands of enzyme functions, cognitive function, prostate health, skin health and immune integrity.

Many people with Parkinson's display a high concentration of copper, above levels recommended for health. While we need trace amounts of copper, higher levels can be damaging. Healthy levels of zinc in our diet or moderate zinc supplementation can block the absorption of copper in the gastrointestinal tract, thus reducing our copper burden.

Where zinc appears low on hair or urine mineral analysis (or copper is high) zinc supplementation is a useful strategy and may obviate the need to remove copper by more assertive means. Take 30mg of elemental zinc or as advised by your healthcare practitioner. Zinc citrate is an easily utilised form.

Probiotic

There is a great deal of focus these days on the performance of our gut microbiome (the bacteria that live in our gastrointestinal tract). The number of bacteria and other microbes existing in our gastrointestinal tract possibly equals, or even outnumbers, the number of cells that compose our body! Trillions of microbes living together in harmony, all working to create a healthy environment for digesting food, creating neurotransmitters and other micronutrients, and keeping us healthy. Or so we hope.

In practice, complete harmony is rare in our modern world. Food production methods, eating habits, stress and pollution all conspire to create imbalance and disharmony in our gut. We often see overgrowth of undesirable microbes, or those that should exist in very small numbers for balance, while more beneficial microbes are destroyed or suppressed.

Microbe numbers can be closely defined through stool tests,

but symptoms of imbalance are often present yet overlooked. Gut imbalance can produce fatigue, digestive discomfort, constipation, diarrhoea, yeast overgrowth (candida is common), increased flatulence, indigestion, reflux, abdominal and back pain, headache, brain fog, reduced production of neurotransmitters (such as dopamine, serotonin, anandamide and others), anxiety, depression, skin disorders, halitosis, body odour and general malaise.

Food is, of course, our first choice to balance our gut function and reduce symptoms. Fermented foods like sauerkraut and kimchi, or yogurt/kefir made from coconut or almond milk (unpasteurised and with no added sugar) may be helpful if consumed regularly to supply health-supporting bacteria.

These foods may be sufficient to rebalance our gut microbiome but, for many of us, probiotic and prebiotic supplementation is required. For mild symptoms and/or suspected imbalance, a general maintenance probiotic from the local health food store may be sufficient. However, where symptoms are significant and are not corrected with dietary adjustments, it is best to consult a healthcare practitioner skilled in the management of gut microbiome. In general, this means a naturopath, holistically trained nutritionist, integrative doctor with training in nutrition and microbiome or a dietitian with post-graduate naturopathic training. Conservative practitioners such as medical doctors, gastroenterologists, conservative dietitians and medically trained nutritionists tend to focus on symptom reduction by using drugs or manipulating the SAD diet, but these approaches are rarely helpful in the long-term.

A recent addition to the available probiotic range of Lactobacillus reuteri DSM 17938 as a single strain in modest numbers is proving to be most helpful in balancing gut and bowel function. L. reuteri DSM17938 has proven helpful for those displaying both constipation and loose stools, plus assisting with general gut dysregulation. There are other L. reuteri supplements marketed, so make sure you get only L. reuteri DSM17938.

Acid/base balance, GORD and ulcers

With the recent discovery that small changes in metabolic pH can significantly change the clearance of amyloid plaque from the brain, our acid/base balance has assumed an even more significant place in our quest for health.[7]

Complementary/alternative medicine practitioners have understood that our post-stomach pH is critical to our health status. The pH in our intestines, interstitium, muscles and blood is very important to maintaining a state of robust health.

For instance, our blood pH is tightly regulated between 7.35 and 7.45. If that pH rises further (alkalosis), we may experience confusion, hand tremor, light-headedness, muscle twitching, nausea, vomiting, numbness or tingling in the face, hands, or feet, prolonged muscle spasms (tetany). Some of these, in mild form, may be mistaken for Parkinson's disease symptoms.

If our blood pH falls below 7.35 (acidosis), we may experience rapid and shallow breathing, confusion, fatigue, headache, sleepiness, lack of appetite, jaundice, increased heart rate, breath that smells fruity, which is a sign of diabetic acidosis (ketoacidosis). Again, some of these symptoms may be mistaken for Parkinson's disease symptoms.

Blood pH is regulated by respiration and mineral levels, particularly potassium. Lung health and good breathing habits are keys to preventing respiratory alkalosis or acidosis. Metabolic pH can be largely regulated by food choices, eating habits and, sometimes, supplements.

Critical to metabolic pH is stomach pH, and this is often forgotten, or mistreated, especially in older patients (although even babies are inappropriately treated for stomach pH sometimes).

We require a pH of 1 to 2 in our stomach in order to successfully break down proteins and solid foods. Once we have thoroughly chewed our food and saliva has done its job, our stomach should reduce it to liquid chyme before releasing it into the small intestine for processing by a wide variety of enzymes which enable us to utilise the nutrients in the food.

If the pH in our stomach rises and moves higher than pH4, we can start to experience very uncomfortable symptoms often attributed to something else and treated inappropriately. The top sphincter of the stomach (the cardiac sphincter or lower oesophageal sphincter) stops food from being regurgitated into the oesophagus, a condition we know as reflux. The correct operation of this sphincter as a one-way valve relies to some extent on an appropriate pH in the stomach. As the pH rises, the sphincter loses integrity and can allow food to be regurgitated.

Conventional Western allopathic medicine looks on reflux (GORD or GERD) as a disease of too much acid. It is true that the regurgitated matter is quite acidic – often with a pH of 4-5 – and this can cause damage to the oesophagus ranging from irritation and inflammation to ulceration. Treatment is generally with proton pump inhibitors (PPI), H2 antagonists or antacid medication. These drugs reduce the amount of acid being produced, so raise the pH of the regurgitated material and ease the symptoms. Over time, oesophageal ulcers may heal and the patient may live in relative comfort while they continue to take the medication. However, they do nothing to correct the cause of the problem and, because the medications also raise the pH in the stomach, digestive dysregulation becomes worse, and attempting to withdraw from the medications can lead to renewed or even worse symptoms. Many patients are told that they will need PPI for life. The big challenge is the body-wide dysregulation this type of treatment causes.[8]

Raising the stomach pH down-regulates our ability to digest food fully, reduces metabolic pH causing symptoms such as fatigue, muscle and joint pain, cloudy thinking, anxiety and depression. Many of these symptoms are related to the reduction in neurotransmitter production in the gut. Dysregulation in the gut may also increase production of misfolded amyloid protein which can be transported to the brain via the vagus nerve and increase cell damage. Amyloid plaque is implicated in Alzheimer's disease and Lewy body diseases, and may be one of the mechanisms causing dopaminergic cell death in the substantia nigra pars compacta.

GORD is not difficult to treat if we work on the cause, particularly if treated when symptoms first appear and before serious damage is caused. Poor food choices, continued stress and failing to support digestive integrity are the causes of GORD, so let's work with those. Changing food choices, improving hydrochloric acid production in the stomach, improving enzyme action in the intestines and making sure our bowels work well are keys for reversing GORD.

Two Australian scientists were awarded a Nobel Prize in 2005 for discovering that Helicobacter pylori was responsible for causing gastric and intestinal ulcers. It was certainly a wonderful discovery and led to a very profitable industry – treating the bug that causes ulcers.

An Australian prime minister at the time proudly announced that we now knew that stress did not cause gastric ulcers, H. pylori did. Western allopathic medicine saw the simple (and very profitable) solution was to give patients large doses of antibiotics to kill the bacteria. When that did not completely suppress the symptoms, they added PPI and this seemed to "cure" the problem.

What the prime minister failed to realise, and the scientists did not explain, was that there are reasons that H. pylori proliferates in some people and not in others. We don't know how many people are infected with H. pylori because most do not have symptoms. While these bacteria can burrow into the stomach wall, hide from the immune system and raise the pH of the stomach contents, most of us successfully suppress the bacterial activity sufficiently to live without any symptoms. However, if our immune system is more-than-usually compromised, H. pylori may proliferate and cause significant damage to the stomach wall and spread down into the small intestine. Circumstances that may suppress our immune system, raise the pH of the stomach and allow H. pylori to "come out and play" include poor food choices, chronic stress, toxins, other illnesses, some medications and surgery. Manufactures of PPI often note that prolonged use of these drugs can cause H. pylori to proliferate, requiring further treatment.[9]

Once again, this condition is not difficult to treat if we deal with the causes rather than an interim symptom – the proliferation of H. pylori. Food choices, reducing stress and supporting the digestive process is key. Of course, we need to kill bacteria, and this can be very successfully accomplished using specific herbal formulas that are highly effective at killing bacteria, have very few adverse effects (except that they tend to taste nasty) and won't create antimicrobial-resistant microbes. Immune-boosting herbs can be included in the one formula, along with herbs that repair the stomach and intestinal lining.

It is vital to treat H. pylori and GORD if present to enable effective digestion and absorption of critical foods for healing. Find an excellent, well-qualified naturopath, herbalist or homeopath to assist you in correcting these symptoms.

CHAPTER 16

ACTIVITY

There is no excuse to be sedentary and inactive. Poor balance, restricted mobility and lack of time are neither reasons nor excuses for sitting around and waiting for the disease symptoms to get worse.

Yet, this is what I see and hear far too often. Patients, at their first consult, will tell me:

"I am so busy with appointments I can't fit anything in like exercising or going to a gym."

"My balance is really bad. I can't exercise for fear I'll fall over."

"I'm too tired to do anything. I'm exhausted all the time."

"I haven't exercised for years. And now I've got this. I'll do something when I get well."

The truth is, we won't get well if we do not become active, exercise regularly and sensibly, and maintain the best possible muscle tone.

There are a few people with Parkinson's who go to the other extreme and exercise themselves into exhaustion – a really bad idea because this pushes us back into fight/flight/freeze response. But these people are a very small minority.

People with Parkinson's at stages one and two on the Hoehn and Yahr scale will have no real difficulty participating in a variety of exercise modalities. There will be lots of excuses – "I'm too tired"; "I'm too busy"; "I work full time"; "I don't know how" – but no legitimate reasons. At stages one and two, we are still able to balance, walk, stand and sit without assistance and generally take care of ourselves.

There are a wide variety of exercise types and regimens that can help us slow the progression of the disease process, increase strength, improve our mental and physical sharpness and, in conjunction with other strategies discussed in this book, reverse the symptoms.

Walking is a good start, but we need to walk with intent and engage in *exercise* while walking; strolling and enjoying the scenery is discussed under meditation – useful but *not* exercise. When walking for exercise, vary the speed and intensity of the action. For instance, walk 100 metres very quickly (so you're puffing), then at a moderate pace for 200 metres, then 100 metres very quickly again, and so on. This will raise your heart and respiration rate, improve circulation and increase muscle tone. This is a useful general exercise, but walking has not been shown to reverse symptoms or slow the disease progress.

Cycling (road or stationary) has been shown to slow symptom progression and, at times, to reverse symptoms. Once again, cycling slowly on flat terrain is unlikely to achieve any significant result except to help maintain balance. Working with a small group of cyclists (who understand that you are a beginner), a personal trainer, an exercise physiologist, occupational therapist or similar can help develop a beneficial regimen of cycling that works with other recovery strategies. Spin cycles (slow-fast-slow-fast, etc.) have proven beneficial.[1]

Before embarking on long and arduous events, such as Melbourne's (Australia) Around the Bay four-day event or the Tour de Fire, 134 miles around Las Vegas, Nevada, make sure of your fitness levels, talk to your healthcare professionals and ensure a high level of support. The idea of exercise is to improve strength, circulation, resilience and muscle tone, not create exhaustion and more fight/flight/freeze response.

Working on an **elliptical cross trainer** can also be of

benefit. Many can be programmed to simulate hilly terrain or change the intensity of work in a set pattern. I have used (in fact, still use) an elliptical cross trainer and, as a 76-year-old with a history of Parkinson's disease and bowel cancer, have found it to work well with a regimen of weights, isometric exercise and brain training.

Boxing is showing good results in mitigating Parkinson's disease symptoms and improving wellbeing. It is very important to engage a competent instructor who understands the limitations your symptoms may create at the time, and is observant enough to see changes/improvements. Properly supervised boxing can improve movement, balance and agility as well as making us feel good. It is also an opportunity to work off any negative emotions – anger, aggression, frustration.

Pilates is fabulous exercise when supervised appropriately and can help reverse symptoms while improving strength, balance, and mobility. Pilates classes can be very beneficial, but it may be useful to engage a clinical Pilates instructor for a few individual sessions initially for accurate assessment of your needs, and to establish a sensible pathway to physical improvements. The instructor can assess each muscle group and develop routines (on the mat or using machines) to develop weaker muscles and stabilise the stronger groups. Most of us develop muscle imbalances because of lifestyle, work or unsupervised exercise regimens.

My personal experience as both a patient and practitioner referring patients to Pilates instructors is that this exercise modality, where available, is high on the list of best exercise for people with Parkinson's.

Swimming, for those with access to a suitable lap pool and who enjoy it, can be useful. Once again, just doing some slow laps won't achieve much, but sprinting, then slow laps, then sprinting again can be helpful. Unfortunately, most pools are chlorinated and this chemical is quite toxic. Make sure you shower thoroughly after swimming in a chlorinated pool. If you have access to the sea, a salt water pool, fresh water lake or river, that is a definite advantage.

Weight training, properly supervised, is very healthy. Work with a qualified personal trainer, neuro-physiotherapist, occupational therapist or neuro-physiologist to develop a weight training program that will enhance your strength, balance and mobility without causing injury or fight/flight/freeze response. Our intention with weight training is to develop a pathway to a healthier life rather than become a dedicated body builder.

High-intensity interval training – the principles of HIIT can be adapted to almost every form of exercise except Pilates and yoga. The basic principle is to be intensely active for 30 seconds, rest for one minute, then repeat. This pattern can be used for walking, cycling, seated exercises and lying exercises, almost without exception. A mix of standard-pace exercise and sessions of high-intensity interval training work very well when restoring good health.

While we have difficulty with standing, walking or general mobility, it is very important – critical, in fact – that we are dedicated to a program of exercise that will increase strength, improve muscle control, enhance balance, and support circulation and normal function. Without appropriate exercise, we cannot increase our mobility.

Body Groove: This is a workout method combining elements from Pilates, yoga, aerobics, dance and strength training. The concept was developed by Misty Tripoli, a Nike elite fitness trainer, who says that she overcame some of her own health problems by getting her groove on.

One of the great things about Body Groove is that it can be done in your own living room at your own pace and level of intensity. All you need is a TV and a DVD player, or a computer with a DVD player installed. There are several DVDs available, each one with several workouts in varying styles and levels of intensity.

All the workouts are done to music (which may not be to your taste but the rhythms are infectious) and you can choose to respond with great enthusiasm or use a more moderate approach. Movements vary from slow to quite quick, and you can participate to the level of your ability on each day.

Even though every track on the DVD is aimed at exercising specific muscle groups or developing better mobility, they are all in the form of free dance so, in the privacy of your home, you can feel comfortable moving as you wish. Don't feel embarrassed if your movements are slow, out of rhythm or asymmetrical; no one is watching. Remember, people with Parkinson's move better with rhythmic music.

There are a number of YouTube sample videos online that are worth checking out to see if this suits you. Just search for BodyGroove.com Once you decide you like it, the DVDs are quite economical as you have a TV Instructor any time you want.

Dancing: Just dancing (without Body Groove) is also excellent exercise for several reasons. Once again, rhythmic music helps us move more fluidly. We can dance with others, or on our own. We can dance in public or in the privacy of our homes. We can dance standing, sitting or lying down.

Yes, it doesn't matter what our levels of balance and mobility are, we can move to music, and that is good exercise for our body, brain and spirit.

Yoga: This has many benefits which vary with the type of yoga practised. One warning, however; I have found that Bikram yoga ("hot yoga") does not necessarily confer any benefits on chronically ill people and may be damaging to the fascia. However, all other schools of yoga can and do bring benefits to those who practise with dedication.

Yoga can bring benefits of improved breathing, improved mobility and balance and increased muscle tone; many yoga schools include meditation which is always of benefit.

Exercise if your balance and mobility are compromised: Many patients have told me that they can't participate in exercise because they need a walking stick or frame for balance and support. Well, that is nonsense.

For mild balance and mobility impairment, Nordic walking, recumbent cycling, weight training and Pilates are some excellent options readily accessible. Dancing with another for support, or while seated, is excellent.

If your mobility and balance are more compromised so that it is difficult to stand or walk, chair exercises such as yoga, weight training, or individually created exercise programs are possible and health-giving. We can dance sitting down too. Moving to music while seated can generate the same neurotransmitters and beneficial chemicals as dancing upright, and give us joy. Even boxing, Pilates and some aerobic exercises can be adapted for being seated. Body Groove, described above, can also be adapted easily for sitting down. Swimming can be great exercise, especially if you have any back pain.

I needed a walking frame for balance and mobility for some weeks several years ago (post bowel surgery). Here is a useful exercise that really helped me to progress towards full mobility.

1. Sit on a firm, straight-backed chair with your walking frame as close as possible with the wheels locked.

2. Using the frame for support and stability, stand up as straight as you can. Try to stand with your back straight using the frame only for balance rather than to hold you up.

3. While standing, "march" on the spot – that is, raise each leg so your knee reaches waist height (or as close as you can manage). Two steps for each leg.

4. Sit down again, take two deep breaths.

5. Then, stand up and repeat the exercise.

6. Do three sets of this routine at least three times each day.

7. As you get stronger, increase the number of marching steps for each set up to ten each leg, then increase the number of sets you do each day. Before too long, you will find your reliance on the walking frame is decreasing, your legs and back are getting stronger, and you feel better.

Once you have mastered this little exercise, you can move on to gym, Pilates, boxing and many other great activities.

Perhaps you feel left out because you spend most of your time lying down, and believe that you are prevented from exercising. Not so! Many exercises can be accomplished while lying down. It is best to be reclined on a semi-firm surface if possible (wide massage table, Feldenkrais table, yoga mat or similar), but even in bed we can exercise. TheraBands resistance bands (or similar) can be utilised to give resistance for stretches and controlled movements; wrist and ankle weights can be attached to improve limb strength; rolling exercises are useful to improve mobility; and partial sit-ups are valuable. We can also dance lying down! Play your favourite rhythmic music and let your body move in any way that feels right to you. Remember, no one is watching.

If you are able to obtain the services of a well-qualified and empathic personal trainer or occupational therapist who has a good understanding of neurodegenerative disorders, they will be able to create an individual exercise program suited to your circumstances to help you move forward.

CHAPTER 17

ENGAGE WITH HEALTHY PEOPLE AND DEVELOP A HEALTHY MINDSET

While we strive to be independent and create our own thoughts, there is no doubt that we are strongly influenced by those with whom we choose to associate.

Some of our habitual thought patterns are developed within the first few weeks and months of childhood. When we hear the sound of people telling us how beautiful we are, how clever, how wanted, this creates neural patterns in our brain that are of benefit for later life.

However, if the sounds we hear are of tired and angry parents, visitors who resent spending their time with your family, or those who don't like having children around, we will develop negative neural patterns that will influence our thoughts as we grow.

Childhood thought patterns are changeable. We may need help from counsellors or other practitioners (psychologists, etc.), but we *can* change our thoughts. Often making decisions to focus on positive aspects of life, and mixing with positive people, will be enough to begin our transition from negative neural patterns to positive.

As we grow and experience life, we will encounter many varied thought patterns, consciously and unconsciously. Decisions about the amount of time we spend with the different people we meet as we move through life will influence the way we deal with challenges, including diagnosed illness.

Mixing with those who see every setback as a tragedy or punishment will create in us thought patterns that are similar. We may see our diagnosis with Parkinson's disease as the end of happiness for us, or retribution for some real or imagined sin from many years ago. We may accept our doctor's prognosis of "progressive, degenerative and incurable" as the only possibility, and give up trying to be well and independent.

These are lessons I had to unlearn. I was taught, from birth, that doctors, bankers and priests were infallible (a little less than God) and, if they said something was true, then it was true. I was also taught (implicitly rather than explicitly) that my worth was measured by what I could do for others, especially if that meant sacrifice for myself.

Through my journey with Parkinson's disease, with the help of those who loved me even at my ugliest, I discovered that I am a beautiful being (albeit one who, sometimes, does less-than-beautiful things), worthy of all the love I receive, and more, without having to pay for that love.

Our attitude towards ourselves changes the way our body produces chemicals. If we are constantly self-critical, we maintain a level of fight/flight/freeze response that suppresses our immune function and production of dopamine (and serotonin and anandamide). If we grant ourselves unconditional love, and see our innate beauty, we enhance immune function and production of dopamine, serotonin and anandamide.

Those around us can reinforce our feeling of worthiness or destroy our ability to be truly well. Our friends can support our determination to be well or belittle our attempts to change and enforce their attitude of medical worship.

Family (sometimes the real "F" word) can be the rock on which we build our recovery, or a destructive force that exacerbates the illness process.

During my journey, I needed to break contact with ("divorce") many friends and family members who felt that their assumed medical knowledge was far more important than my desire to become well. As my health improved over several years, I was able to rebuild my relationship with many of these people, but on a basis that prioritised my need to continue improving my health.

Case history: *Angelo was in his late forties when he was diagnosed with Parkinson's disease. At his first appointment in my clinic, he was puzzled, frustrated, afraid and determined to avoid Western medication if possible. His wife appeared supportive and equally keen to move towards wellness through lifestyle changes and "natural" therapies.*

Angelo made very significant changes, moving away from toxic living circumstances to an area more conducive to a healthy lifestyle, improving his food choices and becoming active in health-improving practices. Over several appointments, we saw symptoms reducing and general improvements in Angelo's health.

There was a gap of about three months in appointments (his choice) and, when I saw Angelo again, I noted that he had commenced taking Parkinson's disease medication. The reason he gave for this was "the tremor was embarrassing". He told me that he was restless at night now and wanted help with this. I suspected that the medication was a culprit but, supporting his desire to try the drug, I prescribed some herbal sleep support and made another appointment.

During the next visit, Angelo told me he was taking a "sleeping pill" from the doctor. It was, in fact, an anticonvulsant drug often prescribed for sleep. However, one of the common adverse effects of this drug is tremor. So Angelo was needing more Parkinson's disease medication to try and suppress tremor while adding a tremor-inducing drug to improve sleep – a circle of negativity.

When I tried to point out the undesirable aspect of this drug combination, his wife broke in angrily, saying, "What about me? If he is restless at night, I can't sleep properly. He disturbs me!" I attempted to discuss the alternative view of emphasising activities and/or drug combinations that would support Angelo's expressed desire to be well, but was roundly chastised by his wife for not considering her health. Her parting shot was, "If I don't sleep well, I won't be able to look after Angelo when he needs it!", not considering the fact that, if Angelo recovered, he would not need looking after.

Many doctors have been party to a negative attitude towards becoming well. I believe that most doctors and medical specialists act with sincerity, in a way that they have been taught (and have come to believe) is world's best practice for people with Parkinson's. However, most use nocebo (negative statements) as a powerful tool to bring patients to "a sense of reality" or avoid "false hope". Their desire to avoid any charge of supporting unrealistic prognoses to patients leads to a habitual use of negative phrases that are designed to squash any hope of wellness. Patients hear statements such as those that I heard when I was unwell, or have been reported to me by patients:

"We don't know what causes Parkinson's disease and there is no cure." (I agree that there is no cure, but this book goes a long way towards showing what causes Parkinson's disease).

"I'll prescribe these drugs to slow the symptoms. They'll only be helpful for about five years, so get your affairs in order."

"Don't waste your money on vitamins, it's quackery."

"There is no such thing as a Parkinson's diet." (I agree, but there is a big difference between healthy food choices and the Standard Australian Diet.)

"There is nothing you can do to help yourself."

"Nobody ever gets well when they have Parkinson's disease."

Statements like this increase the patient's fight/flight/freeze response, suppressing dopamine (well, you know that story already).

Case history: *Edmund was comfortably retired, in his sixties, when he was diagnosed with Parkinson's disease. He was distressed* *but had a strong desire to become well and enjoy his retirement, grandchildren and golf. He accepted a small dose of levodopa drug and found his way to my clinic.*

Over the following two years, Edmund (and I) noticed a slow reduction in symptoms. His tremor reduced, mobility increased, his golf swing improved and he had more energy when playing with his grandchildren. He reduced his medication to a minuscule dose ("non-therapeutic").

Edmund decided he would keep his scheduled annual appointment with his neurologist, despite feeling that he did not really need any help from that quarter, and certainly did not need more medication.

(I support the rationality of maintaining contact with all members of a health team.)

When I saw Edmund next, he looked shattered; his tremor was out of control, he was tired, sad and on the brink of giving up. I asked what had happened and he reported that his neurologist had examined him and agreed that his health had improved significantly and Parkinson's disease symptoms diminished unusually. Then his neurologist said "But you will get worse!" and proceeded to describe the type of degenerative process he (the neurologist) anticipated.

Medical specialists who emphasise the negative and seek to strip patients of any hope of helping themselves to a better life, claim to be adhering to modern medical ethics in that they do not give false hope. However, by purposely destroying any hope of wellness at all, they are, in fact, *part of the patient's illness* – exacerbating their fight/flight/freeze response, inflammation and anxiety/depression, so increasing illness symptoms.

On the other hand, those who support patients' choices for change and self-help are part of the journey to wellness, even if they don't believe in such a thing.

Whenever possible, we should choose medical specialists who support the idea of self-help and the possibility of improvements. Currently (2019) there are some who see the worth of exercise (cycling, boxing, weights, PD Warrior, LSVT BIG – exercise regimens specifically designed to help those diagnosed with Parkinson's disease), dancing and singing. A few even discuss the Mediterranean diet (which they don't really understand or they would not be so enthusiastic), but these specialists are few. The next best possibility is a neurologist who will support our right to make choices about our health, even if they don't agree with those choices, and refrain from bullying tactics or denigrating our efforts to be well.

People who will enhance our pathway to wellness are those who embrace adventure and recognise that our adventure may not be their choice, but support our changes and decisions. People who are happy and laugh a lot are good medicine. Those who have walked a similar journey to wellness (perhaps from a different health crisis) are often very encouraging. These are people who will enhance our journey to wellness, whether they be friends, family or associates whom we meet from time to time.

Many family members will respond positively to open discussion of our choices and progress. One of my family members said to me that they respected my decisions even though it was not what they chose for themselves, while another shouted at me and treated me as if I was lacking in intelligence. I chose to see the former much more often that the latter.

We are, in general, social creatures and crave the company of others. When the company is loving, supportive and open to change, this is healthy and helpful. If, however, the company is that of people who want to mould us into their image and force us to adopt their attitudes of negativity, it is better to be alone.

I spent a great deal of my "illness" time alone, searching within my mind and memories for a true image of me. I was accused of being self-centred, reclusive, becoming a hypochondriac because "you're on your own all the time". But the time alone allowed me to see that I was not the sort of person my closest associates said I was (weak, obedient, clumsy, dishonest and useless), but a person of knowledge and courage who could change the circumstances forced on me. This new awareness enabled many of the changes I made to become well.

The point is that, if the people around you do not support your desire to be well, spend some time alone, then seek new company. Find companionship in books and stories of recovery and courage; look for knowledge in your local library and science-based sites like PubMed rather than Dr Google.

The internet has vastly expanded our access to information but has also expanded our access to misinformation, disinformation, and hopeless negativity. You will find many forums and information sites on the internet offering enormous amounts of unsupported information on how to live with Parkinson's disease (and/or many other diseases). Some are offered by those seeking to exploit misery and our very human desire for instant "cures", while most are presented by good-hearted people who seek to improve our quality of life but accept the inevitability of continued degeneration.

In my opinion, these forums and support sites are not helpful. I have examined many and still belong to one through which I seek to provide information about recovery. The challenge is that the very nature of the site is negative. When I am asked to describe symptoms, there is no provision to indicate "no symptoms". I have to have (or pretend to have) symptoms to give an answer before I can move on.

There are some sites providing stories of "cures" and treatments that do contain some very useful information. However, the people moderating the sites are often inexperienced in Parkinson's disease and/or recovery and/or CAM or WAM, so it is difficult to distinguish between useful and useless information. Some useful criteria to consider when examining these sites are:

- Do they offer a "cure"? (There is no "cure" for Parkinson's disease.)
- Does the story of recovery make sense in the light of

what we know about the causes of Parkinson's disease?

- Is the "cure" or therapy offered very expensive?
- Has the person offering the treatment or therapy walked the journey and become well?

A word on the concept of false hope. In my opinion, false hope does not exist. There is either hope or no hope. Hope is a thought process *and* a chemical process. When we hope, we produce more serotonin, dopamine and anandamide; we digest food better, sleep better, feel more energetic and create health. When hope is removed or destroyed, our neurotransmitter production diminishes, our sleep becomes disturbed and fatigue sets in quickly.

False hope is a term coined by those who choose to be no hopers. These are people who do not understand that hope and courage are twins – courage brings hope and hope increases courage.

Hope is. It either exists or it does not. Hope can never be false.

CHAPTER 18

LAUGH, LOVE AND MEDITATE

We all know that laughing makes us feel good. We enjoy chuckling, giggling, laughing out loud, a good belly laugh. But we don't always realise why we feel good.

Scientists studying the physiology of laughter have found that many of the chemical changes that happen during laughter are the same as those that occur during exercise. Endorphins (our natural painkillers) and many neurotransmitters are boosted during laughter, while stress hormones like cortisol and adrenaline are suppressed.

There's even better news. Laughter improves our immune system. Cells that produce antibodies, T-cells and natural killer cells increase in number while gamma interferon and immunoglobulin A are preserved or increased in production.[1,2]

Laughter not only makes us feel good, it is good for us. Our pain levels may reduce and our immune protection increase if we laugh for just a few minutes each day.[3,4]

Okay, you're feeling pretty down about having Parkinson's disease, you're struggling to do many of the things you used find enjoyable, and you just don't see that there's much to laugh about. Don't worry about it, *pretend* to laugh; even faking a laugh will bring about many of the physiological changes that are good for us. Even better, watching humorous movies, hearing jokes or reading funny books without laughing will still bring some positive changes.

Choosing to watch, hear or read humour also boosts our

sense of control, an important part of feeling healthier. People recovering from surgery in a Florida hospital who were allowed to watch their favourite funny movies needed fewer painkillers than those who watched no humour or who had to watch what they were told.

Laughter can boost our immune system, reduce pain, exercise our body and make us feel good. There are no toxic adverse effects and laughter costs nothing!

What's the catch?

We don't do it enough!

Children playing around in a safe environment laugh between 300 and 400 times each day. As adults, we laugh, perhaps, fifteen to seventeen times daily. What a reduction in self-help that is! Just by laughing, or pretending to laugh thirty times each day, we can double all the benefits. At 30 seconds per pretend laugh, that's only fifteen minutes per day for all those benefits. And we gain a sense of control, which further boosts our feeling of wellbeing.[5]

This all sounds like a hard sell on television, doesn't it? And here are the "steak knives". Laughter may help us look better. Susan Welch, a certified laughter therapist and director of Authentic Happiness Australia, says that "fifteen minutes of laughter stimulates the blood supply to the face"; and "A good laugh oxygenates the body, nourishing the skin and reducing that tired look."[6]

Good news specifically for those of us diagnosed with Parkinson's disease is that laughing can, and will, help us produce more dopamine! In fact, laughing reduces production of all stress hormones (adrenaline, aldosterone, cortisol and testosterone) and increases levels of dopamine, serotonin, glutamine and anandamide. It is truly the second-best medicine; that is, second only to really loving ourselves.

Now you're convinced that laughter is among the best and

cheapest medicine you can get, what are you going to do about it? Here are some suggestions:

- Make a "comedy evening" each week with your family, hire funny videos or DVD's, watch them together with a little of your favourite treat food (vegie sticks with dips, coconut ice-cream with mango, or similar lovely treats). Laugh out loud at the funny bits, even if you don't feel like it.

- Buy a giant joke book and read at least two pages every day. Go back over your favourite jokes twice per week. Laugh out loud, even when people are watching.

- Find a "Laugh Buddy" and make definite dates to see them at least once each week. A laugh buddy is someone who is prepared to help you find laughs, even when you're feeling down. They will smile at you when you frown, they'll laugh when you are clumsy or make mistakes and give you a hug or a pat on the back at the same time. They will find jokes to share with you; maybe they'll forward them via email, but they'll also tell them when you get together. They'll be prepared to look silly so that you can laugh together. Your laugh buddy may be a family member, a friend, brother or sister, your child, or someone new who comes into your life. If you're very lucky, your laugh buddy will be your life-partner/husband/wife. That is indeed a precious gift.

- Everyone can have a laugh buddy, and you can be your own secondary laugh buddy as you talk with yourself in the mirror. Tell some of your favourite jokes and smile, laugh, chuckle at your image. You'll be surprised at how this improves your appearance and your health.

- Get together with family or friends and play "remember when" – *remember when Dad fell in the fish pond* (laugh); *remember when I was learning to ride a horse and I got on one side and fell off the other* (laugh); *remember when Mum accidentally sprayed under her arm with fly spray instead of deodorant* (laugh).

- Meet with three or four friends each week and tell jokes, even the old ones that you have heard over and over for years. Laugh at every joke, even if you don't think it's funny on the day. If the joke is told badly, laugh because it was told so badly (even if you told it).

- Save some of the thousands of funny jokes, pictures and movies that circulate in cyberspace in a special "laugh" folder. Log into this folder every day and read or watch at least five items in there.

- Make faces at yourself in a mirror for three minutes every day.

- Join a laughter workshop. Sounds like hard work, I know, but it is actually hilarious fun to be with a group of people who just want to laugh and be silly.

- If you can't find a laughter workshop convenient to you, get a group of friends together and hire someone to run it for you – check the internet for lots of contacts to help you find a therapist; or ask around, many people who work for children's charities know the value of laughter and can help you.

- Think about children laughing. Happy and healthy kids laugh when they see a butterfly flutter around a flower, when Teddy falls off the couch, when the dog barks at the cat and the cat jumps, when they drop food on the table cloth, when Granny farts. Pretend to be a kid again and laugh at everything.

One last benefit of laughter is that it can, and will, improve your relationships. You can't be angry or bitter at someone if you laugh together. If you laugh a lot, and feel childlike and joyful, you don't even want to feel sad or angry or negative or left-out or any of those other feelings that fracture relationships.

You just want to be with that person who laughs when you do and makes you want to laugh more. Victor Borge, that king of comedy in music, says "Laughter is the closest distance between two people."[7]

Go on, laugh, it can only make you well.

Homework

1. Find a laugh buddy.
2. Start collecting jokes in books, emails, recordings and read/listen to some every day.
3. Laugh at least once each evening before bed (you'll sleep better).

Anandamide

"The Bliss Hormone"

Anandamide is a neurotransmitter (not really a hormone) found in human organs, especially the brain. It is nicknamed the bliss hormone as it was originally postulated to be the natural substance mimicked by THC (Δ^9-tetrahyrocannabinol), the principle psychoactive ingredient in cannabis (marijuana). THC locks onto cannabinoid receptors first discovered in 1988.

THC does not occur naturally in the body, and our body does not create receptors for substances it doesn't produce, so scientists were certain that some sort of endogenous (made in the body) substance was produced to occupy the receptors sites locked onto by cannabis. Israeli scientist Raphael Mechoulam discovered anandamide (more properly named arachidonoylethanolamine or AEA) in 1992.

Anandamide connects with CB1 cannabinoid receptors found in the brain and nervous system, and CB2 receptors found throughout the rest of the body. The difference is quite important as anandamide plays various roles in our health. The CB2 receptors are involved in the health of our immune system, while the CB1 receptors seem to be concerned with a variety of tasks including memory, eating behaviour, sleep and pain relief. They also seem to influence the neural generation of motivation and pleasure. Anandamide is critical in the early development of babies in the uterus (while THC from cannabis may cause disruption or abortion of pregnancy).

We learn to remember new knowledge or carry out new activities by creating new connections between neurons. The more we use each connection – that is, practise the memory or activity – the stronger that connection becomes. If we stop using that connection, it becomes weak and may break. This has profound implications in recovery and we will explore it further in a later chapter. Biochemical evidence suggests that anandamide is involved in creating and breaking short-term neural connections. Moreover, anandamide is synthesised in areas of the brain that are important for memory, higher thought processes and *control of movement.*

With the modest evidence available to date, it seems obvious that production of anandamide is a very important for our health. Much of the evidence so far indicates that it is at least as important as dopamine and serotonin in regulating brain function. It seems to be involved in our movements, memory, sleep, eating, pain control and learning. These are all areas that challenge many of us when diagnosed with Parkinson's disease. Incidentally, there is at least one study showing that anandamide inhibits the proliferation of human breast cancer cells in vitro, so all women could benefit from increased anandamide.

Finding more anandamide

There is scant Western-scientific evidence on improving production of anandamide in our brain and there is little available from our food. However, we have seen very significant increases in anandamide in the blood of long-distance runners during the "runner's high". This state of being among long-distance runners is fascinating as it treads a fine line between the benefits of meditation and the danger of over-stressing our body.[8]

A 2004 study of twenty-four college students who ran or bicycled for 40 minutes at 76 per cent of their maximum heart rate showed an 80 per cent increase in anandamide immediately following exercise. The athletes also reported feelings of relaxation, regulated mood and increased appetite.[9]

Our clinical experience indicates that meditation (relaxation) brings the same benefits of regulated mood and better appetite, plus improved physical performance, so it seems that we can increase anandamide production through meditation. Laughter can produce the same effects, and we know that thinking/speaking lovingly about ourselves increases production of anandamide, dopamine and serotonin. We also now know that appropriate exercise regimens will increase anandamide production.

What we are seeing here is a picture of circular dependence. We need anandamide to assist in the reversal of our symptoms and eventual recovery. We can produce more anandamide with exercise and this will help us relax, meditate, eat better, feel better about ourselves and move more freely.

But ... when we meditate, we produce more anandamide, so we can exercise better, eat better, feel better about ourselves, relax more and laugh more freely.

And ... when we laugh, we produce more anandamide, so we can feel better about ourselves, exercise better, eat better, meditate more easily and look at life more joyfully.

And ... when we think lovingly of ourselves, we produce more anandamide, so we can ... (you fill in the gaps).

Sing and dance

I spoke about dancing earlier but it is worth repeating. Dancing (on your feet, seated or even lying down) will enhance production of dopamine, serotonin, anandamide, endorphins, oxytocin and other endogenous chemicals that will enhance your road to health.

Some studies have shown reduction in cortisol production during group singing (indicating reduced stress response) and participants have reported enhanced feelings of wellbeing.

There are now many centres provided for people with Parkinson's offering choir or group singing. I recently attended a Parkinson's disease support group meeting which started with everyone joining in singing some popular songs.

My clinical experience has shown that, while group singing is very helpful, singing by ourselves can also be health-giving. Many of the same beneficial effects, other than those derived from interaction with others, accrue as we sing along to the radio or our favourite recordings. Singing in the shower, kitchen, bedroom or car can be just as valuable as joining a choir or singing group and is something we can do every day.

Dancing and singing each day is mandatory for patients who want to get well.

CHAPTER 19

HYDRATION

Water is absolutely vital for life. Maintenance of water volume, pH and electrolyte concentrations within narrow limits is essential for survival. Water continuously moves through cell membranes, from blood to lymph to plasma, and through the fascia, transporting nutrients and extracting wastes. About 40 per cent of our body weight is composed of intracellular fluid (fluid inside each cell), which is mainly water. Another 20 per cent of body weight is extracellular fluid (fluid between the cells).

Homeostasis (the efficient balancing of our body's metabolism) requires that our water intake must equal its elimination via kidneys, liver, skin (perspiration) and respiration. This means that we must ingest a relatively large volume of hydrating fluids during each day in addition to the water we gain from food and cell metabolism. *We need to drink between 1.5 and 3 litres of water each day (depending on our level of activity and environment) to maintain this balance.*

Our water intake depends, to a large extent, on our thirst sensation, or our deliberate ingestion of water without prompting by thirst. We live in a very dehydrating society. Chemicals in our food, air pollution, eating and drinking habits, air-conditioning and stress all rob our bodies of vital water. Even the water supplied in many cities is polluted with fluoride and chlorine that rob us of the benefits of water, as these chemicals tend to be dehydrating. These same chemicals also reduce our thirst sensation. In fact, the less we habitually drink, the less we feel thirsty – especially if we try to make ourselves feel "better" by nibbling on biscuits or drinking coffee.

For our bodies to operate efficiently, we must both take in adequate quantities of pure water (*at least six to eight glasses daily*) and be able to utilise this water effectively. This means that our bodies must be able to transport that water right into our cells to ensure the proper production of chemicals, disposal of waste products and transport of the chemicals produced to where they are needed.

By drinking too little water, we reduce the effectiveness of our physical defences. Our skin becomes dry, brittle and porous, so allowing intruders (micro-organisms) to penetrate our first line of defence. Once inside our "fortress", these intruders are faced by a very weakened immune system – weakened by the lack of water. Disease-fighting cells are produced less efficiently and are slow to get to where they are needed because our lymph system and fascia transport systems have slowed down.

Water is the most important nutrient that the body uses. It is correctly thought of as a nutrient as it is a limiting factor in many, if not all, biochemical processes. The correct metabolism of all other nutrients depends on the availability of sufficient water for correct biochemistry to occur. The macronutrients (nutrients required in relatively large amounts on a daily basis) protein, carbohydrate and fat all require water for their correct assimilation and utilisation. All micronutrients (nutrients required in smaller amounts or less frequently) including vitamins and minerals require water for correct uptake and distribution.

The water pathway

It may be useful for us to have a look at what happens to water, and other nutrients, as they enter the body. The first process is digestion. The digestive process is not required for plain water, but every other food or drink that is ingested starts the digestive process. This process depends on the secretion of gastric juices in the stomach and other digestive juices in the small intestine. These juices are largely composed of water, so this initial step of digestion actually requires the body to secrete a considerable quantity of water.

In a poorly hydrated individual, this may compromise an already stressed system. This is especially important in athletes where the temporary loss of circulating water can be critical. Many individuals who experience digestive difficulties may see rapid improvements following some attention to improved hydration. If sufficient water is available, the digestive process continues until the fully digested food finds its way into the part of the small intestine where uptake of nutrients occurs. Here, water again plays its part, as all nutrients are wrapped in a cocoon of water so they can be transported out of the gastrointestinal tract and into the circulation, in some cases this occurs via diffusion – the dissolved nutrient simply moves through the cells of the gut and into surrounding small blood vessels. In other cases, there are specific pumps that select a particular nutrient and actively move it to the circulation where it is picked up by transport mechanisms so that it finds its correct destination. These processes all depend on adequate amounts of water being available at all times and will quickly falter in a dehydrated individual.

The second process is distribution via the circulation. At this point the water from the gut, laden with nutrients, becomes circulating water, now a component of the blood's plasma. This circulating water will take the dissolved nutrients and the specific transporters to the right cell for the nutrients to be used to build new cells, repair damaged cells, nourish existing cells and to create energy and cell products like hormones, electrical activity or immune components. The water, having entered the specific cell to carry its cargo, then leaves the cells, this time carrying a load of waste products or toxins. This is the third and last part of the process – excretion. This cargo of waste product is transported to the organs of excretion (kidneys, gut, skin and lungs) where the waste products are packaged and delivered back to the outside world.

In someone whose hydration is compromised, these transport processes are limited and the whole system becomes compromised. There are many reasons this transport cascade fails but the most common reason is that the transport medium – water – is not present in sufficient quantity. This is the metabolic state usually known as dehydration. In a dehydrated individual, any available water follows a much shorter path and does not facilitate the transport of nutrients or clearance of waste products. Long term or chronic dehydration, even to only a small extent, steadily downgrades the nutrient transport system and progressively degrades the body.

Hydration and thirst

Dehydration also downgrades another system – the thirst reflex. Paradoxically long-term dehydration has the effect of decreasing our sensitivity to the very system that should notify us that all is not right. The reason is that the thirst reflex is a complex behavioural circuit and is actively filtered by our higher brain functions. To understand this, consider the situation where you are at a cocktail party. You are standing speaking to someone and you are able to concentrate on what they are saying without any difficulty because you are able to filter out all of the background noise. Now a few metres away someone says your name and even though you have no idea what else they are saying, you hear your name loud and clear above the noise. This is the filter at work. Normally the background noise is filtered out but when it contains an important piece of information, in this example your name, the filter lets that information get through.

It turns out that the thirst reflex is also filtered. When all is well, like when we are young and well hydrated, the message gets through the filter every time because the filter knows the message to drink is an important one. As we grow older (and, in modern Western society, this can begin at a young age) we start to respond to the thirst message with actions that don't actually do much to hydrate the system. Often we drink soft drinks or milk. Later in life it's caffeinated soft drinks, tea, coffee and alcoholic beverages. These drinks don't do much for our immediate hydration state, because unlike water, they need to be digested or they act as diuretics and actually dehydrate us. The consequence of this is that the message to drink begins to be filtered because, like the boy who cried wolf, our thirst reflex is not being heard. Ultimately the message can be lost altogether and often the profoundly dehydrated individuals will report that they are never thirsty (this isn't always the case as some dehydrated people speak of the unquenchable thirst – the flip side of the same coin). One added consequence of the lost thirst reflex is that many people begin to confuse the thirst message with the huger message. What is really a message to drink finds an answer in eating food. We conjecture that, at least with some people, their tendency to overeat is a consequence of a damaged thirst reflex.

Resetting the reflex is not an easy process and requires attention to drinking water whenever the vaguest thirst is perceived as this will serve to strengthen the reflex. There are specific remedies designed to reset the reflex that can help with this also.

This section above was written and previously published by Dr Jaroslav Boublik.[1]

The **Aqua Hydration Formulas** (Aquas) have been developed to improve hydration by increasing both our sensation of thirst and absorption of water into our cells, thus improving our bodily functions and elimination of wastes. The Aquas consist of four separate formulas specific for males and females, morning and evening. They are composed of homeopathic remedies, Bach Flower Remedies, herbals and, in one case, alpha-tocopherol. These formulas are designed to:

- improve the uptake of water under hypothalamic control

- increase our thirst sensation
- improve the bioavailability of water at cellular level
- improve hydration throughout the body
- work with emotional levels which may affect hydration.

Our hypothalamus holds the major mechanism for indicating thirst and guiding us to quench that thirst. It also has a major role in regulating temperature, sleep and appetite. Hypothalamic sensors are constantly monitoring sodium levels (salinity) and, as salinity increases, our thirst sensation is triggered until we drink sufficient water to reduce salinity to acceptable levels.

As explained above in the section by Dr Jaroslav Boublik, our "noisy" life may cause us to mistake thirst for a need for food, caffeinated drinks or sugar. The Aqua Hydration Formulas help us to discern the thirst signal more accurately, so assisting in increased water intake.

The Aqua Hydration Formulas seem to have a calming effect on the hypothalamus, a boon for those constantly in fight/flight/ freeze response. When combined with activities and strategies described in other chapters, the Aquas may help reduce our stress response and enhance a healing pathway.

Theoretically, there are no contraindications to using the Aqua formulas at the dosages suggested on the containers. In practice, it is not so simple, and I have listed below some rules and guidelines for taking the Aquas that I have found to be useful in my practice, following my personal experience with the Aqua Hydration Formulas (see *Shaky Past* and *Stop Parkin' and Start Livin'*, both available on www.returntostillness.com.au and Amazon).[2,3]

The Aqua Hydration Formulas are a core therapy/remedy to *enhance what you can do for yourself.* Rehydrating our bodies opens the way for the efficient production and utilisation of chemicals required for good health. However, *it is important to be cautious in using the Aquas*; people with chronic disorders are often debilitated and sensitive, no matter how robust and confident they seem.

The particular nature of chronic disorders may bring great sensitivity to all medication, including herbs, homeopathics and flower essences – the components of the Aquas.

My experience in using the Aqua Hydration Formulas in the treatment of chronic disorders indicates that they may bring the following benefits:

- improved bowel and bladder health
- a greater sense of wellbeing
- increased utilisation of any medication you may be taking, bringing faster "kick-in" and greater effect
- improved absorption of food and nutritional supplements
- increased energy levels
- better sleep.

Benefits will vary with each individual, of course, and the full effect of hydration (when treating chronic disorders) will not be felt unless combined with all self-help activities.

Find out more about the Aqua Hydration Formulas on their web site: www.hydration.net.au

Take only as directed by your healthcare practitioner. Start at a VERY low dose.

Buying the Aqua Hydration Formulas

Some health food stores and pharmacies in Australia stock the Aqua Hydration Formulas, so you can buy them locally. If you cannot find a local supplier, you can buy them on a number of websites, depending on your location. There are suppliers in Australia, USA and UK who will ship almost anywhere in the world. Links and addresses are found in Appendix 3, along with suggested doses and titration.

CHAPTER 20

MITIGATING SYMPTOMS

WAM and CAM

The symptoms of Parkinson's disease can vary from uncomfortable and vaguely embarrassing to debilitating and dangerously inhibiting daily function.

For most patients, the temptation is to focus on reducing symptoms, sometimes to the detriment of overall recovery.

Many practitioners also focus on symptom reduction because they are locked into the premise that Parkinson's is an irreversible disease with no known cause. Now that we know so much about the causes of Parkinson's disease, however, it is surely our responsibility to focus on reversing the causes in the long-term rather than simply mitigating symptoms in the short-term.

That does not mean that we should ignore symptoms and allow patients to continue living in debilitating circumstances while we pursue the years-long goal of recovery. Quality of life is undoubtedly important, but not to the detriment of total wellness.

We, patients and practitioners, must strike a balance between enhancing immediate quality of life and establishing patterns of behaviour that will, ultimately, lead to complete wellness. This can be very difficult when the illness process has been allowed to develop to a point where symptoms adversely affect every aspect of daily life. There is an old business adage that *when you're up to your neck in alligators, it is difficult to remember that your goal is to drain the swamp.*

Similarly, when Parkinson's disease symptoms inhibit getting out of bed, showering, dressing, eating, moving around home, driving, socialising and enjoyment, it can be difficult to focus on recovery. Yet this is what we must do to achieve our goal of wellness.

All Western allopathic medicine (WAM) treatments are aimed at reducing the impact of symptoms. Western allopathic medicine practitioners continue to labour under the misapprehension that the causes of Parkinson's disease remain unknown, therefore their task is to decrease the impact of symptoms for as long as possible.[1,2,3,4,5,6]

Western allopathic medicine treatments for the early stages of Parkinson's disease focus on increasing the supply of dopamine in the striatum nigra. This strategy can often provide relief from most symptoms for some time, although one of the most embarrassing symptoms, tremor, is rarely helped. As the disease process advances, pharmaceutical prescriptions are increased to deal with the limits of early intervention and offset adverse effects caused by earlier drug strategies. Over the past decade, Western allopathic medicine practitioners have been more prepared to embrace the concepts of diet (although this has been guided by "experts" with little real knowledge of what is needed) and exercise of various types to supplement pharmaceutical intervention and improve quality of life.

There is no doubt that some pharmaceutical strategies can improve quality of life and should be employed, where really necessary, even during a pathway to wellness. With appropriate management, levodopa drugs can be a useful part of symptom management during the recovery journey until the disease process has been reversed sufficiently to manage without any drug support.

Food choices (appropriately guided) and exercise are, of course, critical to everyone's health and are even more important when faced with a chronic disease diagnosis.[7]

Most complementary/alternative medicine (CAM) practitioners also focus on symptom mitigation or on reversing some interim step in the disease process. Complementary/alternative medicine training still promotes the philosophy of dopamine deficiency being the sole challenge with those diagnosed with Parkinson's disease,[8] but practitioners do, usually, work to improve food choices and activity, and may also advise meditation and inflammation-reducing strategies.

There is certainly a place for symptom mitigation in the treatment of any disease state. Pain, poor mobility, sleep deprivation and social embarrassment can all inhibit the metabolic changes required for wellness. Therefore, it is incumbent upon us to develop strategies that will mitigate symptoms when possible without inhibiting any progress towards wellness.

Tremor

This is the symptom most often complained about and used as a judge of progress. It is also, unfortunately, the symptom least likely to be reduced through pharmaceutical intervention and the one most likely to linger until late in the recovery process. While some pharmaceuticals can reduce tremor for a short time, and this can be tempting, especially in social situations, all tremor-reducing drugs come with a long list of possible adverse effects including fatigue, dizziness, confusion, tinnitus, headache and tachycardia.[9] However, there are strategies that can reduce the impact of tremor and increase comfort during the recovery process.

Meditation – is a requirement for recovery from any chronic disease and can assist in reducing a variety of symptoms. Many patients report tremor reduction during meditation and, in some cases, complete cessation of tremor. In my personal experience, my significant tremor and speech inhibition resolved completely while in a meditative state. Mindfulness and other forms of meditation will, over time, reduce the intensity and impact of tremor.

Exercise – may increase tremor initially or immediately after exercise, but will ultimately reduce tremor. High-intensity interval training is useful for symptom reduction, including tremor, while boxing and circuit training can also be very helpful. Machines such as exercycles, elliptical cross trainers and rowing machines can all be helpful.

Magnesium – magnesium supplementation is important for those diagnosed with Parkinson's disease anyway as part of their nutritional balance. Magnesium as directed/advised may reduce the intensity of tremor. Taken appropriately, it may also assist sleep and this can reduce the intensity of tremor also.

Vitamin B complex (activated) – is useful to support the nervous system and so may assist in reducing the intensity of tremor (see Supplements in Chapter 9).

"Doggy shake" – when tremor becomes more intense, for instance in a social situation, or even at various times during the day, it is useful to take time out and shake the tremoring limb or the whole body vigorously, like a dog shaking off water. This may be best done in private, although making a joke of it can get friends involved in a "doggy shake" dance and supporting the patient with laughter. The vigorous shaking can release tension and reduce tremor for some time. This is similar to the effect of exercise, but used on a more ad hoc basis.

Dancing – dance movements and rhythmic music can improve mobility and reduce the tension component of tremor. Music and dance should be part of every day.

Acceptance – this is, possibly, the most important strategy, even though it is last on my list here. For many people with Parkinson's, tremor is a fact of life every day until they are well again. Tremor is not a disease nor a disaster; it is just an annoying symptom. Accept that tremor is a sign that there is still a way to go in the recovery process and get on with other daily activities. In my personal experience, focusing on each day and the strategies I used to ultimately recover vastly reduced the impact tremor had on my life. I had very severe tremor in both hands and arms, right leg and head. I used all the strategies advised above but also accepted that the intensity of my tremor indicated my level of health. It slowly reduced in intensity and, after a couple of years, became more intermittent than constant, eventually disappearing three years after diagnosis.

Urinary Incontinence/Frequency/Urgency

There are several reasons for urinary dysregulation in people with Parkinson's. Before using pharmaceutical intervention, which may create or increase adverse symptoms,[10] it is important to understand why this is occurring in each individual patient and treat the cause. Adverse effects caused or exacerbated by pharmaceutical intervention for incontinence include constipation, nausea, dry mouth, urinary hesitancy and retention, dizziness, headache, drowsiness, confusion, blurred vison and impotence.[11]

Before beginning any anti-incontinence therapy, it is most important to be assessed by an experienced doctor (preferably a urologist) to make sure there is no mechanical damage or underlying kidney/bladder disease process causing incontinence.

It is also very important to examine any medications you may be taking and make sure that incontinence is not a known adverse effect.

Causes of incontinence and other urinary symptoms (other than above) are varied and can be in combination. One of the most common is dehydration. Many people habitually drink coffee or caffeinated tea rather than water in the mistaken belief that these provide useable fluids for their body. Coffee and tea are, in fact, diuretic and cause loss of fluid, while caffeine stimulates the fight/flight/freeze response causing further dehydration. Dehydrated bladder muscle is unable to hold normal amounts of urine (400 mL or even up to one litre, depending on the individual and circumstances) while dehydrated sphincters become weakened, thus causing urgency, frequency, leakage and incontinence. "Energy drinks" containing caffeine, aspartame and other additives may also be dehydrating.

The answer here is to drink only filtered water, herbal (non-caffeinated) teas, vegetable juices and/or diluted fruit juices (fresh). It is best to slowly increase water intake while reducing intake of coffee and tea to prevent bladder shock. Replacing caffeinated drinks with water over three to four weeks usually works well. Removing refined sugar and grains from the diet will also reduce inflammation. All the food choices discussed in Chapter 12 are important for both bladder and bowel control.

Incontinence may also be caused by constipation when bowel fullness puts pressure on the bladder. Constipation also exacerbates inflammation which can irritate the bladder muscle and disrupt nerve messages. Resolving constipation without harsh laxatives will often reduce or resolve incontinence.

Pelvic floor weakness from sedentary lifestyles may also play a part in incontinence. Activity/exercise is very important for overall health, recovery from chronic disorders and bladder control. Developing strength and control in pelvic muscles will help increase bladder control and capacity, and enable patients to calmly find a bathroom before voiding.

Pelvic floor exercises can become part of the daily routine, many times during each day – while standing, sitting, reading, watching TV, driving (at red lights), lying down. There is no excuse for neglecting pelvic floor exercises. There is a great deal of information online and in many health books on protocols of pelvic floor exercises, and they should be a part of daily routine. Basic instructions are to sit, stand or lie comfortably and squeeze the muscles around your bladder and rectum ten to fifteen times in a row. Don't hold your breath or tighten your stomach, buttock or thigh muscles at the same time. When you get used to doing pelvic floor exercises, start to hold each squeeze for five seconds.

If dietary choices are impeccable, and all other strategies are in place, there are some homeopathic and herbal medicines that can be prescribed prior to resorting to pharmaceutical intervention. While these formulas and remedies lack gold standard evidence (see Chapter 5), they have been successfully and safely used in clinics around the world for many years. It is always best to check with your healthcare practitioner before taking any medicine, but there are no reports of any adverse effects or contraindications for the medicines listed below.

Dr Reckeweg R74 Nocturnin is my first choice. This is a homeopathic complex made in Germany. It is available in many countries through practitioners and, in a few cases, online. In some countries, these complexes are not available direct from the manufacturer, but may be compounded by a suitable pharmacy. R74 should be started at moderate doses and slowly increased as/if required. Ten drops in 20 mL water taken one to two hours before bed is a starting point. Hold the remedy in the mouth for 60 seconds before swallowing. If there is no improvement in fourteen days, increase the dose to fifteen drops. If no improvement after a further fourteen days, add a second dose of fifteen drops during the afternoon.

Heel Plantago Homaccord: Another German homeopathic complex. Again, this is available through practitioners in many countries and, occasionally, online. Doses, times and instructions are exactly the same as for R74. Some patients find that R74 works well and Plantago does not, while others find the opposite. For some, both are effective.

Herbal formulas: These should be created by individual practitioners for each patient based on symptoms, sensitivities and other medicines being used. Astringent herbs can help reduce bladder reactivity, while herbs to support kidney and bladder function are often added. The advantage of herbal formulas is that they can be modified to help each individual with their particular pattern of symptoms or challenges. For instance, if constipation plays a role in incontinence, mild laxative herbs may be added; if a mild infection is suspected, antimicrobial herbs can be used. Western herbal formulations have been safely used for centuries and have been shown, in unbiased research, to be as effective as pharmaceutical medicine without the adverse effects. *All herbal medicines must be supervised by a qualified healthcare practitioner, as there are cases of herb/drug interaction (positive or negative) and there are contraindications for certain herbs in some conditions.*

In summary, incontinence is a symptom and must be addressed by its cause wherever possible. If there is no underlying mechanical challenge or disease, incontinence will resolve as health improves.

Constipation

Constipation often develops during the prodromal period of Parkinson's disease (before other symptoms appear). As a large percentage of dopamine and other neurotransmitters are made in the gut, it is critical to address gut function to improve wellness. Recent medical research has also found misfolded proteins (alpha-synuclein) in the walls of the bowel. These may be transported to the brain via the vagus nerve and are implicated in the development of Parkinson's disease, Alzheimer's and other forms of dementia.

Bowel function is a critical part of our ability to eliminate toxins from our body and affects all aspects of wellness. Causes of bowel dysfunction may be physical or neurological and, occasionally, infectious.

The definition of constipation varies depending on our view of normal function. The Mayo Clinic (Minnesota, USA) defines it as less than three bowel movements per week over a period of several weeks.

In my view, this is extreme constipation. The absolute minimum elimination of waste to prevent reabsorption of toxins and restriction of gut function is, in my opinion, at least one large bowel motion per day. Peak bowel efficiency includes one bowel motion *per meal*.

Bowel motions should be the size and consistency of a large, ripe banana (type 4 on the Bristol Stool Chart). On this stool chart (easily available online) types 1–3 all constitute degrees of constipation while types 5–7 are degrees of diarrhoea.

Bowel health is *very* important, not only for our progress towards good health, but also because it can indicate more serious challenges. If your bowel health changes, suddenly or gradually, have that checked out by a conscientious doctor. Stool tests, while valuable, may not show everything. When my bowel function changed, I had a stool test, blood tests, prostate exam, and other scans. I saw several doctors, naturopaths and physical therapists. It was only after a year of investigation that I was able to get a referral for a colonoscopy which identified a stage 3 adenocarcinoma in my rectum and sigmoid colon.

If you have developed symptoms of Parkinson's disease, your bowel is ineffective, and your bowel health has been thoroughly checked, chances are that the constipation is the result of one or more of the causes listed below. There are strategies shown to assist in correcting bowel balance.

Food choices play a huge role in bowel function. If we choose refined, sugary, over-processed foods, we will, almost inevitably, develop inefficient bowel function. The food choices detailed in Chapter 9 are designed for efficient bowel function as well as good nutrition, so be assiduous in your food choices, including lots of vegetables (raw and steamed), fruit and fibrous foods like quinoa.

Water and other hydrating fluids are critical. We need water in the stool to create the ideal consistency and flush our bowel. Herbal teas and vegetable juices will also help. Dehydration is a primary cause of constipation and water (1.5 to 2 litres per day) is the major remedy for that. Drinking 500 mL to 1 litre of room-temperature water on rising, before eating, may be sufficient to resolve constipation if all other strategies are in place.

Vitamin C powder (which you should be taking anyway) can help to hydrate the bowel and stool. The general advice (as in Chapter 15) is to start vitamin C powder at a low dose (around 1000 mg twice daily) and slowly increase the doses until you reach "bowel tolerance" (when elimination becomes efficient but before it produces excess gas or loose stools).

Magnesium powder (again, a priority) can work with vitamin C to hydrate the bowel and stool. With most magnesium powders, half a teaspoon twice daily (can be taken with the vitamin C) will be sufficient but, as described in Chapter 15, magnesium plays many important roles in our body, so individuals may need more. Diasporal is a very well researched brand of magnesium citrate powder and half a sachet twice daily is usually helpful.

Fermented foods (sauerkraut, kimchi, etc.) can often be helpful for bowel function. Consume these as meals or snacks.

Probiotics are usually important for those who have any significant bowel dysfunction for any reason. Probiotics are expensive, and it is important to choose the ones best suited for you. Many OTC probiotics sold by drug stores, pharmacies or discount stores are of doubtful quality so you may be wasting your money. Your local naturopath or nutritionist will probably be able to advise you on what strains of probiotic bacteria will help you the most. In the absence of this advice, 2018 research has shown that Lactobacillus reuteri DSM17938 is helpful for most people, easy to take (it is chewable) and store (does not need refrigeration), and assists in developing healthy bacterial balance in the bowel. This product, under the name BioGaia Protectis, is widely available through practitioners and online around the world.

Exercise is vital for health and bowel function. If we are sedentary, we are more likely to have reduced peristalsis (movement in the gut wall) and reduced muscle strength in the abdominal area. Movement is vital for the processing of food, stool development and stool movement. Walking, dancing and cycling are useful while more intense exercise like high-intensity interval training, Pilates and boxing will help. Yoga, with its focus on centring and balance, is most useful.

Bowel massage can be very helpful in correcting bowel function. Bowel (also known as the large intestine) massage can be administered by someone helping you, or you can help yourself. If you are constipated, you should be massaging your abdomen and bowel at least once daily. In the illustration below (which is the anterior view – that is seen from the front), you will notice that the bowel has several parts, but is, in reality, a continuous tube. The stool enters at the cecum, moves up the right side of your abdomen, across the transverse colon from right to left, then down the descending colon on your left side, moving more towards the centre in the sigmoid colon (a storage area), through the rectum, then leaves the body via the anus.

Bowel massage should be firm as we are trying to move stationary stool along the tube. Always start on your left side massaging downwards. We want to empty the end of the tube before trying to move more material into the storage area.

Perhaps think of your sigmoid colon as the despatch department of a large manufacturing facility. We must clear the despatch area before the manufacturing plant can send us more goods.

Use firm, downward strokes from just below the bottom rib to the pubic bone for two or three minutes. Then similar strokes under the ribs from right to left to clear the transverse colon. Finally, stroke upward on your right side to clear the ascending colon.

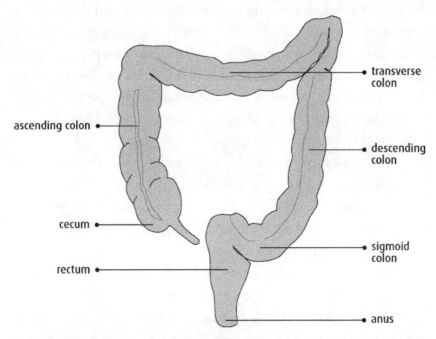

transverse colon

ascending colon

descending colon

cecum

sigmoid colon

rectum

anus

Bowel massage is probably best done while lying on your back, but can also be done while sitting or standing. Food, hydration and supplement strategies detailed above are necessary to make bowel massage most effective.

Sleep

This may be challenging for people with Parkinson's. Diurnal rhythms are often disrupted, stiffness and pain prevent comfort in bed and may wake those who have fallen asleep, and frequent trips to the toilet disrupt sleep significantly.

Sleep is, of course, very important for healing, but sleep patterns tend to change slowly without people with Parkinson's noticing until they become significant, and will take time and effort to correct.

Using pharmaceutical medication to induce sleep is, in my opinion, a last resort. All pharmaceutical medications have some adverse effects and are habit-forming to some degree.[12] Using medication nightly is courting disaster as it will take very little time to become reliant on chemically induced sleep and be unable to rest without. This will slow the healing process, especially as many sleeping medications have adverse effects mimicking the symptoms of Parkinson's disease. Try all the strategies below first then, if sleep is still a real challenge, use medication two or three times per week only to prevent habituation.

Sleep hygiene is vital to good sleep patterns:

- *Exercise* during each day to make sure that you are physically tired when going to bed.

- Eat your *evening meal* as early as possible so digestion is well under way before bed. Eating late in the evening can significantly disturb sleep.

- *Create a habit* of going to bed and rising at the same time each day. This will assist in renewing diurnal rhythms.

- *Turn off the television* one hour before bed. Take time to prepare for bed, changing into sleepwear, toileting and cleaning teeth, then read a calming book, meditate or listen to soft music for a while.

- *Move away from the computer* also at least one hour before bed.

- Make sure your *sleepwear* is comfortable. It doesn't matter what it looks like.

- *Stretch* all your muscles before bed to improve comfort and relaxation.

- *Temperature control* in bed can be problematic and you may find that blankets work better than a doona/duvet. I find that, some nights, I like three blankets, but occasionally need a fourth, while on warmer nights one or two will do. Adjustment is easier with light, microfibre blankets.

- Try to ensure *complete darkness* if you are comfortable with that. This may vary from person to person. However, it is important to prevent outside light from entering the room. Some need the comfort of a *night-light* and, if so, use the faintest light possible and place it close to floor level.

- Make sure the *path to the bathroom* is clear and easy to navigate. A weak night-light in the bathroom may eliminate the need to switch on a bright light when toileting, so preserving some sleep mood.

- *Play soft music* while going to sleep, timed to turn off after one hour or so. I used this strategy (playing classical swoon music) for many months when my sleep patterns were very disrupted.

- Reduce the number of *toilet breaks* at night by using the incontinence strategies above.

- Non-pharmaceutical remedies can help:

- Take *flower essence* sleep mixes for three to four weeks to see if that is sufficient for your needs. These can do no harm and, for many, are all that is needed to begin the sleep process again.

- Take an extra dose of *magnesium* (citrate, malate, glycinate or orotate) with your evening meal. This can help relax muscles (and mind) and enhance sleep.

- The tissue salt, *Mag Phos*, dissolved under your tongue as you are going to bed can help relax muscles, so maintaining comfort for longer. Dissolve one tablet each five minutes for three doses before sleep.

- *Vitamin B6* (50 mg), preferably in the "activated" form of Pyridoxal 5 phosphate (P5P) with your evening meal may help.

- Try *sleep supplements* containing herbs like lavender, valerian, passionflower or Jamaica dogwood that can gently improve sleep patterns. Ask your naturopath or herbalist for recommendations.

- Have your naturopath or herbalist make a *herbal mix* especially for you. They can choose the most suitable herbs by studying your individual sleep pattern.

- Ask your naturopath for *homeopathic* sleep simplexes or complexes. These are chosen for your individual sleep patterns.

- Be *patient*. Sleep patterns will change slowly. Keep your *journal* so you can really know what your sleep patterns are and how they are changing.

Balance

Balance is very important for safety and function through our daily life. Many activities require us to stand, walk, move around or multitask. These functions can be compromised when we develop symptoms of Parkinson's disease.

The reasons for poor balance can be complex; this is not really explained by simply attributing it to dopamine deficiency. Many neural pathways are compromised during the prodromal years, before diagnosis with a disease.

Deficiencies and imbalances in and between various balance system (ocular, vestibular, hypothalamic, muscular) may all contribute to unsteadiness, reduced reflexes and poor balance.

Furthermore, some of the medications used to treat Parkinson's disease and associated disorders (hypertension, hypercholesterolemia, incontinence, reflux, pain) may exacerbate or cause balance issues. Increases in Parkinson's disease medication may be counterproductive until you try all other strategies to enhance balance and security.

Assessing the pathways to poor balance

Check all your medication. Use your pharmacist or local library to thoroughly check the actions and possible adverse effects of all medications you are taking for any reason. If working with a naturopath, ask them to check their drug guides for these details also. Remember that taking more than one drug that has a possible adverse effect of dysregulated posture or balance increases the chances of encountering this adverse effect exponentially. You may be taking a levodopa drug, cholesterol-lowering drug, blood pressure drug and a sleeping drug; all these (depending on your specific prescription) may affect balance,[13] so taking all four increases the chances of the adverse effect.

If your medication may be affecting your balance, discuss this with your doctor and demand a review. Some medications may not be necessary. Sometimes doctors, who are always pressed for time, simply renew prescriptions without reviewing your total drug load and possible synergistic reactions.

Your doctor may not wish to cooperate without more information (and, as I said, they are often pressed for time) so ask your naturopath to chart your drugs, highlighting the adverse effects declared by the manufacturer (or post-marketing) that can affect balance. Or do this yourself if you have access to a good drug guide. Information online is often inadequate, so take the time to research thoroughly.

Take this chart to your doctor and again ask for a review. If there is still no cooperation, you may need to seek another doctor. However, most are prepared to help once the evidence is presented.

> **Case history**: *Bernard presented diagnosed with Parkinson's disease and taking eight different medications, including levodopa, anti-hypertensive, antidepressant, anti-nausea, sleeping drug, proton pump inhibitor, cholesterol-lowering medication and antihistamine. As he displayed a number of distressing symptoms, I charted his drugs as one step forward and found that several caused nausea, others caused headache, some caused depression and most affected posture, balance or could cause postural hypotension. I sent his drug chart, with a letter, to his general practitioner asking for assistance in managing Bernard's drug load. His doctor read the letter, examined*

the chart, then eliminated six of Bernard's drugs immediately. The doctor had realised (without me pointing it out directly) that most of Bernard's drugs had been prescribed to mitigate the adverse effects caused by drugs prescribed earlier. Once Bernard had established good protocols of food choices, lifestyle habits and supplementation, most of the drugs were unnecessary and his doctor was wise enough to see that.

Improve muscle strength and flexibility with exercise

If your balance is compromised, you can exercise with secure support, or seated, but you must exercise, keep those muscles moving and build strength. Part of our ability to maintain balance depends on the interaction of muscles in our feet, legs, hips, pelvis, buttocks and back that make minute adjustments automatically to maintain our upright position.

Have your *ears checked* by your doctor to make sure there is no inner ear disease, infection or dysregulation. Your doctor may refer you to a specialist if there is any doubt.

Be checked for POTS and postural hypotension

POTS (postural orthostatic tachycardia syndrome) symptoms are changes in BP (blood pressure) and pulse measures between lying down and standing. In some circumstances, when you move from lying to standing, your blood pressure will drop and, as a consequence, your heart rate will rise to compensate. Your brain is momentarily deprived of sufficient blood flow and you may experience dizziness, nausea or other symptoms of unwellness. You may fall without warning. The causes of POTS are multifactorial, but some medications can exacerbate this, so add it to your drug chart.

Postural hypotension occurs when your blood pressure drops with change of posture (e.g. from lying to standing, bending down to straightening up) without an increase of heart rate. This often occurs when your circulation system is compromised.

High-intensity interval training, other guided exercises and activities like walking and cross training can help, plus plenty of fluids (especially water), and supplements like vitamin E and CoQ10 that improve circulation.

It is important to have these syndromes monitored by your healthcare practitioners, as sudden changes in blood pressure can cause falls and injuries. Talk to your healthcare practitioner before beginning a new exercise regimen if POTS or postural hypotension are affecting you.

With the support and advice of your healthcare practitioner, begin specific *balance exercises*. **Safety first!** Make sure you are supported and that there is someone close by to steady you if necessary:

High-knee marches – march on the spot bringing each knee above your waist if possible (or as high as you can manage). Make sure you are supported either by standing with your back in a corner of two walls (so being supported at each shoulder) or with a solid support in front of you (rail, sideboard/buffet, etc.) or both. March twenty steps on each leg, rest for one minute, then do it again.

Unsteady base – when you are confident with high knee marches, begin doing this on some thick foam or an old mattress. Again, make sure you are well supported when you start this. The unsteady base will further enhance your ability to balance on uneven surfaces.

Balance board or disc – these are very simple mechanisms to enhance our ability to balance. Both balance boards and balance discs (wobble discs) are available online for moderate cost. It is also easy to make a balance board at home.

Home-made balance board: use a piece of timber a little more than shoulder width long, a little wider than your feet are long, and thick enough to support your weight without bending. Find the centre and firmly attach a fulcrum – this could be a piece of broom handle, dowel about 2.5 cm (one inch) diameter, or a narrow piece of timber rounded at the bottom to allow rocking. The fulcrum is attached to the board across the centre line to make a mini seesaw (teeter totter).

Using solid support which allows you to stand upright, stand on the board with feet near each end, and practise balancing with the board level. Practice for three or four minutes, rest for five minutes, then practise again. Do this at least twice daily; more often is better.

Use the purchased balance boards and balance discs in the same way.

Once you are confident at balancing, start practising without support, but make sure that support is right there if you need it. **Always be safe.** Over time, you will become proficient at balancing without support which will help your general balance and mobility.

Side steps: Using support that allows you to stand upright, start with your feet together. Move your right foot to the right 1.5 times the width of your shoulders, follow with your left foot, then immediately move your left foot to the left 1.5 times the width of your shoulders and follow with your right foot. Practise this movement slowly at first then as you gain coordination and confidence, speed the process up until you can make two to four steps per second securely. This can also be part of your high-intensity interval training regimen.

Standing on one leg: Using support that allows you to stand upright, stand on one leg for five seconds while breathing deeply. Repeat using the other leg. Do ten on each leg then rest by walking around, meditating or singing for ten minutes before practising again.

Walking on rough ground (with support): **Always have someone with you** when walking on rough ground until you are fully confident of your ability to balance. Where possible, walk on grass, sand or rough earth rather than stone or concrete. However, cobblestones can be great practice. Walking on rough, uneven surfaces enhances your ability to balance. Remember, safety first.

Find a functional neurologist if possible: These are chiropractors trained at a special facility in Florida USA, who have received a diploma of functional neurology from the American Chiropractic Neurology Board (ACNB).

Diplomates from the ACNB are spread thinly across the globe and not all continue to practise true functional neurology after graduating. So be aware of what you are looking for.

To find diplomates, check the ACNB website at https:// www.acnb.org/ and use the doctor locator to see if there is a practitioner near you. Check the expiry date of their registration (shown in the far-right column of the list) and it is a good idea to have a short chat with them before making an appointment to make sure they understand that you want help with balance and mobility, not general health advice.

The reason I suggest this is that many chiropractors undertake some post-graduate study in nutrition and/or supplementation, while some are engaged in business ventures producing supplements of questionable value.

However, warnings aside, I have observed excellent progress in patients working with dedicated ACNB diplomates while using all other recovery strategies on their way to better health.

Fine Motor Skills

As the symptoms of Parkinson's disease progress, our ability to write, fasten buttons, tie shoelaces, use small tools and other fine motor skills diminish. This can be very frustrating, especially as we have taken these skills for granted since our arduous learning process in childhood. It is almost like becoming children again and having to learn these basic skills.

The good news is that we *can* relearn these skills with persistence and practice.

1. Firstly, make up your mind that you *can* and *will* restore fine motor skills.

2. List the activities most important to you in priority order (e.g. 1 – fasten buttons; 2 – tie shoelaces; 3 – write notes; etc.).

3. Set aside ten to fifteen minutes each day to practise your most important fine motor skill.

4. Practise slowly and in an easy position – e.g. use an old shirt laid out on a table to practise fastening buttons; put your shoes on a table and sit down calmly to practise tying shoelaces.

5. Find an objective measure for each skill. For instance, use a kitchen timer to note how long it takes you to fasten three buttons. Note this time each day and watch your progress.

6. Be realistic about progress. Each activity will take some time to relearn. By using objective measures, you will be able to see even very small improvements. A one-second improvement in the time taken to fasten three buttons is an improvement – celebrate it.

7. As you see improvements in one activity, start practising another as well.

8. To improve writing, use school exercise book with wide lines as used by children just starting out at school. Then write very slowly filling up the space between the lines; like this:

    a. You want to write like this – writing

    b. But you practise writing like this –

writing.

9. Talk about your priorities and practise with family and loved ones so they can share your progress and celebration.

Remember, reducing or mitigating symptoms is for comfort, but our main objective is to find a pathway to complete wellness.

CHAPTER 21

BODYWORK

There are many forms of excellent bodywork available that can bring comfort and assist mobility for those diagnosed with Parkinson's disease. Some modalities will bring comfort simply because we are receiving loving touch from a caring practitioner, some will generate chemical reactions (e.g. producing endorphins – natural painkillers) that provide physical comfort, and a few modalities will bring positive therapeutic effects to our lives.

During my journey with Parkinson's disease (see Appendix 5 and *Shaky Past*[1]), I experimented with a number of bodywork modalities – massage of various types, craniosacral therapy, Feldenkrais, reflexology, osteopathy and Bowen therapy.[2] I found advantages and disadvantages with most, and it became clear that the most important component in delivering the therapy was the practitioner. If my therapist was of the type who simply sells their therapy or processes their clients, then I rarely gained any benefit and often felt much worse. If, on the other hand, the therapist showed they cared about me and my journey, took time to understand what I and my body needed in the way of duration and intensity of treatment, I always gained some benefit.

It became clear, and this has been confirmed by my experience in practice, that people with Parkinson's disease need *very gentle* bodywork, no matter how robust or confident they may appear. This makes sense when we consider that an underlying condition with Parkinson's disease is cell fragility. If our cell membranes are fragile, they need gentle persuasion to resume their normal function and resilience; hard or rough bodywork is likely to have an adverse effect.

After trying many forms of bodywork during my journey with Parkinson's disease, I found that Bowen therapy, combined with the Aqua Hydration Formulas and self-help activities, brought the greatest benefit, *providing I (or my patients) were fully engaged in all other self-help activities discussed in this book*. However, many forms of bodywork can, and do help those diagnosed with Parkinson's disease, and it is good to try any that seem right to you as a practitioner or patient; I must emphasise again, however, that the therapist must treat each patient with gentleness, respect and compassion.

My observations below are borne from personal experience, clinical observation and discussion with many experienced practitioners.

Bowen therapy: "Pumping water"

Bowen therapy is very gentle bodywork developed by Thomas Ambrose Bowen in Geelong from the 1950s through to his death in 1982. It consists of gentle movements across muscles, tendons and ligaments to relieve pain, spasm and stiffness of movement.

Tom Bowen was intuitive in his diagnosis and could often correct dysfunction with a single treatment or, at the most, three. He was extremely busy, reportedly treating up to fourteen patients per hour at times; this equated to approximately 11,000 patients per year. He successfully treated all sorts of conditions ranging from intractable pain, muscle spasm, sporting injuries, respiratory problems to arthritis and other chronic disorders.[3,4]

Most Bowen therapists today do not see patients at the rate that Tom Bowen did during his busiest years. While some therapists may have two rooms in operation at once, many see one patient only at a time and spend from half an hour to one-and-a-half hours in treatment.

A Bowen therapy session consists of light movements across

the bellies of muscles, tendons or ligaments, then pauses for two or more minutes to allow the patient's body to make adjustments.

There are a number of hypotheses concerning the way Bowen therapy works. Current research indicates that there are probably two major effects created by the therapist's moves during a Bowen therapy session. The first is the movement of water through the fascia (thixotropy – the property of becoming less viscous, or more fluid under the influence of an applied stress such as pressure or movement), and changes in fascia.[5] Fascia is a protein substance, like the white of an egg, made up of proteoglycans and glycosaminoglycans, contains collagen and reticulin fibres, and fills all the apparent spaces in our body between organs, muscles, bones, tendons and ligaments, and the brain (the dura) – the "gaps" between the various parts of our body that appear separate in anatomy charts.[6] Fascia carries fluids, immune system cells and other elements vital to our well-being. During times of illness, injury, fatigue or stress, fascia can become "cooked", like an egg white, and firmly attached to the muscle or bone it surrounds, no longer allowing free movement of fluid and nutrients. This can create discomfort, stiffness or pain and inhibit our return to wellness.[7]

The second major effect of a Bowen therapy treatment is a movement of electrical energy throughout the body. This can be thought of as electrical current, qi, prana or life-energy, depending on the philosophy you accept. However we view it, it is vital to have a balanced electrical energy flow throughout our bodies for us to feel well and satisfied with our life. The moves in a Bowen therapy session serve to remove blockages, correct imbalances and restore free flow of electrical energy over the whole body, even though the moves are made only at specific points. This is similar to the work done in acupuncture or acupressure.

My adventure with Bowen therapy began in 1996 when I read an article about the therapy in the *International Journal of Alternative and Complementary Medicine*.[8] I had never heard of Bowen therapy before, let alone had any Bowen treatment. Despite my ignorance, I intuitively knew that I needed to train as a Bowen therapist, and set about finding a teacher. It took many months before I was able to find a class which would accept me and, in July 1997, I trained with Rick Loader. This began a real love affair with Bowen therapy. Almost immediately, I transferred most of my massage clients to Bowen therapy because I could obtain such great success using this therapy rather than traditional massage. Despite my training, however, I did not have formal treatment from a Bowen therapist until late in 1997 when I went back to Rick for treatment on my frozen right shoulder.

I started treating people with Parkinson's disease using Bowen therapy and Aqua Hydration Formulas in the second half of 1998. This was very much an experiment because I had used a large number of therapies to obtain my own recovery. However, intuitively and intellectually, I believed that Bowen therapy and hydration were the major therapies instrumental in my full recovery (supporting all the self-help activities I employed).

Two years after my first training, I completed a Neurostructural Integration Technique course, and was amazed at the power of this more advanced Bowen therapy. Since then, I have treated people displaying the symptoms of Parkinson's disease, multiple sclerosis, Multiple System Atrophy, motor neurone disease, spasmodic torticollis, lupus, ankylosing spondylitis and a variety of other degenerative disorders, using the combination of Aqua Hydration Formulas and Bowen therapy, plus all the self-help activities as described.

Bowen therapy is very powerful treatment for pain, injury and a number of illnesses. However, I have found that in the treatment of neurological disorders disease, it works best with dedicated self-help and concomitant therapies as described elsewhere. While some improvement in Parkinson's disease symptoms can be obtained by using only Bowen therapy, the results are generally slow and unsatisfying. Using the hydration effect of Aqua Hydration Formulas, plus the hydrating and balancing effect of Bowen therapy, plus self-help and appropriate changes to lifestyle and food, is very powerful medicine indeed. All those who have come to me with Parkinson's disease and persisted with this combination protocol have made great steps forward in returning to health.

Any Bowen therapist treating a patient with neurological disorders needs to remember that the pain and stiffness displayed by their patient is neurological in origin – not necessarily only physical. Therefore, the therapy needs to be gentle and balancing, despite the often-asymmetrical nature of the symptoms displayed. Treatment which is too firm or asymmetrical in approach can be detrimental to the patient's progress, as well as causing unnecessary pain.

The timing of treatments is important also. Many therapists try to see their Parkinson's disease patients frequently in the hope of gaining significant result within a short period. My experience indicates that this is rarely satisfactory. Occasionally, I have seen patients weekly in order to help them over a difficult patch – for instance, when they are reducing medication or experiencing extra stress in their lives. Generally, however, I find that *treatments each two weeks* work well.

Remember, *recovering from Parkinson's disease takes at least three years or more* and requires significant input from the patient as well as other supporting, activities. It is very important to establish a supportive, comforting relationship between Bowen therapist and patient so you can both enjoy and learn from this exciting, challenging journey.

If you are a person suffering from Parkinson's disease, Bowen therapy can open the way to freeing you from many inhibiting issues from the past. **Counselling, kinesiology, hypnotherapy and/or flower essences** are often wonderful accompaniments to Bowen therapy and you may want to work with therapists who are prepared to join you on this adventure.

There are a number of interpretations of Tom Bowen's principles of healing that are now available for study or treatment. Bowtech, Bowen Essentials, Neurostructural Integration Technique, Fascial Kinetics, Smart Bowen and International School of Bowen therapy courses are available throughout Australia, while Bowtech, Neurostructural Integration Technique, Smart Bowen, International School of Bowen therapy and some National Interpretations of Bowen are taught in many countries. There are practitioners, colleges and associations around the world.

Information for Bowen practitioners and therapists

Neurological disorders are difficult to treat for three reasons:

The skeletal and muscular dysfunctions we observe are neurological in origin and do not necessarily respond to Bowen in the same way as injuries and skeletal imbalances.

1. The symptoms occur as a result of damage to, or destruction of brain cells over a wide area. Therefore, long-term or permanent improvement can only result from repair or regeneration of these brain cells.

2. Repair, and consequent resolution of symptoms, takes a very long time, and cannot be hurried.

Each Bowen session serves a number of purposes. Each of these purposes is equally important, and it is vital that we do not concentrate solely on the physical manifestations of the disease.

Practitioners, each time you see your Parkinson's disease patient, you bring to them the following gifts:

3. Contact with a professional health practitioner who believes they can become well.

4. Contact with a health practitioner who gives them time to speak and listens to what they have to say.

5. The knowledge that they are complete, beautiful human beings, worthy of your undivided care and attention.

6. The healing touch of Bowen therapy.

7. The certainty that they will receive the comfort you give them on a regular basis.

8. An assessment of their current condition and progress over time.

9. Even though there are a number of Bowen therapy schools teaching different interpretations of Tom Bowen's work, all are valid, all can help people with Parkinson's disease move toward health. There are, however, principles of treatment which should be observed closely:

If it hurts, it's too hard.

The purpose of Bowen therapy in treating neurological disorders is to move and hydrate fascia, balance energy and encourage regeneration/reactivation of brain cells. Therefore, the therapy does not need to be hard or deep. In my experience, digging too deeply into muscles that are rigid, locked and painful is counter-productive; it causes the muscles to become even more rigid, creates pain, and operates on a physical, rather than a neurological level.

All treatment should be symmetrical, except for the coccyx move, specific neuro balance moves and extraordinary circumstances.

Two of the purposes of using Bowen therapy are to encourage symmetrical energy within the brain and symmetry of physical movement. Therefore, the therapy needs to be symmetrical. The coccyx move is, of its nature, asymmetrical and serves to promote symmetry of energy along and around the spine. Occasionally, there is a need to treat a specific asymmetrical condition such as a frozen shoulder or asymmetrical back pain. Asymmetrical treatment is appropriate here, but it needs to be understood that this is simply treating the physical symptoms of a neurological condition.

Bowen therapy can't do it alone.

It is tempting to think that persistent use of Bowen therapy will eventually create a healing pathway without recourse to any other therapy. In my experience, this is not possible with Parkinson's disease. Bowen therapy can be a critical, integral part of a synergistic recovery program. It helps give mobility and peace as well as the benefits described above.

Many people with Parkinson's disease are old, frail and rigid. All are very sensitive.

It is very important to move each muscle group or limb only as much as is comfortable for the patient. The rigidity, pain and slowness of movement shown by our patients is neurological in origin and we must be patient in re-educating the brain to allow freedom of movement. It has been my personal experience that attempting to create freedom of movement by challenging rigidity is painful, depressing and inclined to set us back or discourage us from trying to get well.

Bowen therapy is one way to assess mobility, flexibility and balance without formal testing and to gain a real appreciation of the progress each person is making toward health.

Is there a standard protocol?

Following the first one or two treatments, I find it most effective to give my clients a complete treatment at each visit. I do not intend to describe specific moves to use during any one treatment – rather, I wish to set down principles of treatment I have found to be effective since 1998. Because each interpretation of Tom Bowen's work names moves differently, I will give general descriptions only.

Each practitioner should assess his or her client on each visit as you do now. Treatments may need to be varied from a set routine because of particular stresses, accidents or changes in your client's condition.

On the first two visits, I suggest that basic moves only be used covering the back, neck and legs. On the second visit, it may be useful to introduce the TMJ move if your client is robust enough. This can assist with balance and mobility.

From the third visit, I like to do a complete Bowen treatment each time. This includes the basic back moves (sometimes freeing the erector spinae muscles) and repeating the lower back, sacrum, piriformis and psoas moves where mobility is a major problem, plus sacrum and hamstrings while prone. I often include pelvic moves including psoas anterior move. In the supine position, I use abdominal/respiratory moves, neck, knee, ankle, shoulder, elbow and wrist (carpal tunnel) and, almost invariably, the TMJ. I work slowly and very lightly, with variable pauses, to let each client relax and gain full benefit from the treatment.

I also incorporate a form of Yin Tui Na on the feet and a specific cranial move; see details at the end of this chapter.

If you are skilled in any other form of foot or cranial work, you may wish to incorporate some individual moves into your routine. However, people receiving basic Bowen therapy from a loving practitioner who uses a **very light** touch make good progress. I cannot emphasise enough how important it is to use **extremely light** touch. Firmness of touch will only result in discomfort and aggravation of symptoms. The maximum weight I suggest for any Bowen therapy move is the pressure you would willingly apply to your closed eye without causing discomfort. This equates to **less than five grams** of weight.

Remember, you are the practitioner your client sees most often. Therefore, you have a unique opportunity to join them on their great adventure. I encourage you to participate fully and enjoy the experience.

A significant symptom of Parkinson's disease is muscular stiffness, rigidity and pain. During my long prodromal period of over thirty years, I had sought therapies other than Bowen therapy to alleviate and/or cure these symptoms which were progressing slowly.

Chiropractic seemed to be a logical choice as most of my pain and stiffness was blamed on posture, work injury or car accidents. I persisted with chiropractic treatment for over twenty years with little success. Certainly, I almost always gained some symptomatic relief after each treatment, but it did not "hold". Within two or three days, the symptoms would return, rapidly reaching the pre-treatment severity. I sometimes had three or four treatments close together to try and consolidate benefits, but the result was the same – a rapid return to pre-treatment status. A number of chiropractors told me that I was a "lifetime chiropractic patient".

Massage: I tried massage on several occasions over the years and enjoyed the experience but, as with chiropractic, gained only short-term alleviation of pain. Neither massage nor chiropractic could do more than lessen the pain level for a short time; they could not take it away.

Early in my Parkinson's disease adventure, I was given fortnightly deep-tissue massages by a colleague. We theorised that the significant muscle movement which occurs during massage would ease rigidity and enhance the work done by craniosacral therapy. We were wrong. While I felt invigorated and encouraged after each massage, my body rebelled within 24 hours by giving me dreadful cramps and pain in all the muscle groups massaged. I persisted for a few weeks hoping that my body would get used to the procedure, as I was in the habit of making my body obey me, but had to give up as the pain was too great.

I later received some gentle relaxation massages from another colleague. While these did little for my rigidity and pain, they definitely increased my sense of wellbeing and helped me reconnect my poor old body with the real person hiding inside.

Greg Morling has written a useful article on massaging Parkinson's disease patients and emphasises the need to be aware of the frailty of the Parkinsonian body.[9] I am convinced that there is a significant place for careful, aware massage in the treatment of Parkinson's disease. Massage will not cure any of the Parkinsonian symptoms, but will enhance the ability of the person with Parkinson's to pursue their goal of recovery.

Acupuncture and **Cupping** were also tried at various times and were successful in easing specific symptoms at specific sites, but, again, brought no long-term relief.

By the time of my crisis in August 1995 (Shaky Past1 and Appendix 5), I had been in escalating pain, with associated rigidity and stiffness, for over thirty years. (In fact, in June 1998, I celebrated my first pain-free birthday in thirty-five years).

My referral to a Craniosacral therapist by my naturopath was fortuitous and a real breakthrough in my health. My therapist's opinion (albeit incorrect) that all my physical symptoms at the time were related to the head injury sustained in childhood modified her approach to my treatment.

My therapist (Julie) used gentle osteopathic and massage techniques to ease the rigidity in muscles with direct influence on the cranial structure, plus others causing pain. While techniques varied from visit to visit, the process did not vary. Julie would first ease rigid muscles, then work on the cranium. This, of course makes sense as muscles directly or indirectly attaching to the cranial structure will influence cranial stress levels, while cranial health and fascial integrity will influence almost the entire body.[10],[11]

Craniosacral Therapy (CST), like all energy-based bodywork techniques, is a comprehensive, holistic therapy that can be used as a stand-alone therapy or in conjunction with any other conventional Western, alternative or complementary modality. My therapist was happy for me to experiment with any other therapy while she was treating me. She said, "You are in charge. You are your own best doctor."

There were three major aims as a focus for my CST:

- free up the skull suture lines and allow normal movement again;
- improve the flow of cerebrospinal fluid (CSF) throughout the central nervous system (CNS);
- improve the vascularity, plasticity and vital strength of the bones in my skull damaged by repeated impacts – especially the left temporal bone.

Conventional Western allopathic medicine accepts that it is normal for the skull's suture lines to become immovable in some adults, especially older adults. Craniosacral therapists disagree. In their view, the sutures need to remain free to make extremely small, but palpable movements in order to allow the CSF to flow freely. The sutures can be felt to move in a rhythmic way, independent of cardiac and respiratory rhythms, which coincides with the production and flow of CSF. If the sutures are completely immovable, the movement of CSF is inhibited, causing nerve dysfunction.

The brain is covered by the dura mater, part of the continuous fascia that surrounds all subcutaneous parts of our body. Lymph and cerebrospinal fluid spread throughout the craniosacral system via channels in the fascia.[12] Inhibition of movement in the skull's sutures also impedes flow of CSF through the fascia. As this is continuous throughout the body, this inhibition can have detrimental effects far from the cause. Areas of particular concern are the tentorium cerebelli and falx cerebri, folds in the dura mater that extend into major brain fissures – the cerebrum/cerebellum fissure and the longitudinal fissure respectively. These folds may be damaged during birth (too fast, too long in the birth canal, or forceps delivery) and are particularly far-reaching in their effect on all body systems.[13] Injuries similar to birthing injuries (e.g. concussion) are likely to cause similar detrimental effects.

My therapist also discovered that the left temporal bone of my skull felt solid and immovable like concrete, unlike the slightly flexible feel of normal living bone. In her opinion, this could only have been the result of repeated impacts against something solid.

For over two years, during fortnightly visits, my therapist worked assiduously to restore free flow of CSF, ease my rigidity and pain, enhance the physical improvements resulting from other therapies, and bring some life back to my left temporal bone. Her care enabled me to keep on working during my journey.

Craniosacral therapy continues to be a nurturing and comforting therapy for many of my clients who often alternate CST treatments with Bowen therapy on a weekly basis.

Feldenkrais is a bodywork modality developed by Moshe Feldenkrais to facilitate the "integration of the skeletal, developmental, environmental and neuromuscular systems".[14] It offers a framework in which the patterns of movement, thought and feeling can be explored.[15]

Moshe Feldenkrais said of his method, "What I'm after isn't flexible bones but flexible brains. What I'm after is to restore each person to their human dignity." [16]

There are two processes in working with Feldenkrais. Awareness Through Movement (ATM) sessions involve the therapist verbally guiding their client through a series of movements, drawing attention to how they move and encouraging them to use their attention, perception and imagination to discover more efficient and effective ways of moving.[17]

In Functional Integration (FI) sessions, the therapist moves the client, or uses their hands to guide the client's movement in patterns that will help restore awareness and balance.[18]

I commenced a series of Functional Integration sessions with a practitioner I had contacted through my work as a massage therapist. At each session, I lay supine on a low padded table while my practitioner moved quietly around me, gently stretching or rearranging my limbs, pushing or just touching head, hands, face, hips. With each move, she tried to bring some balance back to my distorted, frail body while I entered a state close to trance and felt a connection develop between my spirit, mind and body. I often felt quite euphoric as I left a session and had to be particularly careful while driving, as it was easy to "go off with the fairies" until I grounded myself again.

I enjoyed my FI sessions but the results were always temporary. Within a day or two, the sense of wellbeing and reduction in pain would dissipate and I would be back to square one.

I was referred to Basil Glazer (a prominent Feldenkrais teacher) during his visit to Melbourne in 1996. Basil's treatment was much stronger than my practitioner's. He pulled and stretched my body in ways that seemed right and balancing at the time and, because of this, I did not object to the pain caused by the treatment. At the end of the session, I felt taller, stood straighter and moved with more assurance. I thought we had achieved a breakthrough. However, 24 hours later, I was in agonising pain. My whole body seemed to be cramping, aching and burning with deep, deep pain. My body had rebelled again. Some three days later, I was back in my pre-treatment state; very disappointed. I decided not to pursue Feldenkrais as a therapy. However, a number of my patients have participated in Feldenkrais, both FI sessions and ATM sessions, with excellent results.

Alexander Technique

"The Alexander Technique is a way of learning how you can get rid of harmful tension in your body."[19]

Some other definitions:

"The Alexander Technique is a way of learning to move mindfully through life. The Alexander process shines a light on inefficient habits of movement and patterns of accumulated tension, which interferes with our innate ability to move easily and according to how we are designed. It's a simple yet powerful approach that offers the opportunity to take charge of one's own learning and healing process, because it's not a series of passive treatments but an active exploration that changes the way one thinks and

responds in activity. It produces a skill set that can be applied in every situation. Lessons leave one feeling lighter, freer, and more grounded."[20]

"The Alexander Technique is a method that works to change (movement) habits in our everyday activities. It is a simple and practical method for improving ease and freedom of movement, balance, support and coordination. The technique teaches the use of the appropriate amount of effort for a particular activity, giving you more energy for all your activities. It is not a series of treatments or exercises, but rather a re-education of the mind and body. The Alexander Technique is a method which helps a person discover a new balance in the body by releasing unnecessary tension. It can be applied to sitting, lying down, standing, walking, lifting, and other daily activities ..."[21]

There have been several small studies on the benefits of the Alexander Technique for people with Parkinson's, and all have shown that this technique can help mitigate symptoms and improve wellbeing if patients continue to practise the technique (as with all self-help strategies).

My experience with Alexander Technique is limited. In 2005, I thought I could usefully become an Alexander Technique teacher in order to help my patients even more than I was with my current strategies. However, the training was very expensive and I could not afford the cost. I began negotiating with Alexander Technique teachers local to each patient with the intention of working as a team to benefit the patients. Unfortunately, the teachers I encountered were not prepared to work in a team and, again, the cost was prohibitive.

Alexander Technique shows great promise in mitigating some of the symptoms of Parkinson's disease and increasing wellbeing for people with Parkinson's. Teamwork and moderate cost are the keys for any healing strategies.

My experience with all these bodywork modalities emphasises my view that *any and all bodywork for people with Parkinson's disease must be very gentle and nurturing*.

Additional "tools" for Bowen therapists

Incorporating Yin Tui Na

Yin Tui Na, or Child Tuina, is a very ancient Chinese therapy which was developed long before acupuncture, possibly more than 10,000 years ago. It consists of very gentle pressure placed on particular points of the body to influence the subcutaneous areas, muscles and bones, bringing mobility and freedom. The pressure used is, in general, no more than the pressure you would be prepared to place on your own naked eyeball (for instance, when inserting a contact lens)– i.e. about 2 grams. The positive results of this therapy are gained by focusing the mind through our hands placed on our patient's body. This focus and a very gentle pressure can bring powerful benefits for the patient.

Applying Tuina for the benefit of our Parkinson's disease patients requires an even more gentle approach than the use of Bowen therapy. In this regard, it can be related more closely to Craniosacral therapy. The keys to the successful use of Tuina are patience, gentle touch and mind focus. While this method can be applied over the whole of the body, in the treatment of people with neurological and autoimmune disorders, I apply it only to feet. I have found that using Bowen therapy over the rest of the body and, especially, down the legs to the feet, brings balance and mobility. Adding Tuina to the feet assists in bringing balance and grounding, as well as enhancing the mobility of our patients, and improving neurological function.

The traditional method of Tuina is to place the palms of our hands over the area to be influenced. This is highly successful however, in practice, this may be difficult, depending on your hand size and table height.

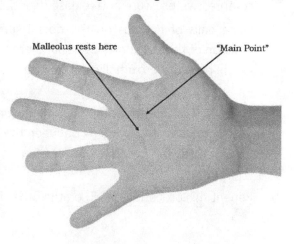

Malleolus rests here

"Main Point"

In my experience, I have found the following procedure to be effective. Start with your foot on the side of the most dominant symptoms or the side where symptoms first appeared:

1. Place hands on either side of the ankle so that the malleoli rest in your palms and the "Main Point" lies level with the navicular bone (fig. 1).

2. Focus your mind through your palms so that you feel or "see" the structure of the ankle. In most cases, the foot structure will feel solid, stuck or "dead". You will not feel any movement or possibility of movement.

3. After holding this position for some minutes so that you feel "at one" with the foot, apply very gentle, opposing pressure, then release (fig. 1). Repeat this several times. The pressure is "thought" more than applied. If your patient notices your pressure, it is too hard.

4. After some minutes, you may feel a response, or you may feel that this is long enough. Follow your intuition.

5. Place the balls of your thumbs centrally below the talus/tibia/fibula junction so that they rest on the top of the talus bone. Place very gentle pressure on the talus bone as if to push it away from the tibia/fibula, then release (fig. 2). Repeat several times.

6. Place "Main Point" or your thumbs (whichever is most comfortable) on either side of the cuneiform/cuboid bones. Apply gentle compressive pressure and release (fig. 3). Repeat several times.

7. Place balls of thumbs on the dorsal surface just distal to the junction of the cuneiform bones and proximal metatarsals. Apply gentle pressure proximally and release. Do this several times (fig. 4).

8. Place balls of thumbs at the talus/fibula junction and draw gently distally towards the webbing between the large and second toes. Do this three or four times to "draw energy" down into the feet (fig. 5).

9. Repeat this procedure (1–8) on the other foot.

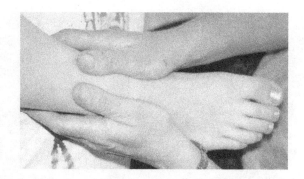

Figure 1: "Main Point" in line with the navicular/cuneiform junction.

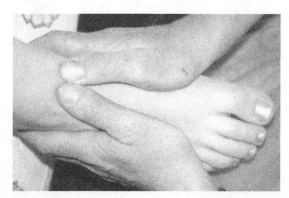

Figure 2: Pulse pressure proximal to the talus bone toward the plantar surface of the foot.

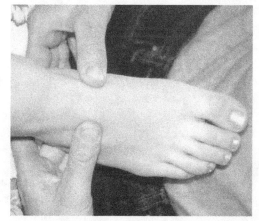

Figure 3: Thumbs or "Main Point" give pulse pressure across cuneiform/cuboid bones.

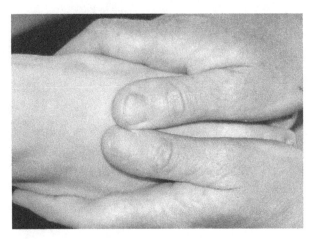

Figure 4: Pulse pressure from distal edge of cuneiforms proximally.

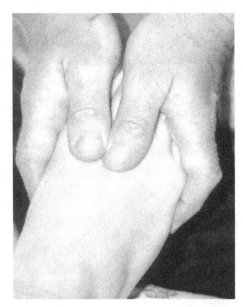

Figure 5: Drawing energy (qi) from talus/fibula junction toward junction of large toe.

Cranial Move

This move has been reported by one or more of Tom Bowen's "Boys" as being used by Tom in treating many patients. It may be completed while the patient is supine or seated. The description below is for supine patients.

1. Support the head with one hand and lift slightly from the pillow.
2. Starting at the occipital process, make firm anterior moves along the line of the sagittal suture until you reach the transverse suture line. Allow your patient's head to rest back on the pillow.
3. With your thumbs, make a single sweeping move in opposing directions along the line of the transverse sutures. Stop at temple level.
4. Return to the centre point and continue anterior moves as if the sagittal suture extended onto the forehead. Stop at the Pineal point/"third eye" on mid forehead.
5. Make another single opposing sweep with your thumbs across the forehead, stopping at the temples.

This move may be applied one to three times in the course of a Bowen treatment.

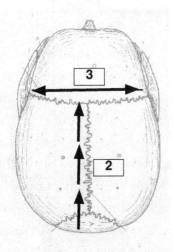 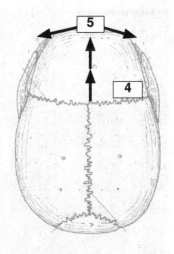

CHAPTER 22

COMORBIDITIES AND CONFLICTING TREATMENTS

Control, intuition, business plan[1]

In previous chapters we have discussed a number of "diseases" or "conditions" that are frequently diagnosed during the prodromal years before diagnosis with Parkinson's disease and are treated as separate illnesses. As we have seen, these diagnoses and treatments may, for some, be part of the aetiological pathway leading to Parkinson's disease symptoms. For others, they may be aggravating factors that exacerbate the onset of Parkinson's disease symptoms.

One of the most difficult healthcare situations we face is the patient with multiple diagnoses, treated by several specialists, all focusing on their area of expertise, and ignoring treatments prescribed for ostensibly separate illnesses outside their perceived purview.

In many cases we see the unfortunate situation of a patient diagnosed with hypertension and hypercholesterolemia, prescribed BP-lowering and serum-cholesterol-lowering medications, and told that they must take these medications for the rest of their lives or they will die. A short time later, the patient develops reflux and is prescribed a proton pump inhibitor (PPI) which relieves the symptoms for some time but reflux eventually returns, and the patient is diagnosed with Helicobacter pylori and treated with "triple therapy", two antibiotics and increased PPI.

So far, the patient's GP/PCP, cardiologist and gastroenterologist have not communicated, as they do not see any connection between the diagnosed illnesses.

Some time later, the patient becomes quite depressed, is referred to a psychiatrist who prescribes an antidepressant long-term. Within twelve months, the patient has developed a hand tremor, their movements have slowed and thoughts are a little cloudy. They are diagnosed with Parkinson's disease and prescribed levodopa medication.

There is no doubt that the patient is unwell, but do they truly have five separate and unrelated illnesses? Is there any relationship between any or all of these "diseases"? Are they, in fact, all stemming from the same aetiological pathways, and part of a syndrome that can be treated effectively by instigating wellness strategies while using minimum intervention to suppress symptoms?

The patient above is "factional", that is, they are not a real person, but based on hundreds of patients I see in my clinic, some with identical aetiological pathways. The "comorbidities" have resulted in conflicting treatments, and poor communication between healthcare practitioners has exacerbated the problem for the patient. In this case, treatments for hypertension and hypercholesterolemia exacerbated an already compromised digestive system, resulting in reflux. The PPI prescribed for reflux increased the risk for H. pylori, resulting in the necessity to treat with antibiotics and increased PPI. Their compromised gut (exacerbated by antibiotics and PPI) reduced production of serotonin, dopamine, anandamide, oxytocin and other neurotransmitters, resulting in depression, while the antidepressant caused tremor, paucity of movement and exacerbated other symptoms, all resulting in a diagnosis of Parkinson's disease.

There are three major challenges for patients and practitioners:

1. Parkinson's disease is seen as a separate disease with a dis-

tinct cause, as yet unknown, and a potential "cure", yet to be discovered;

2. All the "illnesses" mentioned above are seen as separate diseases requiring specialised care and treatment, and of no relevance to neurodegenerative disorders such as Parkinson's disease;

3. Communication between Western allopathic medicine practitioners is ludicrously poor, regimented by healthcare authorities (so doctors must be very careful about any views they may express), and often not read by the recipient. I know this from personal experience when visiting specialists who have received a letter from my referring doctor, but asked me for all the information contained in that letter.

There are three major factors in redressing the frailties of the current system, achieving better health outcomes for patients and satisfaction for practitioners.

Control

Patients – take control of your health and healthcare. Do not abdicate your responsibility and allow authoritative Western allopathic medicine or complementary/alternative medicine to dictate your pathway without questions.

Practitioners with specialist knowledge are available, and responsible for giving you the best advice they can, prescribing the most effective treatments when you ask them to, monitoring your progress (or lack thereof) and discussing that with you, and communicating effectively with other healthcare practitioners on your team, whether they be Western allopathic medicine or complementary/alternative medicine practitioners.

Practitioners – the patient is in charge and has the right to make decisions about their life and treatment. Our job is to present our opinion and advice, discuss that rationally and patiently with each person and, if necessary, their carers. Once we have presented our best advice, without dictatorial demands, it is up to our patient to accept or reject that advice, and that is their right.

No disease is irrelevant! If the patient has a history of any disorders, treated or not, we must factor that into our deliberations on the best way to treat. In the example above, each doctor considered comorbidities to be irrelevant, resulting in an illness pathway leading to "Parkinson's disease".

When presented with another illness that may be less closely related to the original diagnosis of Parkinson's disease, we must still be cognisant of the connection between lifestyle choices, history, environment and all diagnosed diseases.

Case history: *Bella was diagnosed with Parkinson's disease at fifty-six years old and was offered levodopa medication. She was unhappy with what she knew of the balance between benefits and adverse effects of levodopa and, as her symptoms were mild, chose to focus on diet, lifestyle, supplements and other self-help strategies. About a year into her experience with Parkinson's disease, Bella was diagnosed with chronic Borreliosis and, again, chose to use complementary/alternative medicine rather than heavy-duty antibiotics over a long period. Her practitioner explained that, while Borrelia infections did not necessarily "cause" Parkinson's disease, her chronic infection was a major influence on her level of wellness and PD symptoms.*

Bella focused on a program of total wellness – excellent food choices, some supplements, homeopathic medicine, meditation and a variety of self-help strategies. However, two years later, she noticed a lump in her breast and, after many scans, tests, interviews and discussions, was diagnosed with non-Hodgkin lymphoma. She felt that the seriousness of the diagnosis warranted intense Western allopathic medicine treatment and discussed a treatment plan with her oncologist.

The oncologist was totally focused on cancer treatment and refused to allow any other form of treatment for any other disorder while Bella was undergoing chemotherapy, despite there being no evidence that any of her current therapeutic choices would interfere in any way with chemotherapy and, in fact, would, most likely, enhance her ability to endure the rigours of the intended therapy and gain more benefit.

As with much cancer therapy, Bella was frightened by the dramatic prognosis repeatedly given ("do as I say or you will die"), so succumbed to the demands of the oncologist. The result was a short remission from cancer, but a resurgence of Parkinson's disease and Borreliosis symptoms.

The causes of non-Hodgkin lymphoma are yet to be fully elucidated but there is ample evidence that patients who support their immune systems and maintain a sense of control over their health are more likely to find remission over a long period.

Had Bella's Western allopathic medicine and complementary/alternative medicine practitioners been enabled to discuss her treatment and circumstances as peers (i.e. equals), there is no doubt her quality of life would have improved and she may well have responded better to the cancer treatment. Bella continued to struggle with the conflict between the common Western allopathic medicine view of attacking disease, killing cells, and getting worse in the hope that she will get better, and the complementary/alternative medicine focus on supporting her immune system, balancing her nervous system and repairing damaged cells and organs.

About a year after achieving remission from non-Hodgkin lymphoma, Bella again noticed a breast lump and consulted with her oncologist/haematologist. The diagnosis was a relapse and prognosis dire. Bella was told she needed immediate, heavy-duty chemotherapy for some months and that this would be "much worse than last time".

Bella insisted on a PET scan and large biopsy which both showed a cyst with possibly some cancer cells involved.

With this more definite and less frightening diagnosis, Bella undertook significant complementary/alternative medicine treatment for her total wellness with close monitoring by her team of healthcare specialists and GP/PCP.

With this new regimen, Bella's health improved steadily, she became more confident in dealing with her health and life in general, and the breast lump slowly reduced in size.

Bella continues to consult regularly with all Western allopathic medicine and complementary/alternative medicine practitioners on her team, but is enjoying her life of wellness.

Intuition

This is an often-neglected skill we have and can use to our benefit. Both Western allopathic medicine and many complementary/alternative medicine practitioners generally discount the patient's intuition as "ignorance" or "false hope", and push their own agenda of diagnosis and treatment. This attitude may be to the detriment of the patient's long-term health.

Patients – We are often given signals by our body that something is not right, out of balance, not working; we often speak of this as a "gut feeling", or that we "just have a feeling that ..." All too often, we suppress our inner knowledge and rely on outside assessments to decide what is right or wrong for us.

There is no doubt that objective assessment of health status is important and, sometimes, the only way to diagnose an illness process. However, it is vital that we listen to messages that we receive from our body (intuition or "gut feelings") and express our thoughts to our practitioners.

If our practitioners ignore or dismiss our intuition, it is time to find another practitioner. Where objective tests, scans or assessments appear to contradict our intuition, it is up to the practitioner to find the connection and explain how we may be misinterpreting the message, even though it seems accurate to us.

Case history: *Lyndon was concerned that his balance was "off"; he felt that he was being pulled forward and to the left constantly and his knees seemed to collapse without warning. He spoke to several doctors who dismissed his concerns, as there was no objective cause that they could see. Some offered antidepressants while one prescribed an anti-emetic for his dizziness.*

Lyndon "knew" something was seriously wrong and that it may be related to several old head injuries from football, and a more recent fall with concussion. One doctor reluctantly referred him for a CT scan which Lyndon thought was useless and refused. He eventually found a GP who accepted his concerns, examined him thoroughly and referred him for a privately-funded MRI; the results were indeterminate.

Lyndon was persistent as he "knew" something was wrong. He was able to find a functional neurologist who had access to a new scan that was able to map brain activity. This showed damage to Lyndon's brain stem, cerebellum and right frontal lobe, causing dysautonomia and postural orthostatic tachycardia syndrome (POTS).

Lyndon's intuition was right, but he needed specialist practitioner investigation and explanation before he knew exactly what was happening and could start repairs.

Patients, if you feel something is wrong, do not be dismissed. Persist, insist and pursue answers until you find an explanation for your gut feelings. You may not find the answers you expect, but there are always answers.

Practitioners: our patients often know more about their health than we give them credit for. They often do not know ***why***, but usually know ***what*** and, if enabled, will ask telling questions. Sometimes these questions can open up a new line of enquiry for us. For instance, one patient told me, in the middle of a consultation, that they had often felt uncomfortable as a child when they saw aerial crop spraying on a farm in the distance, even though it seemed so far away. They wondered if I thought that had any relationship to their diagnosis of

Parkinson's disease. We now know, of course, that many pesticides can drift as vapour for over thirty kilometres (eighteen miles) and, while it is in tiny amounts at that distance, frequent exposure can lead to toxicity. In my patient's case, the distant aerial spraying almost certainly was one factor in their progress towards Parkinson's disease and their intuition was spot on.

Sometimes our patients' intuition is harder to explain but, rather than dismiss it as irrelevant, we will do well to explore and research to see what relevance there is to their long-term health.

> **Case history**: *Joan was anxious and, at times, felt that she stumbled when out shopping. Her family did not notice any changes and, as they did not accompany her when shopping, did not see her stumble. She saw her GP, who prescribed medicine for her anxiety, but dismissed her other concerns as "ageing" (she was only sixty-three).*
>
> *Joan felt that there was more to her health than simply anxiety and age, and saw several more doctors, who all diagnosed anxiety and ageing.*
>
> *Six months later, she saw an integrative doctor, who gave her a very thorough physical examination and ordered a variety of tests. This doctor diagnosed heavy metal toxicity (Joan had grown up in an old goldmining district) and prodromal Parkinson's disease.*
>
> *The integrative doctor had asked many questions and delved into Joan's life history to find the clues leading to appropriate diagnosis. With chelation, dietary changes and some self-help strategies, Joan's anxiety faded, her walk became sure and stable again and Parkinson's disease did not develop.*
>
> *Joan was persistent, insistent and pursued her questions until she found answers. It should not have been so difficult for her.*

Business plan

So many of us have plans for our homes, work, families, holidays and sporting activities. But we do not have plans for our health.

When diagnosed with a chronic disease, we flounder in confusion and either grab any medication offered, or go on a mad hunt for anything that will save us from the impending doom predicted by medical practitioners, websites and groups raising money for a "cure".

Diagnosis with Parkinson's disease is serious, but it is not urgent. We have time to stop, read, ask questions and consider our options. We have time to develop a business plan for our health that can guide us through the mire of conflicting information flooding our mind. You may find this planning process useful.

1. On diagnosis, ask your doctor as many questions as you can think of about why they have diagnosed Parkinson's disease, what has caused your symptoms, what treatment they suggest and why, and what they suggest that you can do to help yourself. Your doctor may be impatient, not allow time for your questions, not know the cause and say that you can't really help yourself. Don't be upset, your doctor will follow their training and want you to just follow instructions without question.

2. You may be referred to a physiotherapist, dietitian or counsellor, or simply be offered medication.

3. Once you get home, start a planning chart in a way that is easy and meaningful for you. It may look something like this:

Practitioner	Diagonisis	Causes	Treatment	Self-help	Other
Doctor	Parkinson's	Don't know	Levodopa	Stay active	?

4. Start researching stories of people who have reversed Parkinson's disease partly or fully. You may find my story (Appendix 5) resonates with you, or Colin Potter in the UK, or other stories online. If elements of these stories appeal to you, add notes to your chart:

Practitioner	Diagnosis	Causes	Treatment	Self-help	Other
Doctor	Parkinson's	Don't know	Levodopa	Stay active	?
Potter	Parkinson's	Toxins	Diet, detox	Exercise	Positive thinking
Coleman	PD & MSA	Trauma, toxins	Diet, Aquas, etc	Exercise, meditation	Bowen
Harrison	Parkinson's	Unknown	Levodopa, diet	Meditation, detox	Weaned off levodopa

5. As you collect this information, you will start to see commonalities among those who have been able to reverse the illness process.

6. You may find it beneficial to read stories of those who have reversed other serious illness such as multiple sclerosis, diabetes or cancer. Again, chart any story that resonates with you.

7. Prepare a budget, if you do not already have one, and decide how much you can and are willing to spend on getting well. Very few positive therapies are covered by any insurance.

8. Look at the activities listed in your chart and see how many cost little or nothing – meditation, exercise (most types), self-love, laughter, singing, dancing, listening to music, detox activities. Many health-giving activities are free.

9. Select changes you can make that have been of benefit to

most recoverees – food changes, using organic/biodegrad-able cleaners (they may actually be cheaper than your current chemicals), Bowen therapy, meditation class, basic supplements. Cost these out and I think you will be surprised at how little extra these changes cost.

10. Seek practitioners who are prepared to support you in your efforts to be well without promising a "cure" (which does not exist), insisting on blind compliance with their very expensive program of supplements and therapies, or opposing your choices.

11. Develop a daily plan which includes times for health-giving activities, time with family and friends, down time and sleep. You may need to make this a weekly plan (as I do) to cater for different activities each day. Your day might look something like this:

7.30	rise, take Aquas and dry skin brush
7.45	shower
8.15	high-intensity interval training
8.30	breakfast and supplements
9.30	meditation
10.00	gardening
11.30	cuppa with spouse/partner, listening to music
11.45	dance
12.30	more gardening or potter in the shed
1.30	lunch
3.00	Bowen treatment
4.30	take Aquas
5.00	high-intensity interval training then meditation
6.30	dinner

And so on, to suit your plan.

12. Your daily/weekly plan can be on a large sheet of paper, or in a diary, or on the computer. I like to use an A4 diary with one day to a page. That way I have room for variations and

changes as needed, but can flick through the pages quickly to see what is happening days ahead if required.

13. Your plan does need some flexibility to cater for appointments with practitioners, special events and family time.

Developing a business plan, treatment charts and daily activities plan will give you a sense of control and understanding. You will no longer be faced with a runaway train, becoming a victim to illness and standard treatment, but the Chief Executive Officer of your own health business, employing those who bring value to the business and moving away from those who are detrimental to your journey.

Your business plan will also help you more effectively deal with any comorbidities (other diagnoses) that may occur. For instance, my plan was moving on nicely when I noticed symptoms developing that puzzled me, and I intuitively felt that there was something serious causing my discomfort. It took nearly a year of persistence, tests and scans, seeing many doctors and complementary/alternative medicine practitioners before I was diagnosed with bowel cancer. My business plan was flexible enough to cope with all these extra appointments, but allowed me to maintain the most important health-giving activities (meditation, food choices, etc.). Once I received the diagnosis, I revised my business plan to deal with the extra treatments needed (and, yes, I am cancer-free now, thank you for asking).

Take control, use your intuition wisely, and develop a business plan.

CHAPTER 23

REVERSING THE TRAUMA/STRESS PATHWAY

Trauma and/or high, sustained stress is implicated in over 90 per cent of the diagnosed cases of Parkinson's disease that I see in my clinic. In Chapter 8, I described the processes through which trauma/stress can trigger and lead to "dis-ease" – sometimes quickly but, more often, over a very long period.

Many patients deny any sort of trauma or untoward stress in their lives without even reviewing what this may mean. However, the information provided in the questionnaire every patient completes before making an appointment to see me can often tell a different story. Place and time of birth can often give clues to past trauma. Considering the history of the birthplace (country/town), school experiences, career choices, workplace experiences, relationships and social interaction may all be aspects of stress levels evoking a response or reaction. As most of these circumstances are normal parts of life, they are often not identified, by patients or practitioners, as stress triggers.

Let us look at some examples of normal circumstances being a source of stress causing an ongoing fight/flight/freeze response.

Birthplace

Anton was born in Munich in 1944. Munich is a beautiful city with a wonderful music and arts history. But, in 1944, Munich was under attack and bombed heavily. This followed many triumphant and terrifying years of World War II. Anton's parents *were traumatised by the war, and Anton, still a tiny baby, was subjected to the terror of the heavy bombing raids.*

Millie *was born in a small rural township where there were strong community ties and families supported each other. But the local industry was dying. Mum lost her part-time job first but soon Dad had his working hours reduced, then was laid off. While in grade five at school, Millie's family moved to the city and Dad found some work which paid enough to support the family, but he hated the work and was constantly unhappy. Millie found it difficult to fit in after an idyllic childhood in the country, the city life did not suit her and she found it very hard to make new friends. Losing her home, school and friends haunted her for many years.*

Freddy *was born in a busy regional centre with constant traffic through to other big centres, and a moderately profitable tourist industry. His family was in a lower socioeconomic category and their living circumstances were marginal. Their area supported a thriving drug trade which included many police raids and some rather nasty battles between traders. Freddy's family was not involved in the trade, but he was constantly afraid of his neighbours and the ongoing violence until they were able to move out when he was eleven.*

School experiences

Jeffrey *was the oldest son and, as heir, was slated to attend his father's old private boarding school so, at seven years old, he was sent away, to return home only during school holidays. This was his life until he graduated and went on to university (college). His father expected Jeffrey to excel academically at school and was not willing to discuss any other aspect of school life. Jeffrey was not able to tell anyone about the hazing and bullying he experienced until he was old enough to mete it out to the younger students; this he felt guilty about but it was the done thing. He did not speak about his school experiences until after his father died and Jeffrey was diagnosed with Parkinson's disease.*

April *was born to peripatetic parents. Her father changed jobs and locations each two to four years, so the family was uprooted, and April enrolled in a new school – sometimes at the beginning of the year, but often mid-term. She found it really difficult to form friendships and, when she did, they were shattered soon after when the family moved again.*

Career

Gareth *was always going to be a medical practitioner. His family enjoyed only a moderate income, so Gareth worked at many part-time jobs during his high school years and during his medical studies. Medical school was very hard and he continued to work part-time to pay his way.*

During his residency, he loved the work, but was subject to bullying by senior registrars and consultants, and his self-esteem slipped, especially with continuous fatigue.

In due course, he completed his training and joined a thriving general practice where he, again, loved the work and his patients, but writhed under the government regulations governing the length of consults, charges and restrictions on available tests, and insurance companies' restrictions on rebates.

Gareth was surprised when diagnosed with Parkinson's disease but began conservative treatment. Unsatisfied with the answers he received from specialists, he quietly sought my advice and was surprised when I discussed stress levels – he thought the stress levels he had endured for so many years were "normal".

Phillip *loved science and, eventually decided to become a geologist. He did not want to teach, so gained employment with large companies exploring for mineral deposits. He loved the work and, at first, enjoyed the months of travel and living rough. Then he fell in love, married and welcomed two delightful children into his life. He still loved his work but hated being away from his family for long periods. He knew he had to choose between his family, whom he loved very deeply, and work that he loved. He eventually*

228

compromised by accepting an administration position that allowed him to be close to his family but lacked the attraction of the "coal face" exploratory work he had enjoyed for so long.

Workplace

Joseph *was a good provider for his family and was proud of his career success, as he was "old school" – with no university qualifications (in fact, he had left school at fifteen to help his family), he had worked hard to prove himself in each position and receive promotion on merit. His peers were less kind and made it known that they respected university qualifications more than merit. Joseph worked harder for longer to prove his worth.*

In his twentieth year of service to one company, Joseph was retrenched ("laid off") as the company was downsizing. After many months on unemployment, he managed to find menial work on night shift, five nights per week. He was diagnosed with Parkinson's disease about four years later.

Angela *was quiet and unassuming, content to carry out her tasks at work without fuss or complaint, happy to be gainfully employed and earning enough to take care of her own needs and her ageing mother. Her workmates were less content and put pressure on Angela to work more slowly, to complain about her tasks and be as disruptive as they were, and bullied Angela when she refused to comply. Fifteen years of this constant pressure led to disease.*

Relationships

Annie *was born to loving parents in 1973. She felt her life was ideal with lots of games and overt love. However, one day, when Annie was four years old, her dad did not come home. Annie did not know that her parents' marriage had been uncertain for some years and, eventually, they had parted. Annie was not told why Dad was no longer there, and rarely saw him after the separation. By the time I saw her in her mid-twenties, she had realised that Dad leaving was not her fault, but she had spent the bulk of her childhood* and early teenage years feeling guilty, as she believed Dad had left because she was naughty.

James loved his wife and children and, with only primary school education (to eleven years old), did his best to provide. His wife was constantly discontented and made that known with snide remarks and put-downs. James did his best, saw service during a major war, sought work that would give him some satisfaction while providing for his family, and maintained a stoic façade in the face of constant criticism. It was a testament to his strength of character that Parkinson's disease was not diagnosed until his mid-sixties.

Social interaction

Jared grew up knowing only that his family worked hard and he was Catholic. He was not aware of any particular stresses in the family until he was ten years old. It was then that he was told that the family was moving because they were not Catholic, but Jewish, and Jews were not welcome in their social circle.

It was only as he matured that Jared realised the cost of secrecy to the family, and the levels of underlying stress that had enveloped him as he grew through childhood.

Colin always felt that he did not belong in social situations. He would attend school activities, parties and dances but feel awkward, on the "outside". His clothes were usually second-hand, he had no experience in interacting peacefully with peers as an equal (his homelife was not peaceful) and could not converse comfortably with others. Anticipating social occasions would cause anxiety and loss of sleep after the event, Colin would review his behaviour and be very self-critical of his failings.

This lack of confidence, low self-esteem and self-criticism lasted until well into his twenties, when he began to acknowledge his skills and strengths, and created some supportive friendships. His early experience played a role in his ill-health many years later.

The stories above are just a few real-life situations in which the patient did not recognise that they had experienced prolonged states of stress that may have had a role in creating pathology. The situations were, to each patient, normal: events or circumstances they saw around them, or experienced daily, or thought was "just part of life", so they did not note these experiences until directly asked.

The beginning of recovery is to acknowledge that some experiences and circumstances in our life may have created a fight/flight/freeze cycle as described in Chapter 8. As a patient, you may not readily see the relevance of any one experience but, as a practitioner, it is our duty to enquire, probe, prod and dig deep to understand the major influences on the HPA axis (the interaction between the hypothalamus, pituitary gland, and adrenal glands) of each individual so we can guide reversal strategies.

People facing prolonged, unresolved stress or trauma will respond in different ways, possibly dictated by their genetic inheritance and/or environment. Some will develop heart disease, cancer, arthritis, diabetes, skin disorders, depression or other psychological disorders, gastric ulcers or inappropriate behaviours such as substance addictions, compulsive gambling or violent behaviour.

Some will develop neurological and autoimmune disorders. The reprogramming of the hypothalamus and cellular dehydration, as well as many of the other effects shown earlier, allow some brain cells to become damaged or inactive, or even die, over many years, ultimately resulting in the expression of neurological disorder symptoms.

There are many excellent therapeutic options to deal with the emotional cost of prolonged stress/trauma. Therapeutic strategies can provide ways to cope with entrenched feelings, "put the past behind us" and respond more strategically to stressful circumstances rather than reacting instinctively.

We need more. We need strategies that will reprogram the HPA axis from fight/flight/freeze reaction to a response consistent with the fluctuating stress levels of a satisfying life. That means working with physiology to repair or replace neural pathways that have been destroyed or dysregulated by prolonged stress.

Much of this work can be done by the patient themselves under guidance from a skilled and observant practitioner. Once the patient becomes engrossed in the recovery pathway, the practitioner may choose to add homeopathic or flower essence remedies to assist the process.

I do not recommend the use of pharmacological agents in the process of trauma recovery unless the patient is unable to function without some drug assistance. Antidepressant and anti-anxiety drugs can be quite effective at suppressing overwhelming feelings of fear and anxiety, reduce depression and may, in extreme cases, prevent suicide. However, the key here is that drugs suppress the symptoms rather than reversing the causes of those symptoms. Furthermore, many antidepressant and anti-anxiety drugs may cause adverse effects that mimic or exacerbate Parkinson's disease symptoms.[11]

Keys to wellness

In Chapters 12–18, we explored patient strategies to assist recovery no matter what the aetiological pathway. Some of those strategies can help develop new physiological responses to stress and recovery from old, even forgotten stress. Review these chapters for details of the strategies, but here is a summary:

Love of ourselves without condition

To be truly well, we need to reach a state of complete acceptance of ourselves, loving ourselves with all our faults and weaknesses, recognising all our strengths and beauty. To do this, we may need help from counsellors or other therapists of various modalities, and our loved ones. However, our most important and powerful "doctor" is ourselves.

Use this "Mirror Talk" exercise every day until you are completely well:

1. Face yourself in a mirror, and look at your face, into your eyes, see all the features of your face, including all the wrinkles you have worked so hard to achieve.

2. While holding your gaze in the mirror, say, "............. (your name) you are wonderful. You have achieved a great deal in life. I love you completely". You may wish to vary the words, but the meaning needs to be there.

3. You may find this very difficult at first. We are not used to giving ourselves love. But persist; it gets easier and more rewarding over time.

Love yourself without condition. The worst thing that can happen is you will get better.

Laughter

Laughter is still the best medicine, or at least one of the best. Laughter releases endorphins and enkephalins in our brain and helps us to feel good. Laughter also reduces the production of stress hormones from the adrenal glands, and increases production of anandamide, dopamine, serotonin and many more useful, healing chemicals.

Meditation

When we meditate, we reduce the production of stress hormones from the adrenal glands, and increase production of anandamide, dopamine, serotonin, endorphins and many more useful, healing chemicals. That's right, it helps us in the same way as loving and laughing. A powerful trio indeed!

There are hundreds of ways, methods, philosophies and practices to meditate. Choose the one that suits you/your patient – they are all correct if they bring us a sense of peace. Be dedicated and meditate daily.

Singing

Some studies have shown reduction in cortisol production during group singing (indicating reduced stress response) and participants have reported enhanced feelings of wellbeing. Other studies show an increased production of endorphins (endogenous "painkillers") and oxytocin during singing. Increases in these chemicals can improve our sense of wellbeing, reduce pain, and enhance the "reward sections" of our brains. This, in turn, will enhance production of dopamine and serotonin, thus relieving some symptoms of Parkinson's disease for some time.

My clinical experience has shown that, while group singing is very helpful, and the chemical benefits may be optimal in the environment of a choir or singing group (even just one that meets in a garage to sing your favourites once a week), singing by ourselves can also be health-giving. Many of the same beneficial effects, other than those derived from interaction with others, accrue as we sing along to the radio or our favourite recordings. Singing in the shower, kitchen, bedroom or car can be just as valuable as joining a choir or singing group and is something we can do every day.

During my journey from diagnosis with Parkinson's disease to recovery, there were many months when I was unable to speak coherently; even though my brain was engaged and I had clear thoughts about what I intended to say, all I produced was gibberish. However, I found I could sing. I was managing sixteen staff at the time and found that I could issue instructions in "opera form", by singing (albeit with a pretty rough voice). Communicating with friends and family became easier when I discovered this also. Using a sing-song delivery made my words more coherent and communication better.

Now we understand the chemical benefits of singing, we can deduce that my symptoms were, in part, mitigated by my constant singing.

Singing is free medicine. Everybody has the opportunity several times each day so there is no excuse for not singing. Do you love opera or classical music, country, rock, jazz, blues? It doesn't matter what it is, play the music and sing along. Check out choirs and music group near you and join in whenever possible.

Free medicine! No excuse!

Dancing

Once again, rhythmic music helps us move more fluidly. We can dance with others, or on our own. We can dance in public or in the privacy of our homes. We can dance standing, sitting or lying down.

Yes, it doesn't matter what our levels of balance and mobility are, we can move to music, and that is good exercise for our body, brain and spirit.

Ballroom dancing, modern dancing, Latin dancing, rock'n'roll, old-time dancing, line dancing. These are all fabulous if you have the opportunity to join in with others. Like singing, dancing can often be more fun in a group and the social interaction also enhances our wellbeing. But we don't need others to dance, just music and willingness. I often dance as I prepare my breakfast – I have the radio playing songs I can sing along with and rhythms that entice me to move my body. There is nothing formal about this, just movement that expresses how the music affects me.

There is good clinical evidence that dancing will bring many of the same benefits as singing and, again, it is free medicine.[2,3] No excuse!

Dance every day. It does not have to be formal steps or forms of dancing; moving to music is dancing. Play your favourite music and let your body move in rhythm. You can dance upright, sitting or lying – just let the music move you.

Art

Drawing, painting, clay modelling, sculpture and other forms of art are fabulous ways to express feelings in a way that is meaningful to us, yet may be nothing but a lovely work of art to others. Art is something we can do on our own or in the company of others.

Art classes can provide us a way of connecting with others in the pursuit of a common interest yet, at the same time, granting an opportunity to draw, paint or create our expression of anger, sadness, loneliness or despair in the privacy or our creation. Only the artist knows the true meaning of his/her art.

Art is another way to release pent-up emotions in the same way as dancing and singing. Pouring our feelings into a creative work is one powerful way to relieve emotional pressure and move our healing journey forward.

Creating

Creating almost anything is a way to express emotion and release pressure. Working with wood, welding steel, developing a garden or restoring an old car are creative hobbies that can sustain us as we walk the long pathway to recovery.

Trauma/post trauma and flower essences

If we accept the proposition that degenerative disorders may originate in unresolved stress or trauma during childhood or early life, we need to find ways of resolving the initiating trigger. Counselling of various types, hypnotherapy, kinesiology and a wide range of energy and spiritual healing modalities are all useful and will assist is this task.

During my work I have found many people who are not aware of the initiating trauma even though it seems obvious to me, or who are not prepared to recognise the event or circumstance as traumatic. Sometimes the factors causing the initial degeneration were seen as normal – e.g. father away at war, systematic abuse common in the neighbourhood, an emotionally manipulative relationship with one or both parents, inappropriate responsibility for siblings, or trauma occurring before birth. In these cases, we need to find a way to open emotional doorways and allow a change in the way our patient views themselves and their place in the world.

Two very useful therapies to help us are Medicine Tree's Trauma/Post Trauma homeopathic spray, and flower essences.

Trauma/Post Trauma

This homeopathic complex, made in Australia, contains eleven different remedies, some in a range of potencies. The combination is aimed at assisting resolution, at all levels, of traumatic events or circumstances. While it can be of benefit in treating recent traumas, I also find it most useful in assisting the resolution of long past events. The action is often subtle and may not be noticed by our patient for many months. Some have told me that they are gaining no benefit from the remedy, while indicating unconsciously that the remedy is working.

For instance, one patient had spent a year telling me that she was one of those people for whom the treatment would not work. She would like to get better, and would go on trying, but it wouldn't work. Three months after starting Trauma/Post Trauma spray, she was telling me how she gained no benefit from the remedy, while discussing her planned activities when she got well. My patient had not noticed the change in language from "it won't work" to "when I get well". Another patient was very doubtful about the worth of the remedy but explained that she had been experiencing "moments of unexplainable joy" for the first time in her memory.

Trauma/Post Trauma spray seems to open the walls we have built up around unbearably painful memories so we can process them with love and a minimum of pain. I have not had a patient who is confronted with very painful or unmanageable issues while using Trauma/Post Trauma spray. Rather, I find that opportunities arise to either explore past events and/or circumstances or to refer my patients on to empathetic counsellors.

Trauma/Post Trauma spray is available in 20 mL spray bottles. I generally prescribe one spray twice daily for two weeks, then two sprays twice daily. I rarely find the need to prescribe more, despite instructions on the bottle allowing up to four sprays four to six times daily.

Trauma/Post Trauma spray contains homeopathic remedies as follows:

Aconitum napellus (Aconite) 30C, Arnica montana 15C & 205C, Bellis perenis 15C, Gelsemium sempervirens 30C, Porcine adrenal glands 7C, Hypericum perforatum 8C, Strychnos ignatia 15C & 30C, Sodium sulphate 15C, Sodium chloride 30C & LM1 & LM2 & LM3, Phosphoric acid 18C, Delphinium staphisagria LM1 & LM2 & LM3 plus ethanol as a preservative.

It is a patented formula owned by Medicine Tree, a division of bWellness in Australia: support@bwellenss.com.au

Flower essences

These beautiful remedies may be used instead of Trauma/Post Trauma spray or in conjunction with the homeopathic as they work at different levels. I happen to use a combination of Bach Flower Remedies and Australian Bush Flower Essences, but there are many varieties of essences available and all work well when prescribed with love. Find the range that resonates with you and develop a way of choosing that sits well with both you and your patient.

Flower essences can be used to help resolve past trauma and/ or to give support in the present. I often use my range of flower essences to help patients find a positive outlook in their current circumstances and focus on welcoming wellness.

CHAPTER 24

FOR PRACTITIONERS

Dealing with depression

Depression is often quoted as one of the symptoms of neurological and autoimmune disorders. In conservative therapy, this depression is generally treated with antidepressants.

Given the training, culture, network structure and diagnostic criteria of conservative practitioners, this seems to be both a reasonable diagnosis and appropriate treatment. In other words, good medicine.

But is it?

There is no doubt that many people with neurological and autoimmune disorders are depressed at some stage. In fact, I would venture to say that everyone diagnosed with a neurological disorder is depressed at some time, whether they are ever diagnosed as such or not.

I would also venture to say that a few display symptoms of clinical depression and need medication for a short to medium term. But I believe that the number of people with neurological and autoimmune disorders who are clinically depressed is far fewer than diagnosed.

Clinical depression is marked by a number of common symptoms:[1]

- Mood change – despondency, despair, loss of interest in people, activities, sex and personal care
- Sleep disturbance
- Anorexia
- Either suicidal ideation or delusional ideation
- Difficulty in thought and concentration
- Anxiety, irritability and/or aggression
- Physical conditions such as fatigue, tiredness, loss of appetite,

weight loss, constipation, bodily aches and pains, headaches, respiratory problems, dryness in the mouth and unusual sensations in chest or abdomen

- A depressed facial expression – frown, immobile face, down-turned mouth, troubled expression.

Many people with neurological and autoimmune disorders exhibit some or most of these symptoms. In fact, I have observed all the symptoms in the above list to some degree in patients at some time during their journey.

Does this mean they are depressed and require antidepressants medication? I believe that this is very rare.

Neurological and autoimmune disorders are frustrating, humiliating, imprisoning, and sometimes painful. Even before diagnosis, we are aware that we can no longer perform to our usual standard in areas of our daily life. As the disorder progresses, we lose energy, become clumsy, perhaps shake, find it difficult to walk, move, sit comfortably, sleep, and relate to our loved ones. We may have difficulty in eating, become constipated, lose our libido or suffer impotence. Some of us have to give up work and become dependent on others for our care.

Of course we feel depressed sometimes!

We don't need drugs to suppress our feelings. We need support, counselling, strategies and therapies that will give us a sense of worth, help us focus on the positive aspects of our life, and give us hope of something better.

It is important to remember that many antidepressant drugs used today can exacerbate some of the symptoms of neurological and autoimmune disorders (read MIMS or a similar drug guide for an understanding of adverse effects). I often see patients who have been given antidepressants for anxiety, find their tremor worsening (for instance), so have their levodopa medication increased, which increases dyskinesia, which makes them more anxious because they feel they are getting worse.

Let's break the cycle.

How to help a patient who seems depressed

There are a number of strategies and therapies that can help your patients move from a negative, hopeless, depressed state into a more positive and motivated emotional state.

1. **Keeping journals and notes.** Your patient's weekly journal will help them understand that they really are making inroads against this debilitating disorder. Your notes will give you the information you need to show them how they have progressed.Remember, progress will be slow and in small steps, so it is vital to keep detailed notes.

2. **Setting goals.** Set easily achievable goals with your patient. Once they realise that they are really achieving something, their mood will change.

3. **Exercise.** Regular, rhythmic exercise like walking, swimming, water aerobics, cross crawling, bike riding (even on an exercise bike) and high-intensity interval training will help produce chemicals in the brain which give us feelings of pleasure. Encourage your patient to undertake regular exercise and, if possible, enlist the aid of a carer or family member to exercise with them. If your patient is not ambulatory, work on exercises that involve rhythmically tensing and relaxing muscles, or other simple, rhythmic movements that can be done two or three times daily.

4. **Counselling.** It is often useful for a person with a neurological disorder to talk to someone outside of their daily circle about the issues that worry them. This may be their health practitioner, or someone trained in counselling – psychologist, psychotherapist, family counsellor, hypnotherapist or similar. Often just explaining our frustrations to someone who knows how to listen will relieve tension and lift depression.

5. **Other modalities** such as kinesiology, art, dance and visualisation can help find the source of the depressed feelings, identify other events or situations that are exacerbating the feelings, and initiate reversal.

6. **Flower essence therapy.** Flower essences are a subtle, yet powerful means of bringing a positive emotional change. If you do not have experience in this type of therapy, network with a local practitioner who can help you.

7. **Emotional Freedom Technique (EFT)** is a system of tapping acupuncture or trigger points while repeating a positive affirmation that can help change negative emotional states to positive. There are many excellent books available on this technique plus online information and demonstrations. EFT can be used on a regular programmed basis, or ad hoc. I certainly found it a most useful technique for changing my own emotional state in times of crisis.

8. **Work with family and carers whenever possible.** Ask them to observe your patient and take note of any progress, however tiny. Ask them to talk about your patient's progress both with your patient, and in company where your patient can hear. The more encouraging remarks that are made, the more your patient will see how well they are doing.

9. **Use supplements or herbs.** There are a number of excellent dietary supplements and herbal combinations that can give emotional support to your patient while they deal with appropriate issues, without causing untoward adverse effects. If you are not qualified to prescribe these, refer your patient to another health practitioner who is.

10. **Laugh.** Laughter is still "the best medicine" (apart from self-love, of course). Laughter releases endorphins and enkephalins in our brain and helps us to "feel good". We can sometimes lift the gloom covering our patients by generating laughter in our treatment room. I often tell the story of acting as drink waiter at a friend's wedding while I still had very severe Parkinsonian tremor; it always gets a laugh. I tell jokes, talk about comedies on television and comment on funny happenings in my life. It is even better when we can talk about funny things happening in the patient's life. One patient was feeling down about his clumsiness with belts, laces, and general dressing problems. He then told me, as an example, how he went to the toilet and couldn't work

out why he couldn't find the fly until he realised he had put his pyjama pants on back to front. We all laughed and he felt much better about his progress.

I am not implying that we should take our patients' challenges lightly. Their struggle to get well is serious business. But sometimes we forget that serious business can include serious laughter, and laughter can flatten out the steepest hill.

In my experience, depression is usually a result of being trapped in a neurological disorder, rather than an endogenous symptom. We can help our patients conquer this unwelcome visitor.

CHAPTER 25

REVERSING THE TOXIN PATHWAY

There are a number of "classes" of toxins we must consider and eliminate when working to reverse the symptoms of Parkinson's disease and walking a pathway to wellness. They are:

1. What we put in our body – food, drink, supplements, medication, recreational drugs

2. What we put on our body – clothes, personal care products, make-up, body decorations

3. Toxic substances in our immediate environment – home, work, recreation areas, shops, vehicles

4. Toxic substances in the wider environment.

The major strategies we can use to reduce the impact of toxins on our health are:

1. Avoidance

2. Mitigation

3. Elimination of accumulated toxins.

In most cases, exposure to a single toxin once or even several times will not cause Parkinson's disease. We have already discussed the probability that Parkinson's disease symptoms are caused by a number of triggers affecting two or more aetiological pathways.

The toxic influences discussed in this chapter can either accumulate in tissue or cells over time, so reaching critical level, or have long-term effects on metabolic systems creating illness symptoms.

In certain circumstances (for instance, shopping in a large supermarket) we may encounter over 1000 toxic chemicals in an hour. Each has a tiny adverse influence on our body, but our immune system and innate protective mechanisms deal with them. However, some chemicals stay locked in tissue or cells and accumulate with other chemicals encountered on our last visit, and the visit before, and our many visits over time.

One small encounter with pesticide or application of a neurotoxic body care product will, most likely, not create any noticeable sickness symptoms. However, repeated and/or constant exposure can cause an ever-increasing burden of wellness disruption, resulting in an identifiable "disease".

What we put in our body

Food: For the vast majority of patients, their food intake is completely under their control. Even if they do not prepare their own meals, being lucky enough to have a spouse, partner or carer to do that, they can negotiate appropriate food choices with the food preparer. A few of my patients have lived in assisted living facilities and it is very difficult to obtain healthy food in such places but, sometimes, some negotiation is possible.

Food is the source of energy and nourishment, but may also be the source of very damaging toxins. We explored this in detail in Chapter 13.

It is critical that all food choices are nourishing, supportive, "clean", healthy and tasty. All inflammatory, toxic and damaging food *must* be eliminated from your diet.

Except in the rare cases of people in assisted living facilities, there is no excuse for consuming toxic or harmful food.

Avoidance is the primary strategy here.

Drink: We also discussed drink in Chapter 13. Water is the prime hydrator and best drink for most of our needs. Many herbal teas can be enjoyable and also have some therapeutic value. Rooibos tea is an example of this.

There is no excuse for consuming caffeine, sugary drinks, drinks with artificial sweeteners or alkaline water.

Once again, avoidance is the best strategy.

Supplements: There are many nutritional supplements that are useful and helpful, especially during our journey to wellness. However, there are some that are useless and some that may cause harm.

In Chapter 15, we discussed the basic supplements that can help most people on their journey, and questions of quality.

Before adding other supplements to your regimen, it is best to seek advice from a well-qualified and open-minded practitioner. Most really good supplements are available only from practitioners or on prescription anyway, so having a nutritionally aware practitioner on your team is very valuable.

Good quality nutritional supplements, selected for your particular needs, can be very helpful on your journey. However, buying just any old brand over the counter (OTC), because of rampant advertising, promotion by a sporting hero or celebrity, because your friend Daisy says it's good, or because it is the cheapest is usually a waste of money because the supplement will not yield the material advertised and/or it will not bring the advantages claimed. Furthermore, some contain adjuvants, emulsifiers, preservatives, colourings and flavours that are actually harmful.

Forums are, in general, a really bad source of information as you will never know whether the person posting information about some "wonder supplement" or "super food" has any training, clinical experience, or is supported/sponsored by the company producing the supplement concerned.

In my experience, Multilevel Marketing (MLM) supplements are rarely worth considering – they are inevitably too expensive because of all the levels of commissions to be paid; most "distributors" have no training except by the manufacturer or their upline contact and have a vested interest in sales rather than your health; practitioners involved often have a strong interest in promoting MLM products over other practitioner-only products because of the commission structure versus wholesale/retail margins; MLM companies are sometimes single-product or single resource manufacturers – i.e. they have access to limited raw materials and seek to exploit the profit potential of that material as far as possible.

Nutritional supplements, if selected for your particular needs, can be valuable in your journey. However, unwisely chosen supplements will waste your money and may harm you.

Medication: There is no doubt that Western allopathic medicine drugs can be lifesaving, life-giving and life-enhancing. On the other hand, inappropriately prescribed drugs can be anything from mildly harmful to deadly.

The challenge with Western pharmaceutical medication is that so much of our Western allopathic medical care is compartmentalised. We may see a general practitioner (or PCP), neurologist, cardiologist, psychiatrist, urologist, gastroenterologist and/or any number of other specialists.

Again, there is no doubt that each of our practitioners will do their best to quell the symptoms pertinent to their speciality. This may include prescribing one or more drugs.

In theory, each specialist should read all the notes made by other specialists and be aware of all our prescribed drugs (and supplements if they are to be very thorough). In practice, this rarely happens.

Again, in theory, our GP/PCP should be aware of all prescriptions by other specialists and assess likely interactions and accumulation of adverse effects. In my experience, this is tragically rare.

Our challenge is to negotiate the labyrinth of medical appointment, tests, diagnoses, prognoses, prescriptions and pronouncements while unwell, often tired, and untrained in medical jargon. We trust our doctors to have our best interests at heart (or we would not be there) and accept that any drugs prescribed are necessary, will improve our health, and not cause harm either as prescribed or in conjunction with any other medication we may be taking.

Real life can be somewhat different from theory. If our specialist is busy and anxious to move on to the next patient, they may not notice that, while the drug they are prescribing with a common adverse effect of headache is unlikely to adversely affect us on its own, we are already taking two other drugs with headache as a common adverse effect so we are much more likely to develop a headache. Then, when we do develop a persistent headache, our GP/PCP may suggest more frequent paracetamol or refer us to a migraine specialist, rather than first examining our drug load.

Two case histories

Alfred was an elderly gentleman diagnosed with Parkinson's disease after a long history with anxiety and hypertension. He was prescribed levodopa in addition to his anti-anxiety and anti-hypertensive medication. Because his doctor was concerned that the levodopa may create some nausea, he also prescribed an anticholinergic antiemetic. Alfred developed sleep disturbances and became quite depressed, so was prescribed a sleeping drug and antidepressant.

When Alfred first contacted me, he was in a state of mind that saw no hope for a better life or return to good health. He felt nauseous all the time, despite the antiemetic drug, had frequent reflux and constant headaches and, because of this, was quite depressed and anxious. He was taking nine drugs as prescribed by three different doctors and specialists.

To gain an understanding of what was happening, I drew up a chart of all his prescribed medication and very common or common adverse effects. This chart showed that, of his nine drugs, all commonly caused nausea (even the antiemetic), seven commonly caused headache, five commonly caused depression or anxiety, a different five could cause sleep dysregulation and three could cause reflux.

Over the next two years, we very carefully and slowly reduced Alfred's drug load. Each time he reduced a drug dose a little, he advised the relevant specialist and his GP. At the end of that two-year process, Alfred no longer had headaches or reflux and was no longer depressed, but still suffered daily nausea. I wrote to his GP pointing out that his remaining four drugs could all cause nausea and, in my opinion, only one was necessary for his health. The GP agreed and supervised Alfred's withdrawal from three of those drugs, which resolved his nausea almost immediately.

At our last contact, Alfred was well, energetic, and free from all Parkinson's disease symptoms as well as drug adverse effects.

Belinda was in her mid-eighties when she called me with a real challenge. She said she had a rash on her legs that was dreadfully itchy and a constant headache that did not respond to analgesia. Belinda was anxious to make an appointment as she had been told that I could possibly help her with these persistent symptoms that severely reduced her quality of life. She had consulted all her current specialists plus dermatologists, neurologists and other doctors to no avail.

As Belinda lived alone and needed help with transport to see me, I asked her to, first, send me a detailed history with a list of all medications she was taking (this is standard procedure for my clinic).

Her letter arrived within a few days, including a list of fourteen drugs prescribed by five different doctors and specialists. Once again, I charted the very common and common adverse effects of all her prescribed drugs. Of the fourteen, eleven commonly caused rash and nine commonly caused headache.

I called Belinda and asked her to speak with her GP about the drug chart I was about to send her, and request a drug review and reduction. I said that, without that, there was nothing I could do to help her.

Belinda's reply was, "My doctor would not give me anything that would harm me!" Then she disconnected the call and I have never heard from her since.

I am sure she was correct. Her doctor would never give her anything that would obviously harm her if he was aware of that potential harm. But none of her doctors had taken the time to explore the possibility of accumulative adverse effects from the drugs prescribed by all her doctors and, as Belinda was a very compliant patient and had almost reverend faith in the wisdom of Western allopathic medicine practitioners, she refused to question a prescription.

Adverse effects from a single drug are unlikely to cause distress or harm in most cases. But, where there are similar/identical adverse effects common to two or more drugs, the likelihood of adverse effects increases exponentially. At least one in three of my new patients are victims of polypharmacy without regulation. In many cases, doctors refuse to cooperate in seeking alternative medications or working to reduce the drug load, so we need to take control, increase wellness using all the strategies in this book, and reduce the drug support as it is safe.

It is vital for practitioners and patients to be aware of accumulative adverse effects from polypharmacy, and all interactions between drugs and food and drugs and supplements. Appendix 4 shows a drug chart with very common or common adverse effects. Many of these drugs have alternatives that may not display the same adverse effects (all Western pharmaceutical medication has some adverse effects) so can be prescribed to lessen the risk of those adverse effects. In many cases, cooperation with and communication between Western allopathic medicine and complementary/alternative medicine practitioners will discover a combination of care strategies that lessens or eliminates the risk of adverse effects. Perhaps this is idealistic (I have experienced only two cases of medical cooperation in my twenty plus years of practice), but it is, by far, the preferred strategy for patient care.

Patients must be willing to ask "why?"

"I accept that you are prescribing this drug/supplement because you feel it is good for me. But why is it good for me? What adverse effects might occur? Are any of these adverse effects the same as for other drugs I am taking?"

I recently visited a cardiologist because my blood pressure had remained consistently high since surgery for cancer. He suggested that I take medication. My first question was "Why is my BP high? Before this, I always had low BP." He said that he did not know but I should take medication. I said, "Why? What is the alternative?" He did not know.

I have chosen to not take medication but to work with other strategies (food, of course, exercise, meditation and stress reduction) and can see my average BP slowly reducing. Taking drugs is easy. Using non-drug strategies is often healthier.

I do not suggest that we should eschew all Western pharmaceutical medication; much is useful, helpful and, in some cases, life-saving. We should accept, with gratitude, prescriptions that will improve our lives. However, we must be aware that not all medication is helpful and not all prescriptions are appropriately researched before being written. Even some old standards are now coming under scrutiny. For instance, aspirin, long held as a life saver by preventing heart attacks and strokes, has been examined in a 4.7-year trial of over 19,000 participants and, later, in a meta-analysis of thirteen clinical trials with a total of over 164,000 participants. These studies found that the harm caused by aspirin in elderly people outweighed any advantages. In fact, the mortality rate was higher in the aspirin group that in the placebo group.[1] We need to ask questions!

Ask your doctor about cumulative adverse effects and do not leave his/her office without an answer.

Ask your pharmacist to check the common adverse effects of all the drugs you are taking (have a list with you) and, if they cannot or will not, ask for a loan of their drug guide and chart adverse effects.

If all else fails, go to your local library and borrow a drug guide, or even go online and chart all common adverse effects.

Once you have your drug chart and you see that there could be problems with common adverse effects, go back to your doctor and demand changes. Many studies in developed countries (primarily USA, Canada, Australia and European countries) have shown that medical error is the third leading cause of death in those societies. Approximately one in five people will be harmed or killed by hospital mistakes or carelessly prescribed medication.[23] As a practitioner (Western allopathic medicine or complementary/alternative medicine) it is our responsibility to do no harm and correct inappropriate prescriptions when we notice them, while patients have a responsibility to ask lots of questions and make sure that your practitioner is certain that all the medicines and supplements prescribed are needed, safe, effective and will not interact with any other prescribed substances or accumulate adverse effects.

Western pharmaceutical medication can help us in many ways but can also be the source of life-damaging toxins. Avoid if possible; otherwise use wisely.

Dental treatments: There is no doubt that dentistry has improved remarkably over the past seventy years. My memories of dental treatments in childhood are the stuff of nightmares, but more modern treatments have reduced pain and improved outcomes. Healthy teeth and good dental care are vital to our health.

All dental treatments have the possibility of toxic absorption no matter how holistic your dentist may be. Antiseptics, cleaning compounds, X-rays and a multitude of EMFs accumulate to challenge our body.

However, dental care is critical and, in most cases, we can be assiduous in detox protocols before and after dental treatments to offset any disadvantages and health challenges.

Fluoride treatments are contentious and problematic. Fluoride, in appropriate forms (e.g. calcium fluoride), may be helpful for tooth mineralisation in very low doses (0.7-1.2 ppm) but, in higher doses, can cause health challenges, sometimes severe.

Some studies have found that tea drinkers (all black, white and green teas contain fluoride) using fluoridated water are vulnerable to fluorosis. Excess fluoride can also lead to discolouration and weakening of tooth enamel.[4]

Strong teeth can be maintained in most cases with great food choices as in Chapter 13, vitamin C intake and, where required, calcium citrate/hydroxyapatite and boron, thorough and regular cleaning with herbal-based toothpastes and, where tooth enamel seems weak, coconut oil pulling (see detox section in Chapter 26).

Fillings are another critical dental treatment where cavities have formed. Amalgam fillings have been used for over 150 years and are still considered safe by dental and health authorities. However, this finding has been questioned by many researchers.

Amalgam is a mix of mercury, silver, copper and tin. Other metals such as indium, zinc or palladium may also be added. Mercury liquid is added to the metal powders to bind them and render the mix flexible for working, shaping and inserting in cavities. It then helps the mix harden.

It is difficult to measure the absorption of mercury from amalgam fillings. Conservative authorities claim that any mercury absorption is below the safety threshold and does not adversely affect health. However, the vagueness of these claims (e.g. "below the safety threshold") implies that there is at least some mercury absorbed during placement and, possibly, as fillings age.

For patients, one amalgam filling, while strong and secure, will probably not cause any adverse effects. Multiple fillings, ageing fillings and teeth requiring repair from time to time, are likely to exacerbate mercury absorption, which will accumulate with other neurotoxins and, eventually, reach a critical level.

This is one toxic influence for which there are less toxic alternatives.

There is a trend among health-conscious people, or those diagnosed with neurodegenerative disorders anxious to help themselves, to have all amalgam fillings removed by "holistic dentists" who claim to prevent mercury pollution during the process by using mouth dams and strong suction. In my clinical experience, this is rarely a good idea. The process is very expensive, can be quite traumatic and, with all the best equipment, still exposes the patient to mercury fumes via the tooth root – a direct passage to the bloodstream.

My advice is to leave amalgams where they are unless or until they need repair, then use less-toxic material.

No dental filling is completely non-toxic, but they are critical to our health in that we must have strong effective teeth if we are to eat healthy food.

Root canal fillings are also problematic as they can create inflammation, insert toxins quickly into the bloodstream, be the seat for chronic infection that remains undetected for years and, in general, are best avoided.

Recreational drugs: In my view, recreational drugs are never a good choice. They are uncontrolled, all have adverse effects, may interfere with other medications or even interact with food, and all the common ones have significant effects on the nervous system. Avoid them.

What we put on our body

Clothes: We need clothes. The primary aim of clothes is protection from weather, excess sunlight (but not all sunlight), impact hazards like sand particles in high wind or other wind-carried objects, to keep us warm in cold conditions or stop rough surfaces abrading our skin.

A secondary purpose is decoration. We like to look acceptable to our peers and comply with social expectations. Sometimes we choose to rebel and dress to excite, annoy or express independence.

Unlike in Elizabethan times, our clothes are very unlikely to kill us. Back then it was not uncommon to find arsenic or lead in fabrics, or other toxic dyes. As clothes were often worn for long periods (washing once per year was common), poisons were sometimes absorbed transdermally to a fatal extent.

Despite much better control of clothing materials nowadays, we can sometimes make choices that are detrimental to health.

Natural materials such as wool, cotton and hemp are kinder to our bodies than materials made from petrochemicals, such as nylon and polyester. Natural materials allow better air circulation so aiding expulsion of gaseous toxins and wicking sweat away from our skin. However, even these materials, especially wool and cotton, may contain some chemicals from production and processing. It is always best to wash new wool and cotton clothes before wearing.

Cotton clothes are particularly problematic as non-organic cotton is grown using a huge amount of pesticide spray (which can, of course, drift for thirty kilometres). Aldicarb is a highly toxic pesticide widely used in cotton production. Many workers, including children, are harmed and killed by this chemical each year. It is presumed that all pesticides are removed from the cotton during processing, but not from batting (cotton used for mattress covers, including baby mattresses). The pesticides used in cotton production can also enter ground water and waterways, as well as polluting other food sources through drift.

It is always best to buy organic cotton clothing whenever possible. However, even then there may be chemical challenges. Some dyes are not fast, so can be absorbed through the skin. Permanent-press/no-iron chemicals do not wash out and may be toxic over a long period. Be prepared to iron your cotton clothes rather than purchasing non-iron examples, and check that the dye is fast (by washing before use).

While wool is not so chemically loaded during growing, wool clothing may contain dye and permanent-press chemicals, so always check this.

Hemp clothing is often produced organically with non-toxic dyes, but always ask.

Another natural material, leather, is wonderful for shoes, gloves, hats, etc. but, again, we must check for dyes and processing chemicals before wearing next to our skin. Leather pants, for instance, may cause sweating and enhance absorption of any chemicals transdermally. Organically produced leather is wonderful material.

From a practical point of view, sometimes nylon or polyester is what we can afford. If we love sports, the team shirts or fan materials are often produced from polyester (it's much cheaper than cotton). This material tends to exacerbate sweating but does not wick sweat away from the body as well as natural materials so, during strenuous activity, we may be bathed in our own toxic sweat as our body strives to eliminate toxins through the skin.

If you need to wear polyester, look for clothing that allows "breathing" in critical areas such as armpits. Nylon/polyester underwear is never really appropriate (no matter how sexy it might look).

For women, underwire bras may give lift and shape to the breasts, but the pressure from the underwire is one of the aggravating triggers for tissue damage that may lead to breast cancer if other triggers are there. Organic cotton "body form" bras are much healthier, and a healthy breast is a sexy breast.

Personal care products: We have total control over which personal care products we use. While there may be pressure from family and friends to use products other than our own choices, it is our personal responsibility to choose those products which, at least, will not harm us.

Most personal care products are applied directly to our skin; some, like toothpaste and mouth wash, are applied directly to our mucus membrane. Absorption through the skin and mucus membranes is very efficient and many toxins enter our blood-stream rapidly after application and can disrupt many vital functions such as hormone production, digestion or nerve messaging.

Appendix 1 gives details of many human-created or extracted materials that can cause long-term damage and exacerbate the pathway to chronic disease. The list of chemicals in Appendix 1 is not complete. It cannot be. Every year, there are more man-made chemicals released into our environment in foods, drinks, cleaning products, aroma accessories (air fresheners), personal care products and others. Most of these chemicals are possibly safe if applied strictly in accordance with the testing process – that is, short-term application on intact skin/membranes in healthy subjects. There is no testing on fragile individuals with broken or dehydrated skin, or who already struggle with compromised immune systems and chronic inflammatory response. But we can both estimate the likely damage and observe different health outcomes in those populations using toxic personal care products and those avoiding them.

The primary strategy to prevent damage from personal care products is to avoid all the toxic ones and carefully choose products that are neutral or healthy. Let's start at the top:

Hair colour – pure henna is the only safe hair colour to use. But even better, why not celebrate the wisdom and experience reflected in our grey hair? Despite claims to the contrary, all other hair colours contain some toxic products that are readily absorbed through the scalp and skull. When diagnosed with Parkinson's disease, we are fully aware of disrupted neural pathways in our brain, so it seems foolish to risk disrupting those pathways further with hair colour.

Shampoo and conditioner – often contain toxic chemicals to assist in dissolving grease or to aid the application of the detergents/conditioners used. Again, these are readily absorbed through the scalp and skull. There are safe/harmless products available in ethical health food stores or through healthcare practitioners. Always read the labels and, if you do not understand what some of the ingredients are, ask questions or look them up. Some people find that washing their hair with just bicarb is satisfying and using white vinegar as a conditioner works really well. Using non-toxic shampoos and conditioners has the extra benefit of enhancing the health of your hair without all those expensive treatments, and healthy hair not only makes us look good, but feel good as well.

Make-up – many women (and a few men) feel that they cannot face the world without a mask of make-up on their faces. Foundation, blush, eyeliner and colour, lipstick and other covers, colours and attachments are all designed to change the way we look to others while giving us a barrier against revealing our true nature.

Most make-up manufacturers make no attempt to hide the toxic nature of their products nor the long-term damage they can cause; they simply choose to not mention it in any advertising or instructions, and there is no law to force them to reveal the possible health challenges caused by repeated and long-term use of make-up. There are a few (very few) companies producing make-up products that are possibly safe if used occasionally but, even in these cases, there are some doubts about long-term use and whether all ingredients have been revealed.

The best make-up is healthy skin and that results from a healthy body. Excellent food choices, adequate hydration, exercise and plenty of fresh air will ensure that your skin reflects your true health. The state of our skin (soft/dry, clear/damaged) can often be a guide to necessary changes to diet, hydration, supplementation or treatments required.

Our skin is a semipermeable membrane designed to protect us against attack and abrasion, but can, and must be able to transfer helpful materials inward (moisture, oxygen, oils) and toxins out (via sweat). Once we block the skin with make-up, it can no longer do its job and starts to lose integrity.

The most beautiful people I know wear no make-up.

Cleansers and moisturisers – are often created with chemicals designed to remove grease and toxic make-up easily, and represent another assault on the health of our skin. Many soaps are drying and can also damage skin, so we need to search out mild soaps or washing liquids, perhaps use herbal-based products with no chemicals added, or wash with water only. If the water is "hard" (highly mineralised), add a little bicarb to soften it, or some apple cider vinegar.

Moisturise (if necessary) with pure coconut oil; add a drop of very pure essential oil (lavender, frankincense, German chamomile, tea tree, geranium, rosemary, peppermint, lemon, neroli, rose, myrrh, patchouli, tangerine, cypress) chosen for your personal skin needs. There is lots of information available on what oils are best for different skin needs. Choose essential oils that are at least 99.9 per cent pure and, if possible, made in your country or continent. MLM products usually make unprovable claims of purity and tend to be very expensive for the quality and quantity received. Use just one or two drops of essential oil and/or five or six drops of water-miscible vitamin E in 30-50 mL pure coconut oil, massage into your skin and allow that to stay overnight.

Sunscreens – of course it is important to avoid serious over-heating and sunburn. Overexposure to sun, especially in hot, dry areas like central Australia and American desert areas, can lead to skin damage and metabolic consequences caused by dehydration and hyperthermia.

However, there is doubt about the common belief that sun exposure alone causes cancer (melanoma). Most thorough research shows that melanoma requires toxic triggers as well as sun exposure, or toxic triggers only. Otherwise, the majority of rural and outside construction workers exposed to sun most of the day with only partial protection and constant sun on arms, would be diagnosed with melanoma. Yet only a minority receive this diagnosis, with more developing basal cell carcinoma and squamous cell carcinoma but, as these latter two diagnoses are not confined to those exposed to sunlight, it seems wise to avoid carcinogens on our skin. Others with very little sun exposure may also develop melanoma.

Those who avoid sunlight or who are unable to enjoy sun exposure through work schedules or because they live in the northern hemisphere where there is little winter sun, are plagued with disorders such as seasonal affective disorder and vitamin D deficiencies.

The most sensible approach is to enjoy morning sun when temperatures range up to 25° Celsius (80° Fahrenheit) and avoid the hotter parts of the day. Dr George Jelinek has calculated that an ideal exposure is ten to fifteen minutes of morning sun to 90 per cent of our body at least five days per week. While this is simply not possible for many because of work or family commitments, or because there is no sun on many days, sensible sun exposure is definitely healthy and helpful for mood and metabolic functions.

Cancer associations/councils in many countries advocate either complete avoidance of sun exposure or covering up with hats, clothing and sunscreen. Many of these associations/councils have instigated fear campaigns encouraging people to avoid the sun altogether and to use sunscreen when outside. And here is the challenge. Many sunscreens are made with chemicals that are more carcinogenic than sunlight. And some are neurotoxic.

Ideally, we will enjoy time in morning sun as often as possible with the least acceptable clothing and no sunscreen. This will enhance our mood, develop vitamin D, balance hormone production, control blood pressure and may, in fact, reduce your risk of melanoma.

If you anticipate being exposed to sunlight above ideal temperatures or for longer than fifteen minutes, wear a hat and long-sleeved shirt/top and use a sunscreen that is organic and does not contain carcinogenic or neurotoxic chemicals. You will need to research sunscreen ingredients in your country to make sure your sunscreen is not poisoning you.

Do not accept that sunscreens produced or sponsored by cancer associations/councils are safe. I have examined several sunscreens branded by a large cancer organisation and found that nearly half the chemicals included are carcinogenic. It seems that profits speak louder than health.

In summary, choose sensible exposure to sunlight and avoid toxic sunscreens.

Deodorants – body odour is not acceptable in many developed societies and we seek to reduce this with antiperspirant deodorants and disguise it with perfumes. Many of these accessory products are neurotoxic.

It is never okay to use an antiperspirant. Our body needs to perspire to cool and eradicate accumulated toxins. When we block perspiration, we may artificially elevate our temperature which, in extreme weather, can lead to serious injury. We also block the elimination of some toxic waste that then accumulates in our body to cause health issues.

Body odour is caused by bacteria that thrive in warm moist

areas like armpits and crotch. Our first line of protection against odour, therefore, is cleanliness. Most have time for only one shower or bath per day, but we may be able to have an "APC" (armpits and crotch) wash sometimes in addition.

Some of us, however, need a deodorant to remain pleasantly fragrant when close to others. Unfortunately, many commercial deodorants contain neurotoxic (and sometimes carcinogenic) chemicals. Probably the best known is aluminium, implicated in the development of Alzheimer's disease. We now know that there are many similar features in the aetiological pathways leading to Alzheimer's and Parkinson's disease, and aluminium is implicated as a neurotoxin. There is some research also showing that constant application of aluminium deodorants under arm is implicated in the development of breast cancer.

Avoid these toxic deodorants even at the risk of displaying body odour. Body odour is better than cancer or Parkinson's disease.

Where we need a deodorant (as I do) there are a number of excellent alternatives available in most countries, and we can select the one that suits our needs and convenience.

- Clean living (food choices and lifestyle) will reduce body odour.
- Avoid polyester and lycra clothing which do not allow your body to breathe normally.
- Use witch hazel (herbal extract) to clean your armpits – this is an astringent to clean the pores.
- Crystal deodorants work well for many people who do not perspire heavily. These are available in many health food stores and alternative shops.
- Essentials oils can be used individually or in combination. They may be combined with a light carrier oil or with an organic grape alcohol (or similar) as a refreshing deodorant. Some of the essential oils suitable for deodorants are

Bergamot FCF, lavender, thyme, Litsea cubeba, juniper berry, cypress, lemongrass, clary sage, and peppermint. There are many recipes for making deodorants available online and I encourage you to be adventurous in caring for yourself. Make sure you purchase only essential oils guaranteed to be 99.9 per cent pure.

- For those lacking time or energy, there are safe and effective deodorants available from health food and specialty stores. Before purchasing, make sure you ask for a complete list of ingredients to make sure it actually is healthy. If the shop assistant can't tell you, take the details and contact the manufacturer directly. Remember, goods are produced to generate profits; it is our responsibility to make sure those products will not harm us.

The strategies for body odour are cleanliness, mitigation of bacteria, avoiding toxic chemicals and using alternatives.

Perfumes – nearly all perfumes contain petrochemicals that are toxic. The most expensive and exclusive tend to be the most engineered and, consequently, the most toxic. However, on special occasions we may want to present a delightful aroma to attract others or simply feel great.

Here are some healthy alternatives to dousing yourself in toxic perfume which, incidentally, will save you money:

- Carry some fresh herbs with you. Pop a few leaves of rosemary, mint, lavender or any other herb you like into your pocket or purse. Every now and then, give them a gentle squeeze to release their natural aroma. You will smell like a fresh garden – delightful!

- Crush some herb leaves and rub on your skin. Test each herb first by applying a tiny amount to your skin to make sure you do not react to the "leaf juice". If you have some fresh herbs growing at your home (in pots if you don't have a garden), you have a continuous supply of personal aroma plus some healthy herbs for your meals.

- Essential oils – a dab or two of your favourite essential oil will give you a delightful aroma. Again, test the oil on the inside of your wrist before applying more liberally. Essential oil aroma will not last as long as expensive perfumes (because they lack some of the nasty chemicals that make the aroma last) but can be applied frequently to refresh the aroma if needed. They may be more effective if applied with an organic carrier oil like almond or avocado.

The strategies for perfumes are to avoid commercial perfumes and use fresh herbs or essential oils.

Tattoos –Tattoos are problematic, not because of any social stigma, but because we deliberately inject potentially toxic substances into the subdermal layer and so increase absorption into the bloodstream and cell structure. Blood and hair tests have shown increased heavy metal concentration in those with a significant tattoo burden.

The best strategy is avoidance. If you are not yet tattooed, don't.

If you already have tattoos, even for many years, be tested for mineral balance and heavy metal pollution, then apply appropriate support and detox strategies as required. This is really important as toxins in tattoo ink can stay in cells for many years and may be neurotoxic, hormone disruptors or interfere with metabolic function.

Tattoo removal can be expensive and not always successful, but is worth discussing with a well-qualified and experienced physician if your heavy metal burden is high. There are inevitable adverse effects such as skin sensitivity, vulnerability to local infection and possible skin colour change. Each tattoo will require several treatments for complete removal and the number of treatments required increases the possibility of adverse effects, so this must be weighed against the adverse effects of heavy metals in the system.

Toxins in our immediate environment

We looked at our frequent encounters with environmental toxins in Chapter 9. Without isolating ourselves on a pristine island far away from Western civilisation, it is impossible to avoid all these toxins, so our task is to reduce exposure as much as possible and mitigate the adverse influence of these toxins.

Employing constant detox strategies will always help. Daily dry skin brushing, warm lemon water, consuming detox teas or green drinks (*not* green tea though), high-dose vitamin C and consistent water intake will all help to remove toxins as we encounter them.

At home, we have many healthier choices than those products promoted on TV and radio. We can create a much healthier environment and support wellness for ourselves and our families.

Cleaning products are sometimes more toxic than the contaminants they claim to remove. One exposure, or even several months of use, may not lead to any obvious damage, but continual use over years means ongoing damage to cell structures.

"Cutting through grease and grime" means using really strong chemicals that can disrupt metabolic functions in humans. Better alternatives are hot water, white vinegar, lemon juice, eucalyptus oil or bicarb.

"Kills 99.9 per cent of germs" means that the chemicals used are able to break open the cell membranes of the bacteria and/ or disrupt the membranes of viruses. Chemicals that can do that can also destroy the membranes of many cells in our body, causing damage to immune function, nervous system, or causing cell damage that may lead to a variety of cancers. Again, hot water, white vinegar, lemon juice and/or eucalyptus oil will remove sufficient bacteria and viruses for safety, while helping us maintain immune integrity to ward of infections and microbial assaults.

Microfibre cleaning cloths are very useful for removing dust with no adverse effects. They attract and hold dust particles then may be shaken outside to release the dust. There are very expensive cloths sold via multilevel marketing, but I have found much cheaper cloths sold in supermarkets to be just as effective for general cleaning in the house and motor vehicles.

Windows can be effectively cleaned without nasty chemicals sprays by using water with the following recipe – 2 litres clean water, ½ teaspoon organic biodegradable dishwashing liquid, one teaspoon methylated spirits. Wash and then squeegee the glass for a lovely shine.

Out-gassing from new furniture and/or *mould* build-up can exacerbate illness symptoms, especially if we are already fragile. Open windows that promote air flow and house plants, such as succulents, can help to alleviate these dangers.

Electromagnetic frequencies are known to adversely affect cell function. While the full effects of EMF are still being explored, there is no doubt that they can and do cause disruption to electrical signalling in the brain and nervous system, so exacerbating neural dysregulation. Radiofrequency electromagnetic field (RF-EMF) waves can be reduced or blocked by a Faraday cage, that is, a box or cage of material that will block and repel EMF. These cages may be made from aluminium foil, fine aluminium mesh or fine copper mesh (such as insect screens on windows).[5]

Faraday cages or screens will not absorb EMF but block and repel them. When attempting to protect yourself from outside radiation, a screen between you and the source will be effective. However, if the source is in your home (e.g. wi-fi modem), you will need to fully enclose the source in a Faraday cage when not in use, as any screening from outside radiation will bounce internal radiation around the space. A box or cage made from aluminium foil will do the job, but make sure the source is standing on a sheet of foil before placing the cage over it, otherwise it can radiate downwards through the shelf and cause EMF challenges.

In our modern society, we cannot eliminate EMF; communication, financial control, education and research rely very heavily on mechanisms driven by EMF – computers, cell phones, measuring devices and many variations on these themes. We can, however, reduce the impact with care.

Some other strategies to avoid toxins include:

- Shop at farmers markets or at small local shopping centres, which are less likely to be polluted with heavy-duty cleaning chemicals than big shopping malls or supermarkets.

- Discuss with your local merchants the type of cleaning products they use and see if they are open to taking a more organic approach.

- Drink plenty of water while travelling on public transport to flush out toxins in the air and to assist your immune system.

- Speak to your local council about any spraying scheduled on streets and in parks that you frequent. See if they are open to taking a more natural approach to pest control (companion planting, encourage natural pest predators, using vinegar instead of pesticide). If not, ask for dates when they will be spraying and avoid that area for a week afterwards.

- Open windows and doors as often as possible to flush out any gases released from furniture, carpets, paints and adhesives used in house construction.

- Fresh air will also reduce dangers from moulds. Dead mould spores can move around in the air, invisible to the naked eye. When inhaled, they may cling to cells and disrupt function.

- Switch off electronic devices when not in use. Televisions, radios, recording devices, computers and modems should be switched off at the power source rather than simply placed into "sleep" or "standby" mode.

- "Smart meters" – that is, electric meters measuring usage and transmitting data to the provider – are constant emitters of EMF and, in many countries, we have no choice but to try and reduce the damage they cause. Build a Faraday cage around three sides of the meter, only leaving the front of the meter accessible to the provider.

- Use aluminium or copper insect screens on windows to reduce EMF impact from outside sources. However, these screens will also bounce your own EMF back into the room, so reduce the emissions in your home at the same time.

- Use house plants to absorb radiation from a specific source or general household emissions. NASA researched cactus and found that these plants were effective at absorbing EMF. Other useful plants include snake plant (Sansevieria trifaciata), other succulents, aloe vera, asparagus fern and other fleshy-leaf plants. They have the added bonus of increasing the oxygen supply in the room. Another advantage of caring for house plants is that they enhance the look and friendliness of the room with variegated leaf colours, different forms, and sometimes flowers.

- Growing organic wheat in trays or pots can also help to absorb radiation while increasing oxygen. Use only organic wheat seed and harvest the grass when it reaches 100-150 mm, then let it regrow. The harvested grass can be juiced and consumed in green smoothies (a useful detox product), fed to domestic chickens (chooks) or other grass-eating pets, or used in compost and mulch. You will be able to harvest the wheat four or five times before needing to replace the seed.

- Store any necessary toxins like paint, mower fuel or motor oil as far from the house as possible, in a secure storage. Only visit that area when absolutely necessary to use that material, wear protective clothing while using them, and drink lots of water before and after.

- Dispose of any empty paint, oil or fuel containers at your nearest toxic garbage site, then shower and drink lots of water.

Eliminating persistent toxins

Some lipid-soluble toxins will lodge inside cells and persist in the body even if we employ all avoidance and self-help detox strategies.

These are materials that are likely to show up in a hair analysis or challenge urine test as being "high in range" or "out of range". They could include arsenic, aluminium, mercury, cadmium, lead, nickel, silver, tin and titanium; there could be others. Copper is a necessary trace mineral but, if in excess can cause health challenges (as in Wilson's disease, for instance). Pesticides and herbicides may also show up as persistent toxins.

Where toxic minerals are persistent, it is important to use gentle but effective strategies to move these out of cells, into the bloodstream, then eliminate them entirely. This can be a delicate operation as many people with Parkinson's are quite fragile and do not respond well to rigorous detoxification programs.

There is no doubt that chelation therapy can be effective at removing lipid soluble heavy metals from the body. This therapy involves ingesting a drug that will bind to the metal and prevent it from binding to other materials in the bloodstream. Theoretically, the liver and other elimination organs are used to remove the toxic metal.

Drugs used (orally or intravenously) include Dimercaptosuccinic acid (DMSA), 2,3-dimercaptopropanesulfonic acid (DMPS), alpha lipoic acid (ALA), ethylenediaminetetraacetic acid (EDTA), and thiamine tetrahydrofurfuryl disulfide (TTFD).

The two main disadvantages of chelation therapy are cost (patients require constant supervision by a suitably qualified healthcare professional to ensure efficient detox and no adverse reactions), and the possibility of severe adverse reactions because of the rigorous nature of the therapy.

Fragile people may react badly to either the drug used (all have some adverse effects) or the extra load of heavy metals being quickly pulled from cells and circulated in the bloodstream while awaiting elimination.

A two-step process of removing heavy metal and other lipid-soluble toxins may be a better choice. Using specific herbs and/ or nutritional supplements while supporting the methylation cycle to remove toxins from cells, then binding them in the bloodstream with a low-reactive material to facilitate elimination is often easier for patients to tolerate and, while slower than chelation, is as effective in the long term. Another advantage is that this protocol can be used with minimal supervision and is otherwise less costly than chelation.

It is important to support the methylation cycle with folate (5-formyltetrahydrofolate or 5-methyltetrahydrofolate) and other B group vitamins in their activated forms. Vitamin C and magnesium are also important in this protocol.

"Cell cleaning" formulas are usually powders, either taken in water or as capsules, that will include some or all of the following: broccoli sprout powder, organic barley grass, coriander, Organic cracked-cell Chlorella, spirulina, milk thistle (Silybum marianum), Schisandra (S. chinensis), rosemary (Rosmarinus officinalis), Cleavers (Galium aparine), globe artichoke (Cynara scolymus), Lipoic acid, glutamine, Trimethylglycine (TMG),

Methylsulfonylmethane (MSM), calcium glucarate, Taurine, cysteine, zinc citrate.

The formulas will vary from product to product, but will include "greens" and supplements that will render lipid-soluble toxins water-soluble for the purpose of removing them from cells into the bloodstream.

The critical element in this process is to stop any toxins from re-entering cells or circulating in the bloodstream for too long and causing illness symptoms. There are a variety of clays (e.g. "diatomaceous earth") and herbs. One of the most efficient binders is Modified Activated Clinoptilolite (MAC), which is a highly refined form of zeolite. MAC has been cleaned to remove any potential toxins, heat treated to eliminate any possible microbes and presented as powder or capsules.

MAC is not considered a nutritional supplement as it cannot enter the bloodstream, staying within the gut. Its negative polarity attracts positively-charged metals and toxins flowing past the gut in the bloodstream like a magnet. Toxins exit the bloodstream and bind to the MAC, enabling elimination via the bowel and bladder. Powdered MAC is used to clear the small intestine (as in small intestine bacterial overgrowth [SIBO], for instance) while the capsules are created to open only low in the digestive tract, removing toxins from the hepatic blood system, relieving stress from the liver, and aiding elimination.

This system of clearing cells then binding and eliminating toxins can be modified to best suit the health/robustness of each person. Those with high strength and resilience can detox quite quickly, while those who are more fragile can slow the process down to allow their organ systems to cope with the extra load without creating more illness symptoms. It is possible to take holidays from the process if people feel overwhelmed. Some practitioners advise using this type of protocol for three months, then stopping for one month while maintaining strategies of avoidance and general detoxification. Then repeat the protocol as often as necessary to remove all toxic minerals.

A hair mineral analysis from a reputable laboratory can be a useful guide to progress and not expensive.

Detoxing and removal of heavy metals is vital to recovery, but must be approached in ways best suited to each individual.

Active detoxification – self-help strategies

Warm lemon water before meals. This simple activity stimulates production of hydrochloric acid in our stomach (needed for protein digestion and systemic alkalising), and a variety of digestive enzymes in our gut. It can contribute to improved bowel function as well. This strategy also invigorates liver and gall bladder activity. Use a minimum of half a lemon in a small glass of water. A stronger mix is even more effective.

At least 2 litres of "clean" water daily. Dehydration is the enemy of wellness. Drinking adequate water daily flushes our system, hydrates tissues and organs, softens stools and assists with bowel function. We need at least two (preferably three) good bowel evacuations daily for good health.

Chia seeds. Soak in water overnight (or at least eight hours) and add some lemon juice in the morning before drinking. Chia seeds must be soaked for eight hours to be effective. They will bulk up and hydrate stools and assist bowel function without the adverse effects of harsh laxatives. Chia seeds are also a good source of protein, omega 3 fatty acids (anti-inflammatory) and a number of trace minerals. They bind gut toxins (including heavy metals) and can mitigate "Herxheimer" reactions.

Dry skin brushing. Use a natural bristle brush only. Always skin brush before showering or bathing or before bed. Start at the periphery (hands/feet) and brush firmly in small circular motions moving towards the heart. Brush your thorax and back towards the heart as well (it's great if you have a partner to brush your back). Brushing removes dead skin and superficial toxins, stimulates blood and lymph flow, and makes you feel great.

Epsom salts (magnesium sulphate) baths and foot baths. Put two tablespoons in a basin with comfortably warm (not hot water) and soak your feet for twenty minutes. Or put two cups of Epsom salts in your bath (again, comfortably warm, not hot) and soak luxuriously for fifteen to twenty minutes. The Epsom salts will draw toxins out through our skin. However, if we soak for too long, we start to reabsorb the toxins floating in the water. If the water is too hot for immediate comfort, it can affect fascia function and reduce our detoxing efficiency. We must rinse off our feet after foot baths or our whole body after baths using fresh water (warm or cold) to remove any toxins left on the skin.

Oil pulling. To oil pull, slowly swish your choice of unrefined, high-quality organic oil in your mouth (similar to the way you would use a mouthwash only slower) for five to twenty minutes. The process attracts and removes bacteria, toxins and parasites that live in your mouth or lymph system, and also pulls congestion and mucus from your throat and loosens up your sinuses. With the help of your saliva, toxins and microbes bind with the oil, ready to be disposed of. Pulling also helps re-mineralise your teeth and strengthen your gums by thoroughly cleansing the area.

Coconut oil is probably the best to use because it has antimicrobial, anti-inflammatory, and enzymatic properties. This provides the added benefit of killing unwanted bacteria that may be residing in the mouth, while leaving behind healthy probiotic strains.

To start, scoop half to one full teaspoon of coconut oil into the mouth; if it's cold, allow the oil to melt. Now push, swirl, and pull the oil between your teeth, around your gums, and allow it to touch every part of your mouth except your throat. You don't want the oil getting in contact with your throat because it's now carrying toxic material. No gargling!

Stay calm, practise deep breathing through your nose, move quietly through other morning duties. Make this a morning ritual several times each week and enjoy the feeling of cleansing and the relaxation with the absence of talking. Or use bath time to oil pull – multitasking at its best. Some oil pull while showering but, remember, coconut oil must be disposed of in the trash not down the drain.

Once your time of oil pulling is over, spit into the trash, but never the sink — the oil could solidify and clog your drain. Now rinse your mouth out with clean water two or three times. Finally, drink a glass of water and relax. You should be feeling fresh and rejuvenated.

As an added bonus, coconut oil pulling may help remineralise your teeth while removing plaque.

Hydrogen peroxide pulling – this is done in exactly the same way as oil pulling and gives some of the same benefit and some different benefits. Peroxide will kill microbes, remove tooth plaque and really cleanse your mouth. Use 3 per cent or 6 per cent hydrogen peroxide (readily available from pharmacies). Put one capful/one teaspoonful into your mouth and swish around. It will foam and bubble. You can spit into the sink as the peroxide will not clog the drain. Rinse your mouth several times with water and enjoy the lovely, squeaky-clean feeling and the knowledge that many pathogens have just died.

Far/near infrared saunas (with caution). Correctly constructed infrared saunas use panels that remain cool while heating the body. Other saunas heat the air within the sauna enclosure. Theoretically (as yet unproven), increased sweating removes more toxins from the body. We must be very careful, however, not to overheat the body, as this can reduce the effectiveness of fascia function and, over time, cause serious inhibition to health. *Five to ten minutes* in a properly constructed far/near infrared sauna *twice weekly* is probably as much as is healthy.

Sauna time must be followed with a *cold* shower.

General detox

Vitamin C: High dose (10,000 – 30,000 mg daily) enhances immune activity, improves bowel function and reduces inflammation. Vitamin C deficiency is one of the two most common deficiencies in the Western world[6,7] (the other being dehydration from refusing to drink water). Our hunter/gatherer ancestors gained *20,000 to 50,000 mg of* vitamin C daily from their food and may have been able to synthesise ascorbic acid in the same way as most animals.[8] We gain up to 200 mg with an excellent diet (only one-hundredth of the minimum our healthy ancestors consumed). Supplementing to bowel tolerance (when your bowel movements become loose) will assist in killing pathogens via immune function, act as a powerful antioxidant, enhance production of glutathione and coenzyme Q10, and increase bowel function to remove toxins.

Use a good quality vitamin C powder that has three or more mineral ascorbates plus bioflavonoids, and start with half a teaspoon twice daily. Increase by a quarter teaspoon each three to seven days to bowel tolerance, then maintain an intake just below bowel tolerance each day.

Vitamin C supplementation may reduce your requirement for other, more expensive, supplements while enhancing your detoxing program.

Magnesium powder: Improves bowel function and reduces inflammation. Magnesium is often deficient in debilitated people because of the stress of illness and poor dietary habits. Magnesium powder can be taken with vitamin C powder to enhance bowel function, reduce muscle tension and mitigate inflammation. Magnesium citrate is the most researched form of magnesium, but there are other excellent powders available that contain a mix of magnesium forms, or magnesium threonate that is showing promise in neuro dysregulation.[9] If one of your symptoms is chronic or frequent headaches, magnesium citrate is probably the best form unless otherwise advised by your health practitioner.

BioPractica Matrix Phase Detox: Assists with phases I, II and III detox pathways. It may be taken alone or with other powders at one level to heaped teaspoon daily, or in divided doses twice daily. It is particularly useful where constipation is a continuing challenge. This product is made in Australia so may not be available in other countries; if not, find an organic product that has similar ingredients to those shown below.

Serving size approximately one heaped teaspoon.

- Trimethylglycien (TMG) 300 mg
- Methylsulfonylmethane (MSM) 100 mg
- Calcium glucarate 100 mg
- Taurine 60 mg
- Cysteine 50 mg
- Vitamin C (Ascorbic acid) 80 mg
- Magnesium (as citrate) 50 mg
- Zinc (as citrate) 5 mg
- Broccoli sprout powder 100 mg
- Organic barley grass 883 mg
- Coriander 50 mg
- Organic cracked Chlorella 100 mg
- Spirulina 643 mg
- Milk thistle (Silybum marianum) 500 mg
- Schisandra (S. chinensis) 200 mg
- Rosemary (Rosmarinus officinalis) 50 mg
- Cleavers (Galium aparine) 80 mg
- Globe artichoke (Cynara scolymus) 80 mg
- Apple pectin 320 mg

Modified Activated Clinoptilolite (MAC) (Froximun ToxaPrevent Pure): Clinoptilolite is a natural zeolite comprising a microporous arrangement of silica and alumina tetrahedra. It has the complex formula: $(Na,K,Ca)_{2-3}Al_3(Al,Si)_2Si_{13}O_{36}\cdot 12H_2O$. It forms as white to reddish tabular monoclinic tectosilicate crystals with a Mohs hardness of 3.5 to 4 and a specific gravity of 2.1 to 2.2. Zeolites have been used for many years with, sometimes exaggerated, claims of amazing detoxification properties and miraculous "cures". Froximun have modified zeolite with a refining and heat process to develop what is essentially a medical device as the product never enters the bloodstream.

MAC has a negative polarity so attracts toxins with a positive polarity as they pass through the vascular system surrounding the GIT. Once toxins have been pulled into the gut, MAC binds to it and assists elimination.

Heel Galium-Heel: Assists in removing toxins from within cells and boosts immune function. Use at very low dose if ill. Start at one drop per day only in one litre+ of water and move upwards very slowly. Galium Heel is a very powerful remedy and may cause some aggravation in very sensitive people. It can be diluted successfully using K dilutions (Chapter 26) and still be effective. Available in most countries.

Heel Detox Kit: Three remedies that enhance elimination and detoxification via liver, kidneys and lymph. Again, use at very low dose if unwell. Start one remedy at one drop per day and move very slowly upwards. A low-dose protocol is included as Appendix 2.

Aqua Hydration Formulas: By increasing cell hydration via the HPA axis, the Aquas can assist all detox protocols, as well as improve absorption of food, supplements and medications. Use at very low doses (one to three drops daily as opposed to the recommended dose). See Appendix 3 for details.

Medicine Tree Organo LiverGall Tone: Supports liver and gall bladder function. This homeopathic spray can be successfully used at doses much lower than recommended by the manufacturer and is sprayed directly under the tongue. Made in Australia.

Colonic Irrigation/Hydrotherapy: May assist in clearing impacted faecal matter from the colon and improving overall bowel function. Two or three treatments one week apart will give a good clean out. Monthly treatments for maintenance are useful.

Bowen therapy (discussed in Chapter 21) may improve elimination via fascia, lymph, kidneys and bowel. Find a Bowen therapist who works gently and gives plenty of time for each treatment.

Lymph Drainage Massage: Improves elimination via lymph. This specialist massage technique requires lengthy training. Make sure you choose a practitioner who is appropriately qualified.

We live in a very toxic world, primarily made so by the unfettered efforts of mankind to create financial profit or power. Most toxins we encounter will not, by themselves with one encounter, cause great damage, but repeated and/or continued contact with toxic substances, gases and EMF will cause damage over time and inhibit our health.

CHAPTER 26

REVERSING THE INFECTION PATHWAY

What infections?

Infections that may be misdiagnosed as other chronic disorders (including Parkinson's disease) or psychosomatic disorders include Borrelia species, Bartonella and many "co-infections". These may be called Lyme disease or Multisystemic Infectious Diseases Syndrome (MSIDS).

Diagnosis

The vast majority of MSIDS/Lyme patients have been misdiagnosed and mistreated for so long that their disease has become chronic and disseminated through their system. The first point of diagnosis is usually a clinic where an aware practitioner starts to put the pieces of their patient's health puzzle together, and suspects Lyme and/or co-infections; or patients, tired of vague diagnosis or practitioners/specialists who will not entertain any but the most limited diagnosis (e.g. Parkinson's disease), start to explore other explanations for their symptoms. Patients often find their first information from friends or online where chronic infections and their ability to mimic other chronic disorders are discussed.

Patients have usually been unwell for a long time and may have been diagnosed with any of a wide variety of chronic disorders, or not diagnosed and told to seek counselling. "It's all in your head" is a common "diagnosis" by ignorant and arrogant healthcare practitioners. Patients may have been treated for multiple sclerosis (MS), Multiple System Atrophy (MSA), chronic fatigue syndrome (CFS), adrenal exhaustion, thyroid dysfunction, hormone imbalances – or not treated at all. Many have been diagnosed with Parkinson's disease (and/or "atypical Parkinson's disease") and treated with Parkinson's disease medication for a few to many years.[1,2,3]

There are no standard blood tests or scans anywhere in the world that will identify Lyme disease or co-infections with certainty. A number of pathology laboratories are working hard to develop an accurate Borrelia test, but serological testing is still problematic. There are very few testing laboratories in the world that can test for these infections with even reasonable surety. In fact, the best Lyme disease testing laboratories – Igenex in USA, Armin Labs and Infectolab in Germany, Australian Biologics in Australia – can only guarantee between 50 per cent and 70 per cent accuracy, and all include a waiver in their reports encouraging practitioners to use their clinical skills to identify specific infections and use laboratory testing as confirmation only.

The most accurate diagnostic techniques at this stage (2019) are:

- clinical diagnosis by an experience practitioner
- challenge testing (see below).

In short, if practitioners want to help "Lymies" and/or identify the aetiological pathways for those diagnosed with Parkinson's disease, we must become familiar with symptom patterns, and keep our "Lyme Eyes" open all the time.

The symptom pictures below are "bare bones" only as these infections can mimic many other disorders, and each patient will have an individual set of symptoms dependant on health history, predominant infection, co-infections and other comorbidities. The list may help practitioners assess the need for further investigation or referral.

I have listed only the major infections that I see in my clinic. Patients may show symptoms of other co-infections or opportunistic infections that develop because of their compromised immune system.

Symptom pictures

Borrelia (spirochetal bacteria that can exist as spirochete, L-form and cyst).

- Symptoms come on gradually and may not seem related to an obvious cause.
- Only around 30-40 per cent of patients remember or display a rash. The definitive erythema migrans (bulls-eye rash) is a definite sign of Borrelia and may be seen shortly after initial infection/bite, but may appear weeks or months after initial infection;
- The majority of patients *do not* remember a tick bite or serious event before symptoms appear;
- There are many vectors including ticks of various species, mosquitoes, flies and other sanguinivorous creatures;
- Can affect many systems – joints, muscles, cognition, cardiac function;
- Can cause short-term memory loss, poor judgement, loss of ability to solve complex problems;
- May display four-week cycles of symptoms.

Symptoms may include:
- Great fatigue that may get worse in the afternoon, great lethargy
- disturbed vision with loss of acuity, photophobia, floaters, drooping lids
- headaches with stiff neck
- hyperacuity of hearing with pain from sound and tinnitus

- depression, irritability, rage, sadness
- cramps, spasms, weakness or partial paralysis of limbs
- unexplained fevers, sweats, chills, or flushing
- unexplained hair loss
- unexplained menstrual irregularity
- change in bowel function: constipation, diarrhoea
- shortness of breath, cough
- heart palpitations, pulse skips, heart block
- joint pain or swelling
- muscle pain or cramps
- twitching of the face or other muscles
- difficulty with speech or writing
- mood swings, irritability, depression
- disturbed sleep; too much, too little, early awakening.

Borrelia key symptoms:
- arthritic type symptoms with malaise, great fatigue and low mood
- neuro symptoms often mimicking MS, Parkinson's or MND/ALS
- stiffness, paucity of movement, word loss, poor memory with or without dull, persistent pain.

Bartonella (gram negative bacteria that are intracellular parasites generally showing preference for erythrocytes and endothelial cells in humans). Symptoms may include:

- fatigue, restlessness, combative behaviour, anger, rage, suicidal ideation
- myalgias, malaise
- sharp stabbing or burning pain anywhere but often in the feet and/or lower legs – pain may "shoot" from heel to knee
- burning or painful soles of feet; sensation as if walking on glass, stones or hot coals

- sensation as if feet are being crushed or "exploded" outwards
- liver and/or spleen involvement, abdominal pain
- infectious mononucleosis-like syndrome
- conjunctivitis, Bartonella neuroretinitis, loss of vision, flame-shaped haemorrhages, branch retinal artery occlusion with vision loss, cotton wool exudates
- osteomyelitis, myositis, osteolytic lesions (softening of bone), myelitis, radiculitis, transverse myelitis, arthritis, chronic demyelinating polyneuropathy
- endocarditis, cardiomegaly

Other symptoms:

- biopsies of lymph nodes reveal pathology often indistin-guishable from sarcoidosis;
- encephalopathy may occur one to six weeks after the initial infection;
- headaches, cognitive dysfunction, and CNS lesions may be evident;
- rash and lymphadenitis: erythematous papules (red splotches or slightly raised red spots) may develop. Such papules occasionally occur on the lower limbs but are more common on the upper limbs, the head, and neck. The papules may appear on the skin or mucous membranes. Bartonella may also cause subcutaneous nodules, with some bone involvement possible. The nodules may show some hyperpigmentation, be tender, fester, and/or be enlarged or swollen, but not always; unexplained "stretch marks" that may be red/purple in colour and look as if an animal has scratched the skin, but there is no broken skin, hence the common name of "cat scratch fever".

Dr Joseph Burrascano (a leading world authority on Lyme disease and co-infections) suspects Bartonellosis when neurologic symptoms are out of proportion to the other systemic symptoms of chronic Lyme.

Bartonella key symptoms:

° Sharp, burning pains anywhere – may move around body
° Painful soles of feet, especially burning pain
° Shooting or electric pain through feet and lower legs
° Pain and restriction in one or both shoulders, usually with neck involvement
° "Stretch marks" unexplained
° Anger, rage and/or suicidal ideation with depression
° Almost uncontrollable urges to harm themselves or others, even those they love.

Babesia (protozoa similar to malaria – lives within cells).

Symptoms include:

- fatigue
- arthralgias, myalgia, neck and back stiffness
- drenching sweats, night sweats
- headaches – like a vice
- emotional lability, depression
- dizziness, feeling of imbalance
- nausea and vomiting, reduced appetite
- cough, dry and chronic
- dyspnoea, air hunger, shortness of breath
- severe chest wall pain, sharp stabbing pain
- fever, chills
- malaise
- bleeding tendencies, bruising
- symptoms flare every four to six days
- disruptive sleep
- tachycardia, severe low BP, heart problems, pressure around heart.

***Babesia* key symptoms:**
- ○ air hunger
- ○ dry, unproductive cough
- ○ drenching night sweats (whole body; may need to change clothes/sheets more than once during night).

Chlamydia pneumoniae (obligate intracellular gram-negative bacterium).

Description of symptoms:
- spectrum of illness may vary from mild and self-limited to severe pneumonia;
- onset is often gradual with delayed presentation;
- sore throat and hoarseness may precede cough by a week or more, giving biphasic appearance to illness (uncommon in *Legionella*, less common in *mycoplasma, Streptococcus pneumoniae*, and *Haemophilus influenzae*)

Other symptoms:
- dry cough, dryness of the mucous membranes of the mouth, nose, eyes, itching of the ears, irritation of the urinary tract and the rectum
- low grade fever (usually early in illness)
- chills
- rhinitis, sinus congestion
- headache
- malaise
- myalgias
- pain in the tendons, frequent localisation: upper arms, heels (Achilles tendon), soles of feet
- "burning" in the stomach area (sometimes dull pain), bloating
- nausea
- altered mental status.

Mycoplasma (a mollicute genus of bacteria lacking a cell wall around their cell membranes. This can make them naturally resistant to many common antibiotics such as penicillin or other beta-lactam antibiotics that target cell wall synthesis. They can be parasitic or saprotrophic.)

- there are at least five species of Mycoplasma infectious to humans;
- mycoplasma infections may be "coinfections" in patients diagnosed with Parkinson's disease or other neurodegenerative disorders;
- symptoms may include mild pneumonia or genital irritation;
- serology testing is quite accurate;
- mycoplasma are resistant to many antibiotics but can be successfully treated with appropriate herbal formulas.

Other co/opportunistic infections may include Ehrlichia, Anaplasma, Rickettsias, Epstein-Barr virus, Ross River fever, Q fever and system-wide Candida.

Dr Richard Horowitz has included a most useful questionnaire in his book *Why Can't I Get Better?* (St. Martin's Press, New York). He has given permission for all readers to use it as a clinical diagnostic tool or for self-assessment.[4]

Challenge test diagnosis

This is considered by some Lyme Literate Medical Doctors (LLMDs) to be the most accurate diagnostic technique for chronic Lyme disease and co-infections.

Theoretically, if we begin to kill the infectious agent without appropriate detoxification protocols in place, our patient will "herx" (develop a Jarisch-Herxheimer reaction) because of excessive endotoxin release.

Therefore, if we choose a specifically aimed antimicrobial (herbal or antibiotic), prescribe at a low dose, then titrate each

3-4 days, and our patient develops a Herxheimer reaction, we have proven the existence of that infectious agent.

In clinical practice, a positive challenge test has often been confirmed by blood tests when taken. We sometimes forgo the cost of blood tests if the challenge test result is very positive.

Procedure

1. A thorough clinical assessment is vital to identify pathogenic suspects. Compare your patient's symptom picture with the descriptions given earlier or the symptom charts noted. *Test on the basis of the predominant symptom picture.*

2. Choose a specific antimicrobial for the suspected infectious agent. I use Byron White Formulas – A-L for Borrelia, A-Bart for Bartonella, A-Bab for Babesia. There are other herbal formulas available.

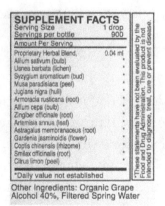
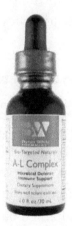

3. Prescribe starting at low dose and titrate each 3-4 days until a mild herx is displayed. I start at one drop daily and increase by one drop each 3-4 days.

4. Your patient makes NO OTHER CHANGES during this test.

5. Once a herx is displayed, confirm by symptom picture that it is the suspected pathogen, stop the remedy and allow 2-5 days wash-out period using some of the detox protocols described later (especially soaked chia seeds, lemon water and Epsom salts baths).

6. Then institute detox protocols, immune support remedies, antimicrobials and proceed with your healing program.

Once a chronic infection has been identified, it MUST be treated. It is critical that thorough detox protocols are developed and adhered to in order to recover with the minimum of distress (see below).

Does the diagnosis of a chronic infection mean that the patient does not have Parkinson's disease? No; it does mean, however, that we have identified one of the aetiological pathways that resulted in Parkinson's disease symptoms, so giving an opportunity to reverse that aetiological pathway and open the way to remove symptoms caused by or exacerbated by that infection.

Detox, detox, detox

"It has been said that the longer one is ill with Lyme, the more neurotoxin is present in the body. It probably is stored in fatty tissues, and once present, persists for a very long time. This may be because of enterohepatic circulation, where the toxin is excreted via the bile into the intestinal tract, but then is reabsorbed from the intestinal tract back into the bloodstream." – Dr Joseph Burrascano, Jr. MD, *Advanced Topics in Lyme Disease: Diagnostic Hints and Treatment Guidelines for Lyme and Other Tick Borne Illnesses*, sixteenth edition, copyright October, 2008.

Neurotoxins and cytokines are what largely make people feel sick. It is not necessarily the microbes themselves, as we live in symbiosis with many different microorganisms in our bodies at all times. It is when the microorganisms produce neurotoxins and cytokines in elevated amounts that patients manifest with "sickness behavior" such as fatigue, arthralgias, flu-like symptoms, and cognitive issues often seen in those with MSIDS. – Dr Richard Horowitz.[5]

Comprehensive detoxification programs are vital if we are to truly regain wellness. When infected with Lyme or co-infections, we have already been burdened with a heavy load of modern civilisation toxins – petrochemicals, herbicides, pesticides, preservatives and other food additives, plastics, and many other immunosuppressive and neurotoxic chemicals that are hidden in our modern environment.

As soon as we begin attacking the infectious pathogens, a variety of endo/exotoxins are released into the bloodstream and it often seems that we become sicker with treatment. Within the Lyme "community", this is described as a Jarisch-Herxheimer reaction, or herx.

In order to maximise immune function, optimise antimicrobial activity, and maintain a reasonable level of wellness during recovery, every patient with Lyme and/or co-infections MUST be active in removing toxins from their body and environment every day.

Environmental detox

We are exposed to chemicals every day: in the air we breathe, the food we eat, products we put on our body, cleaning products, products we use in the garden, the cars that we drive and other forms of transport. Chemicals are not intrinsically bad for us; in fact, our bodies are made up of millions of different chemicals. However, humans have managed to create hundreds of thousands of synthetic chemicals, and often use heavy metals that we need to avoid in our day-to-day lives. Some neurologists estimate that we may contact over 500,000 neurotoxic man-made chemicals during our daily routines.

We must be active in removing toxins from our homes, workplaces and personal use products if we are to live well.

For more details, see Chapter 25 on "Reversing the Toxin Pathway", and "Low-Toxicity Living" – Appendix 1.

Personal detox

"Clean diet": Free from gluten/grains, dairy (cows, sheep and goats), refined sugar, caffeine, aspartame, additives. We should eat lots of fresh vegetables and living food, plus lots of parsley and coriander.

Our diet can be a source of toxins (and probably has been for most of our lives) because of Western eating habits (grain, dairy, sweeteners, colours, sugar, caffeine, etc.), and thousands of preservatives, emulsifiers, excipients, colours, flavours and modified particles added to foods. Even "fresh" foods often contain chemicals used in production that are considered "safe" but can cause real health challenges while accumulating in our body.

In Chapter 25, we discussed many ways to help remove toxic waste from your body. Removal of toxins is always critical to good health, but even more important when we begin killing pathogens which will dump endotoxins into our system as they die. We need to kill the pathogens, but MUST, be assiduous in removing their waste products.

Read Chapter 25 again and adopt all those strategies before proceeding further with antimicrobial activity, or talk to your skilled healthcare professional about a detox program suitable just for you.

Specific detox

Note: Byron White Formulas were stocked and retailed in Australia until late 2018. They are now available to Australian patients via VitaHealth in New York. Patients in USA and other countries should contact Byron White Formulas direct at http://www.byronwhiteformulas.com/

Byron White Formulas (BWF) Detox formulas are designed to work via all elimination pathways; they support the immune system, reduce inflammation, mitigate Herxheimer reactions and maintain an efficient healing pathway.

Byron White Formulas are manufactured in USA and available only on prescription from a qualified healthcare practitioner. A list of BWF practitioners in USA is available on their website (www.byronwhiteformulas.com) but you may need to contact them directly for details of availability in your country. In Australia, they are currently (2019) available via New York using a special order form from your registered practitioner. Byron White Formulas can provide those specific order forms for Australian practitioners.

While there can be difficulties in obtaining appropriate Byron White Formulas, they are worth the effort as the benefits gained from appropriate use are beyond other formulas and/or antibiotics tried to date.

When using antimicrobials (antibiotics or herbals), it is vital to support the body in its ability to release, bind and eliminate toxins, at all levels or layers of the body. BWF Detox formulas can support detoxing in any protocol. They all have the ability to bind and detoxify.

Whole body detox

BWF Detox 1 (drops) is comprised of 17 herbs that have been historically shown to gently support all the detox systems in the body as well as help detox and bind to many of the common toxins found in chronic Lyme and other chronic illness.

Gastrointestinal and neurotoxin detox

BWF Detox 2 (powder) is a companion formula for Detox 1, designed to help bind to toxins in the GI system. It utilises two assayed French clays that have a sieve rating of 325, very fine. It can capture and bind to thousands of toxins, among them mould and fungal and neurotoxins, preventing them from recirculating. It also has activated willow charcoal and many herbs to help further bind, detox and support the GI system.

Soaked Chia seeds and Modified Activated Clinoptilolite are good alternatives.

Lymph and biotoxin detox

BWF BT-Detox (drops) is a bio toxin detox formula that helps with removing bio toxins, biofilm toxins, neuro toxins, chemicals, ammonia and aldehydes. It is especially designed to help with the lymph system's removal of toxins and is suggested whenever there is lymph congestion. Used at very low dose.

Neurological and tissue detox

BWF NT-Detox (drops) utilises 24 herbs and is designed to bind and remove neurotoxins (resulting from cell apoptosis) from the tissues and neurologic systems. This formula helps to draw toxins from the kidneys, lymph, tissues, liver and neurological system, supports the liver and elimination systems. It uses herbs that have historical benefit against gram positive and negative bacteria, viruses, mycoplasma, Borrelia, Babesia, fungi and Bartonella, and helps to remove toxins associated with these pathogens. *This is a prime detox remedy where the dominant symptoms are neurological. Use at low dose only – up to 5 drops twice daily.*

Radiation and environmental detox

BWF Envi-Rad (drops): Radiation can prevent the body from dealing with pathogens and healing. The Envi-Rad detox formula was created out of the need to help the body decrease environmental and radiation toxicity. The environmental toxicity and radiation load that we are being exposed to has increased dramatically over the past 60 years, and strongly affects the body's ability to heal itself and deal with pathogens. Before creating the formula, practitioners took water and air samples from various parts of the United States in a combined effort. The information BWF obtained was used to help target the toxins found, including various forms of radiation, petrochemicals, lead, heavy metals, pesticides, herbicides, solvents and other environmental chemicals.

How to use Byron White Detox Formulas

Note: *BWF Detox Formulas are appropriate for use in conjunction with any form of antimicrobial – antibiotics, BWF antimicrobial formulas or other herbal antimicrobials.*

The appropriate BWF Detox Formula is chosen by observing the dominant symptoms for each patient. Dosage should be adjusted to ensure clearance of toxins in line with microbial die off and endotoxin load.

Patients are unlikely to herx on Detox Formulas but can develop sensitivity reactions such as loose bowels/diarrhoea, stomach ache, or vague feelings of unwellness. Reducing the dose by one drop (or 1/8 teaspoon for powder) will alleviate these reactions.

In general, I have started by killing microbes in the morning and detoxing in the afternoon. This may be varied to suit your patients' particular antimicrobial protocols. However, the principle is to create cell death, then clear out the resultant endotoxins.

Anti microbials

For Lyme disease and co-infections

The International Lyme and Associated Diseases Society (ILADS) published their "Evidence-based guidelines for the management of Lyme disease" in 2004. Their firm recommendation is vigorous antibiotic treatment over an extended period of time. ILADS guidelines are available for free download from http://www.ilads.org/files/ILADS_Guidelines.pdf

Antibiotics are a valid and often effective choice for those resilient enough to withstand the rigors of two to ten years continuous antibiotic use. Antibiotics are particularly effective for acute early Lyme disease, that is, within a few weeks of infection. Three to six months of heavy-duty antibiotics may resolve the infectious effects of Lyme or a co-infection, but will not make you or your patient well.

During and after antibiotic treatments, detoxification is critical, while vigorous support of gut function, liver and other organs must be maintained. High-quality vitamin C supplements, plus probiotics and immune support may ensure that patients do not relapse after antibiotic treatment or suffer from post-antibiotic malaise.

The aim here is to provide alternatives to antibiotics and/or remedies that may be used in conjunction with antibiotics. Each practitioner may choose a different approach for each patient, depending on stage of disease, resilience, patient compliance and response; some patients have definite ideas about how they wish to be treated. For instance, I have seen several patients who absolutely refused to consider antibiotics, even in conjunction with herbals and immune/gut support. They were only willing to use herbal antimicrobials with detox protocols. Those who were dedicated to wellness did very well and many are now free from symptoms (and no longer need herbals or medication).

The list of remedies below is not exhaustive, but I have focused on those I have used in my clinic and are reasonable in cost. Some are made in Australia and may be unavailable in other countries, while others are available world-wide.

Other alternatives are available for private import and from compounding chemists. Private import remedies lack supervision and evidence (unless, like BWF, they are prescribed by an experienced practitioner), while those prepared by compounding chemists tend to be very expensive and not necessarily any more effective than those remedies available "off the shelf". In general terms, most herbals, homeopathics and supplements provided by a qualified healthcare professional tend to be more effective and of higher quality than over the counter products.

Herbals

Antimicrobial herbs have been used successfully for centuries. Herbals are generally best used in combination to achieve an optimal state of health. Herbal antimicrobials may be selected from immune support herbs, antimicrobials and synergistic herbs. In each case, clinical experience and patient presentation will guide the choice of effective herbal combinations.

Immune support is vital when treating any chronic disease. Therefore immune support herbs are a first line treatment, once effective detox protocols have been established. Immune support herbs include Andrographis, Astragalus, Baptisia, Boneset, Cat's Claw, Echinacea, Elderberry, Pau d'Arco, Reishi and Rhodiola.

Antimicrobial herbs may be selected for general, system-wide activity, or more focused activity for particular organ systems or microbial identification. Antimicrobial herbs may be specific for antibacterial, anti-viral or anti-parasitic activity. The first two are useful against Borrelia species ("Lyme"), Bartonella and other bacterial/viral co-infections, while the third class is useful against Babesia and similar protozoa. Some herbs are effective against all microbes, reducing the number of herbs required for treatment.

Antibacterial/viral: Barberry, Elderberry, Elecampane, Garlic, Golden Seal, Lomatium, Myrrh, Oregano, Pau d'Arco, Pelargonium, Propolis, Thuja and Thyme.

Anti-parasitic: Barberry, Euphorbia, Garlic, Pau d'Arco, Propolis and Wormwood.

Homeopathics

Homeopathic remedies are very useful for immune support, particularly when patients are debilitated and fragile. While homeopathic remedies may not have the immediate impact of some herbals, they function to enhance natural body function, so benefits are long lasting.

Homeopathic Simplexes: May be used in conjunction with all other healing activities, even though Classical Homeopathic Training says that we should use only one remedy in isolation from other medicines. My experience has shown that, in fact, a wide range of dietary and lifestyle changes, plus sympathetic prescription of supplements, herbals and homeopathic complexes may enhance the effectiveness of a well-chosen simplex. Prescribing homeopathic simplexes requires great skill after many years of training and experience.

Homeopathic Complexes: May be useful to enhance antimicrobial activity and immune function. Some of my favourites are:

Heel Engystol – 1 tablet one to three times daily away from food. For general immune enhancement.

Galium Heel – 1 to 20 drops in water daily.

Heel Lymphomyosot – 1 to 15 drops in water daily. Useful where lymph stasis and edema is a challenge.

Heel Ubichinon compositum – 1 tablet one to three times daily for general immune enhancement.

Heel Metabolic Kit – a combination of Coenzyme compositum and Ubichinon compositum.

Other remedies

High-dose vitamin C is a must, in my opinion. As well as supporting the immune system and assisting detoxification, it may act as an antimicrobial and anti-inflammatory. High-dose vitamin C is also an effective antioxidant, especially for brain and nervous system.

Byron White Formulas

"Many of my Chronic Lyme disease patients relapse once they are taken off antibiotics, so herbal protocols are essential for them to maintain a sense of wellness. I have used the Byron White Formulas with well over a thousand patients over the past several years. They are an excellent option because of the wide range of treatment options they offer for Lyme disease and coinfections, as well as their superior efficacy and purity. I highly recommend using

them in an integrated treatment approach."

– Dr Richard Horowitz, MD, Hyde Park, NY

Byron White Formulas are used by many LLMDs and Lyme-aware doctors in USA and Australia. They are effective as standalone therapies or in combination with antibiotics or other antimicrobials.

Useful information is available at www.byronwhiteformulas.com If you are qualified to sign up as a practitioner, you can access webinars and other practitioner-only information.

Common BWF antimicrobials used in clinical practice include A-L Complex for Borrelia infections, A-Bab for Babesia, A-Bart for Bartonella, A-EB/H6 for all species of herpes, A-Myco for a wide range of mycoplasma infections, A-CPn for Chlamydia pneumoniae, and A-P Complex for many parasitic infections. A-FNG is particularly useful for biotoxins.

Biofilm

This is a polysaccharide matrix that many bacteria can produce to protect and hide them from attack. Antibiotics may, initially, kill most bacteria within a Biofilm "colony", but organisms known as "persisters" remain and reform the biofilm. If antibiotics are given in high doses over a long period, the sequestered bacteria seem to mutate into a resistant form within weeks. However, if antibiotics are given at a relatively low dose and pulsed, bacteria are less likely to become resistant and treatment may be more successful.

Alternatively, "biofilm busters" can be used to destroy biofilm, thus rendering bacteria vulnerable to antimicrobials. Lumbrokinase is a fibrinolytic enzyme that has some good research to back up claims of reducing fibrin and fibrinogen. It is available in Buluoke®, a product distributed by Researched Nutritionals in USA.

Byron White Formulas A-Bio utilises a combination of herbs

to break down biofilm and is very effective at relatively low doses.

Once "busted", biofilm releases many microbes into surrounding tissue, so patients may experience exacerbated symptoms. It is vital to maintain vigorous detox protocol and gut support as well as antimicrobial activity while destroying biofilm.

Is herxing healthy?

The short answer is NO!

Herxing (Jarisch-Herxheimer reaction) is our body's inflammatory response to endotoxins released by dying bacteria.

The good news about herxing is that it indicates that an antimicrobial medicine (antibiotics or herbal) is working and bacteria are dying.

The BAD NEWS is that herxing damages your body. The process of illness caused by herxing throws your body back into fight/flight/freeze response, creates further inflammation and reduces our ability to eliminate toxins. **Stress caused by severe herxing suppresses our immune system and slows healing.**

LLMDs around the world now know that we can use the beginning of a mild herx reaction as a guide to the pace of antimicrobial activity. When the herx reaction begins, detox protocols can be increased while adjusting antimicrobial activity to just below herx level.

When using Byron White Formulas antimicrobials, the developer (Byron White) strongly advises against allowing herx reactions to continue or become severe. As soon as any herx signs appear, the protocol is to reduce antimicrobial by 1-3 drops per dose while increasing detoxification activity.

It may be necessary to stop antimicrobials altogether for 3-4 days before beginning again at a lower dose.

Severe herxing is dangerous and slows progress towards recovery.

Stop herxing and start recovering!

Increased detox activity, both personally and with detox remedies, can reduce the risk of herxing. Detox is critical to recovery!

Mitigating herxing

When using any antimicrobial against any Lyme-like infection, most patients will herx at some stage. Vigorous detox routines will defer their "herx level" and there are some strategies to mitigate the intensity and length of the herx:

1. Prepare 3 glasses of chia seeds, take one each day in rotation. If a herx begins, take the three glasses throughout a single day (preparing new glasses each time) to mop up endotoxins and reduce the herx intensity.

2. Take lemon water several times each day of herxing.

3. Take 20 drops of good quality Smilax tincture (1:2 or 1:1) 2-3 times daily. However, be cautious as some patients react adversely to Smilax.

4. Increase doses or frequency of currently prescribed detox herbals.

5. Increase dose and/or frequency of detox greens like BioPractica Matrix Phase Detox plus MAC to bind toxins.

6. Make a fresh green juice including coriander and parsley.

7. Soak in an Epsom salts bath for twenty minutes, then rinse off (should be doing this anyway).

8. Drink 2.5 litres/6 pints of water during the day and rest as much as possible.

9. Use a clay-based detox formula like the Byron White Detox 2 powder.

Prescribing for very sensitive patients

"K" dilutions

No matter how careful we are at selecting suitable dosage levels, some patients will aggravate/herx after a few days to a few weeks.

Signs of aggravation/herxing include exacerbation of "normal" symptoms, fatigue, irritability, new or strange symptoms appearing, or a feeling of being "not quite right".

Some people are extremely sensitive to herbal/homeopathic medicines at any time, and the onset of a chronic disorder seems to enhance that sensitivity. In fact, patients may be up to 100 times more sensitive than the "normal" population. If they have reacted to herbal remedies in the past, or have difficulty in taking pharmaceutical medication, it may be wise to start antimicrobials at these dilutions.

Aggravation of symptoms when using appropriately chosen antimicrobials does not indicate any toxic or dangerous condition. However, continuous or uncontrolled herxing is a sign that you need to change your treatment regimen which may be damaging if allowed to continue unchecked.

Herbal and homeopathic medicines are rarely toxic or dangerous. The aggravation/herxing indicates that patients are responding positively to the medicine but need only a tiny dose to achieve the desired result.

"K" dilutions are one useful way to gain this balance between benefit and aggravation. Here's how it works.

K1

1. Put one drop of the appropriate remedy into a glass of water.
2. Throw the water out but do not dry the glass.
3. Refill the glass with water and take a sip of that solution. Does that seem too dilute to be any good? It works!

K2

1. Prepare a K1 dilution.
2. Throw away the water.
3. Refill the glass and take a sip.

Yes, this dilution works too.

To prepare **K3** and **K4** dilutions, repeat the steps above until you have thrown away the **number of glasses coinciding with the dilution number.**

The solution remaining in the glass may be stored in the refrigerator for use on ensuing days. Make sure your patients mark the solutions with the name of the remedy being taken so there is no confusion as they may need to dilute more than one remedy. Generally, each preparation of a K dilution lasts about a week, depending on the size of the glass and how much is sipped each time.

> **Case history: *Martha*** *was very sensitive to her anti-Borrelia herbal formula. A single drop caused severe herx reactions. She tried K4 dilutions, then K8, then K14. Even that caused a herx. She then started putting one drop of K14 on her wrist. After two months, she was able to tolerate a K14 drop orally. Over the next year, Martha slowly reduced the dilution, moving to K13, K12, and so on. Eighteen months after commencing her "wrist treatment", Martha was able to tolerate one full drop orally. Now, after over three years of dedicated self-help and treatment, she is almost symptom-free and needing very little medicine/treatment.*

Quantity dilution

If your patient is somewhat sensitive, but does not need a K dilution, a quantity dilution may serve to start them well with antimicrobials.

- Place one drop of the selected remedy into a glass (about 150 mL) of water.
- The patient can then take any quantity from a teaspoon, ¼ glass, ½ glass etc. to give a proportion of one drop.
- This is often a good way to transition from K dilutions to a full drop and onwards.

Practitioner strategies summary

- Be alert for aberrant symptoms, atypical illness onset or history, or non-responsive patients. These may indicate an infectious aetiological pathway.
- Consider the Horowitz questionnaire.[1]
- Check the patient's symptom picture against Borrelia ("Lyme") and/or other infections.

Other things to check:

- challenge test and/or blood test?
- lifestyle choices
- food choices
- detox protocols
- detox remedies
- antimicrobials.

The presence of a "stealth infection" (Borrelia and/or co-infections) does NOT mean that the diagnosis of Parkinson's disease was wrong. It DOES mean that the infection is one of the aetiological pathways leading to that diagnosis and must be addressed effectively.

CHAPTER 27

CAN WAM and CAM CO-EXIST IN ONE PATIENT?

Indications and contraindications[1]

One of the great tragedies for patients since the rise in power of Western allopathic medicine following World War II is the increasing divide between what is perceived as "evidence-based" medicine and what is often labelled "alternative medicine".

In Chapter 34, I have explained why both these perceptions or labels are incorrect and deliberately misleading. However, those more interested in money or power than patient care continue to propagate fear and misunderstanding to the detriment of patient outcomes and wellbeing.

There is no doubt that individual patients can choose a combination of Western allopathic medicine and complementary/alternative medicine, and this may be the most effective choice for them.

Patients and practitioners need to make therapeutic choices based on immediate intention, long-term goals, safety and proven efficacy. This may mean that individual patients require some support from Western allopathic medicine while developing strategies for recovery, or may rely on Western allopathic medicine completely, or may wish to pursue complementary/alternative medicine strategies only.

Patient A, a 58-year-old woman with stage 2 Parkinson's disease (Hoehn & Yahr Scale), is frustrated with her loss of dexterity, especially fine motor skills, and wishes to continue working in her office job to fund both therapies and an adventurous lifestyle, including travel and bushwalking. She decides that she will take low-dose levodopa drugs to mitigate symptoms while improving her food choices, taking a number of nutritional supplements and therapeutic remedies and herbs. She also begins clinical Pilates classes, boxing sessions and dances daily at home while doing her chores. She later adds meditation classes plus daily meditation at home, works through some stressful issues from childhood and, critically, reconstructs her current marriage relationship with the help of a counsellor.

Patient A finds that, as she improves her lifestyle, immune function and core strength, she needs her levodopa drugs less and less and, in fact, sometimes forgets to take them because she is feeling so good. After two years, she begins to deliberately wean herself of the levodopa and, nearly four years after diagnosis, finds that she is symptom-free and no longer needs any levodopa drugs. She is also able to reduce her supplement and therapeutic remedy intake to some "basic essentials", but continues her meditation and physical activities.

Patient B is a vigorous businessman, 47 years old and self-employed in a successful business. He feels he required his personal input every day. He is frustrated at his declining dexterity and energy, and afraid of the future. His doctors have told him that he has only a few years before his medication stops being effective and he needs to "get his affairs in order" soon.

Patient B begins some complementary/alternative medicine strategies, changes some food choices, takes some supplements and remedies, and promises to meditate. However, he "can't give up coffee" (he loves the adrenal boost), rarely finds time to meditate and pushes his body to the extreme in an effort to ward off his progressive degeneration. He loves cycling and, instead of riding 10-20 kilometres two or three times each week, rides only on Sundays and then covers 150-200 kilometres, ending the day exhausted. He becomes angry when challenged about his choices, feels that his wife expects a comfortable/luxurious lifestyle, and finds it difficult to delegate responsibility in his business.

As his symptoms progress, he increases his Western allopathic medicine intake, reaching maximum intake of levodopa, adding a dopamine agonist and then an MAO-B inhibiter. After a little over two years of "fiddling" with complementary/alternative medicine, he declares that it doesn't work, focuses on drug therapy and gets involved with fundraising for research to "find a cure" for Parkinson's disease. He becomes a "poster boy" for fundraising for a short time, which he finds pleasing.

Within five years, Patient B undergoes Deep Brain Stimulation in an effort to reduce the adverse effects of the high-dose drug therapy he has chosen. It is moderately effective, but he is forced to retire from his business (at 52 years old) and lapses into obscurity. His immediate intent to mitigate symptoms overwhelmed his long-term goal of recovery, to his detriment.

Patient C is 83 years old, retired, and struggling with life. He has diagnosed Parkinson's disease (stage 4.5), hypertension, anxiety, depression, migraine and constant nausea. He feels tired, down and sick all day, every day, and has stopped all social contact and activities outside the home. He is unable to walk without a walking frame and, even with that support, his balance and mobility are severely compromised. His wife is worn out from caring for him. Patient C takes a cocktail of fourteen different Western allopathic medications for his various diagnosed "diseases" but is not showing any improvement.

With encouragement from friends, family, a massage therapist and his wife, Patient C begins a slow introduction of complementary/ alternative medicine strategies. At first, the intention is to mitigate symptoms and improve his quality of life, but the longer-term goal is to reduce his reliance on Western allopathic medication to a minimum, in order to reduce the risk of accumulated adverse effects.

He begins with changing food choices, introducing three basic supplements and one homeopathic remedy. A little later, he adds some gentle exercise and weekly Bowen therapy. After some months, he agrees to basic meditation for a few minutes each day and some social activity outside the home.

Two years after commencing his complementary/alternative medicine strategies, Patient C is able to walk unaided, and has much more energy. However, he still feels nauseous all day, has frequent headaches, and is quite anxious. His complementary/alternative medicine practitioner creates a chart of all his medications, including actions and adverse effects. The chart shows that most of his medications are prescribed to offset the adverse effects of other medications and that, of the fourteen drugs, eleven may cause nausea, nine headache and eight anxiety. With the help of his general practitioner (primary care practitioner), Patient C reduces his medication intake over just a few months and this transforms his life. He no longer feels nauseous, his headaches disappear and he begins to feel confident.

Six years after commencing complementary/alternative medicine, Patient C is free from Parkinson's disease symptoms and feels energetic and confident. He continues to need low-dose antihypertension medication and an occasional sleeping pill. He also continues to take some basic supplements and one homeopathic remedy, plus he continues to exercise and meditate.

Patient C lived into his late nineties, confident, happy and free from Parkinson's disease symptoms.

The choice of Western allopathic medicine or complementary/alternative medicine or some combination is dependent on these four questions:

1. Immediate intention: does the patient want to mitigate symptoms only or begin the process of recovery?

2. Long-term goals: does the patient want to feel better now or recover in the future?

3. Self-importance/love: does the patient care about themselves sufficiently to make the changes and sacrifices need to create a pathway to wellness?

4. Support: does the patient have people around them who will support them through the long journey to wellness, and ward off the opposition (sometimes vicious) from those dedicated to Western allopathic medicine who will attempt to persuade or bully the patient into Western allopathic medicine only?

Once these questions are answered, the patient can make a rational decision about Western allopathic medicine, complementary/alternative medicine or a combination.

CHAPTER 28

STRATEGIES TO AVOID

(if you really want to recover)

There are some prominent complementary/alternative medicine therapies offered for Parkinson's disease with promises varying from symptom reduction to "cure" or "fixing your whole life".

In some cases, there are some benefits from these therapies, but they are often more than offset by adverse effects or the necessity to neglect other, more effective treatments.

In the interests of avoiding defamatory comments, I will be brief, but urge readers to take note of my warnings and investigate thoroughly before spending time and money on these therapies.

Alkaline water is touted as a solution for many illnesses and, if not a complete solution, a priority adjunctive therapy. Alkaline water is proposed to solve metabolic acidosis, chronic inflammation, digestive dysregulation and dehydration, amongst many other claims.[1]

The principle put forward is that, if we drink water with a pH of 8-9, we will reduce acidosis and improve all the other matters mentioned above. However, this just does not make sense.

We require a pH of 1-2 in our stomach for efficient digestion of protein and solid foods. This very low pH also assists in maintaining a tight seal at the pyloric sphincter (the top sphincter where food enters the stomach).

When we drink alkaline water, we raise the pH of our stomach and, incidentally, lower the pH of the water consumed. Our stomach pH gradually rises to above 4, at which stage we stop digesting proteins and solid food efficiently and the pyloric sphincter begins to leak, creating symptoms of reflux. Far from resolving metabolic acidosis, this digestive dysregulation actually exacerbates acidosis.

Drinking water is vital to life and health. However, "natural water" (water from springs, streams and rain in pristine areas) tends to have a pH of 6.5 (slightly acid) to 7.5 (slightly alkaline). Whenever possible, we should drink water within this pH range.

"Cures" for nearly everything are offered online or in books. In my view, there is no "cure" for any disease or disorder. A light-hearted look at "cure" can be seen here:

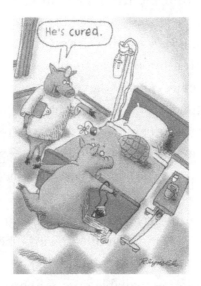

Sites and books offering cures, usually with some sort of supplement/pill/drink, and often at a high cost, need to be treated with wariness and investigation. We should be especially wary if the cure does not demand any changes on our part or promises very fast results.

Developing symptoms of a chronic disorder takes many years and affects most parts of our body, therefore it is likely to take many months (or longer) to reverse the effects and will require us to make changes.

In general, be very wary of anyone offering a cure, whether they be complementary/alternative medicine practitioners, Western allopathic medicine practitioners or researchers, or complete quacks.

Medical marijuana and CBD (cannabidiol) oil: These herbs and extracts are gaining a reputation as panaceas for almost everything.

Marijuana has been consumed in various ways for hundreds, if not thousands of years, and promoters claim that this fact alone lends legitimacy to their claims of efficacy and safety. Nothing could be further from the truth, of course, as many toxic and dangerous substances have been used traditionally with proven ill effects. Fermented grains, herbs and fruits can be as addictive and dangerous as modern alcoholic beverages, intoxicating mushrooms have caused brain damage over thousands of years. Arsenic was routinely used as medicine for over 2,400 years, right through the 19th century. Arsenic was reintroduced as a cancer treatment in 1931 and is still sometimes prescribed today, even though we are aware of its carcinogenic and neurotoxic properties.

With traditional use rendered inoperative as supportive evidence, we must look at modern research into the effects, benefits and adverse effects of marijuana and CBD oil.

Much information is available on marijuana or CBD forums and blogs, and it is telling that many people on these sites are now warning about the dopamine-reducing effects of long-term marijuana usage. THC, the most prevalent cannabinoid in marijuana, stimulates production of dopamine for a short time; this is one of the reasons for the "high" achieved by consuming marijuana. Hyperstimulation of dopamine has a similar effect as levodopa drugs; they bring comfort and symptom relief for some time but, ultimately, reduce endogenous dopamine production, so are drugs of dependence.

There is ample research showing that long-term consumption of marijuana may lead to depression, anxiety, paranoia and other mental disorders which tend to be intractable to standard treatments. There is some research on deaths caused by medicinal and recreational use of marijuana and, while the numbers fall short of deaths caused by many pharmaceutical drugs, it is far from safe.[2,3]

CBD poses a more difficult problem when deciding whether it is useful, damaging or somewhere in between. There is no doubt that CBD oil, used wisely, can bring temporary relief of some very serious symptoms that are debilitating and distressing. It is difficult to ignore spectacular videos of seizures being relieved and almost total relief from excruciating pain.

But what is the long-term effect of CBD oil? Will it, like the THC in marijuana, reduce endogenous dopamine production? At this time (2019) there seems to be disagreement on this point, even among CBD promoters and supporters. On one hand, supporters claim that CBD works "inside the cell", thus bypassing the CB1 receptor that is the primary receptor for dopamine. On the other hand, some CBD blogs state that CBD can be addictive because of its indirect down-regulation of dopamine production.[4]

The most pragmatic opinion I can form from the information currently at hand is that, at best, CBD oil may grant some moderate relief from some symptoms on a temporary basis, providing it is taken/used regularly, but will not reverse the process of illness at all. CBD and marijuana may be helpful to relieve pain and other distressing symptoms in extreme circumstances when all other strategies have failed (unlikely if you are dedicated), and both may be useful at end-stage disease where pain and misery are unbearable, and there is no hope for recovery. For people with Parkinson's, THC and CBD are likely to reduce endogenous production of dopamine, so are counter-productive in the long term.

Anandamide or marijuana?

Anandamide is a neurotransmitter (not really a hormone at all) found in human organs, especially the brain. It is nicknamed "the bliss hormone", as it was originally postulated to be the natural substance mimicked by THC (Delta9-tetrahydrocannabinol), the principal psychoactive ingredient in cannabis (marijuana). THC locks onto the cannabinoid receptors first discovered in 1988.

THC does not occur naturally in the body, and our body does not create receptors for substances it doesn't produce. Scientists were certain that some sort of endogenous (made in the body) substance was produced to occupy the receptors sites locked onto by cannabis. Israeli scientist, Raphael Mechoulam, discovered anandamide (more properly named arachidonoylethanolamine or AEA) in 1992.

Anandamide connects with CB1 cannabinoid receptors found in the brain and nervous system, and CB2 receptors found throughout the rest of the body. The difference is quite important, as anandamide plays various roles in our health. The CB2 receptors are involved in the health of our immune system, while the CB1 receptors seem to be concerned with a variety of tasks including memory, eating behaviour, sleep and pain relief. They also seem to influence the neural generation of motivation and pleasure. Anandamide is critical in the early development of babies in the uterus (while THC from cannabis may cause disruption or abortion of pregnancy).

We learn to remember new knowledge or carry out new activities by creating new connections between neurons. The more we use each connection – that is, practise the memory or activity – the stronger that connection becomes. If we stop using that connection, it becomes weak and may break. This has profound implications in recovery and we will explore it further in other chapters. Biochemical evidence suggests that anandamide is involved in creating and breaking short-term neural connections. Moreover, anandamide is synthesised in areas of the brain that are important for memory, higher thought processes and **control of movement**.

Strategies to increase endogenous production of anandamide will bring long-term benefits similar to the short-term relief obtained from THC or CBD.

We always have choices when we treat diagnosed disorders. If we wish to mitigate symptoms and live comfortably for a while longer without thought to recovery, we can choose treatments like medical marijuana and CBD oil. However, if we wish to recover and live life without symptoms or treatments, we must seek the causes of our symptoms and reverse those.

There is current (2019) research into the application of other cannabinoids (there are over 30) in the treatment of diagnosed Parkinson's disease. The hope is that these cannabinoids will provide some of the benefits of THC and CBD without the adverse effects or dependency properties. It will be some years before we see the results of this research.

Light therapy (phototherapy): There is a great deal written about bright light therapy in various forms, and many claims of benefits in a wide range of illness conditions.

Light, especially sunlight, plays a very important role in promoting health and wellbeing. Seasonal affective disorder is well known, especially in areas far from the equator where seasonal light variations are more extreme, and light therapy (phototherapy) can be very helpful in resolving this.

Ideal sun exposure is around fifteen minutes per day during the morning while exposing 90 per cent of our body. This produces sufficient vitamin D, serotonin, melatonin and other neurotransmitters for our needs. Of course, it is very rare to find people with sufficient time and courage to sunbathe almost nude in the early morning. More often, I see people who have been discouraged from sun exposure by cancer authorities who say that we must shun the sun because of the fear of melanoma.[5]

Of course, we must avoid exposure during the hottest hours of the day and avoid sunburn at all times. However, the fear of sun exposure created by anti-cancer campaigns (as opposed to sensible education strategies) has led to an increase in a number of sun-deficiency syndromes, including osteoporosis and mood disorders. Many sunscreens also contain chemicals that are either carcinogenic or neurotoxic, or both.

Light, in sunlight frequencies, affects production of serotonin, melatonin and, indirectly, a number of other neurotransmitters, hormones and enzymes. This, in turn, affects production of ATP, our energy "packages".

When we are deprived of sunlight – either because we live in areas with long, dark winters, or we are confined indoors for some reason (perhaps working long hours in a windowless office, or our home is an apartment with difficult access and little natural light) – chemical changes may present as depression, fatigue, loss of motivation, withdrawal from social interaction or even increased symptoms of illness.

These are circumstances in which it is important to take action and increase light exposure. The first choice, of course, is to increase natural sun exposure when that is possible. If this cannot be achieved, an appropriate "light box" or mechanism can be usefully applied to substitute for the sun (albeit incompletely).

Light therapy for the above circumstances and symptoms has been shown to be successful and helpful.

However, light therapy, as a treatment for Parkinson's disease, can only reduce some symptoms, and will not slow or reverse the illness process. A number of claims have been made in journals and learned publications that phototherapy will reverse the Parkinson's disease process and may represent a "cure". This is simply not the case. Used as directed, phototherapy may relieve some symptoms related to serotonin and melatonin production, and that may be helpful as part of an overall package of recovery strategies, but will not cure or permanently "fix" your health.

Light boxes/mechanisms are, occasionally, available on loan from hospitals or universities that have an interest in this therapy. However, those available at retail are often quite expensive to achieve the light frequencies and lumen output required. If you are handy in the workshop, there are details online for making efficient light boxes/mechanisms for a fraction of the purchase cost.

Light therapy may help you if you are unable to achieve appropriate sun exposure, but will not cure or fix your health.

Rigorous detox/saunas: Removing toxins from our body is very important (see Chapter 25). We are constantly bombarded with toxic chemicals used for a variety of useful and not-so-useful purposes and may have inherited a toxic load from our parents. Add to this our lifestyle choices that may include foods that are harmful, recreational chemicals (alcohol, nicotine, others), pharmaceuticals for minor ills, household toxins and inadvertent exposure to cleaning and agrochemicals, and there is no doubt that our toxic load may inhibit our recovery.

However, we must temper necessity with caution. Removing toxins quickly and rigorously may exacerbate symptoms or even make us more ill. Many toxins are locked in cells where they inhibit cell function and create or exacerbate symptoms, but do so at a moderate and steady rate. If we quickly extract those toxins from cells and dump them into our bloodstream for processing by our liver, our elimination systems may not be able to cope, and we may feel as if we are being poisoned all over again.

We have a number of elimination pathways – bowels, bladder, skin, respiration – and these are served by organs and systems such as liver, lymph, fascia and blood circulation. All these systems and support systems must be efficiently supported and improved to effectively remove toxins.

We must also remember that diagnosis with Parkinson's disease implies significant inefficiency and sensitivity of many body systems, including elimination.

Rigorous liver detox protocols may overstress other systems. Aggressive herbal detox protocols may create more illness symptoms and discourage patients from moving towards wellness. Assertive chelation therapies may present a number of adverse effects that discourage wellness.

Saunas (direct heat, far infrared and near infrared) can be a useful part of a thorough detoxification protocol, but only if used cautiously. The heat of saunas encourages sweating, which is one way for our body to eliminate toxins, especially when bowel and bladder are less than fully functional.

However, excessive heat can adversely affect fascia, which is an important part of our elimination system. In fact, fascia plays a critical role in health, being the largest organ in our body (larger than the skin, for instance), and is intimately involved in blood and lymph circulation, hydration, temperature control, movement (giving lubrication and supporting posture), immune support and inflammation.

If fascia is overheated, it becomes "sticky", inhibiting many of its functions and exacerbating illness. When saunas are part of a detox protocol, they should be used for ten to fifteen minutes only and immediately followed by a COLD shower (not lukewarm or tepid, but cold) to help fascia recover its jelly-like state.[6]

All detox and sauna protocols must be created with the fragility of the patient and complexity of the illness process in mind. Gentle and long-term works better than short and aggressive.

Amino acid therapy: This is not a therapy to necessarily avoid completely, but comes with some cautions about effectiveness and costs.

According to Dr Marty Hinz, creator of the Amino Acid Protocol for Parkinson's disease:

> The Hinz protocol is a scientifically based Amino Acid protocol. It uses a natural form of L-dopa which wipes out Parkinson's symptoms and balances blood levels of amino acids with other neurotransmitters. Giving too much L-Dopa, whether it's with pharmaceutical drugs like Sinemet or even a natural form will cause an imbalance of neurotransmitters and can cause symptoms like nausea and depression. You must carefully balance neurotransmitters with other amino acids like 5-HTP. You should not attempt this protocol on your own without medical supervision. It is a very specific process that requires skilled professional help. (https://www.theparkinsonsplan.com/hinz-protocol/).

Dr Hinz says that:

> Parkinson's disease is associated with depletion of tyrosine hydroxylase, dopamine, serotonin, and norepinephrine. Exacerbating this is the fact that administration of L-dopa may deplete l-tyrosine, l-tryptophan, 5-hydroxytryptophan (5-HTP), serotonin, and sulfur amino acids. The properly balanced administration of L-dopa in conjunction with 5-HTP, l-tyrosine, l-cysteine, and cofactors under the guidance of organic cation transporter functional status determination (herein referred to as "OCT assay interpretation") of urinary serotonin and dopamine, is at the heart of this novel treatment protocol.

This approach seems logical and firmly based in science rarely visited by conservative Western allopathic medicine practitioners or Parkinson's disease researchers.

In reading Dr Hinz's work more thoroughly, however, we can see that this therapy is not addressing the initiating causes (aetiological pathways) of Parkinson's disease and is really looking only at dopamine deficiency, rather than the reasons for the dopamine deficit. While this may bring significant relief of symptoms (and obviously can do this if we are to believe the many testimonials online), it cannot help where Parkinson's disease symptoms are caused by something other than dopamine deficit.

Some clinics promoting Dr Hinz's amino acid therapy (AAT) take a more holistic approach and construct lifestyle changes to support physical and emotional health while supplying the supplements for the AAT protocol. This seems likely to be of more benefit long-term.

Another caution is the cost of this protocol. Dr Hinz says there is a one-off cost of around US$8000 (in 2018), plus the cost of lab tests (urine and blood), then monthly costs for supplements of US$300-600, plus repeat visits to consulting doctors and lab tests as required. These costs are ongoing for the foreseeable future, according to Dr Hinz's website.

Dr Hinz replaces synthetic levodopa/carbidopa drugs with a "natural" form of levodopa (Mucuna puriens) which is certainly more "natural" than synthesised pharmaceuticals, but still processed and not packaged with a decarboxylase inhibitor, so may be poorly absorbed. Dr Hinz claims that packaging the Mucuna with 5-HTP assists absorption, while balancing with other supplements to promote other neurotransmitters will eliminate many of the adverse effects of conservative Parkinson's disease treatment.

Other than the ongoing costs, cautions include the probability that supplementation with Mucuna (levodopa) will, over time, reduce endogenous production of dopamine (as do levodopa drugs), thus creating dependency on the supplements for wellbeing.

More importantly, this protocol does not address the aetiological pathways leading to a diagnosis of Parkinson's disease, so can only be considered as a supportive therapy rather than a way to reverse the causes.

Aggressive/extreme bodywork: There are many excellent forms of bodywork that can alleviate symptoms in a wide range of circumstances.

For people with Parkinson's, we must consider not only the type of bodywork, but the way it is delivered. People with Parkinson's are quite fragile, even when appearing robust, and bodywork practitioners must be aware of this fragility when assessing how to treat.

As we have seen earlier, developing symptoms of Parkinson's disease is akin to running a continuous marathon for many years, exhausting our reserves of neurotransmitters and creating cell damage. Delivering bodywork as if we are "attacking" the symptoms of stiffness, rigidity and pain can only bring discomfort and, possibly, more cellular damage in the long term.

On the other hand, by approaching each fragile body with gentleness and patience, we bring comfort and may assist in reversing symptoms or even causes.

Case history: *Walter was in his late 70s when he attended my clinic, diagnosed with Parkinson's disease some three years earlier. A major symptom was a very rigid neck which prevented him from turning his head at all and caused great discomfort.*

On palpation, the sternocleidomastoid and scalene muscles were so rigid that I was unable to compress the muscle body at all. It felt as if his neck muscles were steel, surrounded by steel cords. A number of physiotherapists, massage therapists and kind friends had attempted to release the muscles by using very firm to hard pressure, with techniques varying from standard massage to Rolfing-type moves. He had also seen a chiropractor who had attempted a neck adjustment, causing severe pain and no improvement.

I commenced using standard Bowen moves, but using extremely light pressure – equivalent to the pressure used when inserting a contact lens. Each time I saw him (generally each two weeks), I would commence with this very gently work on his neck muscles.

Within three months, Walter could turn his head 30 degrees each way and no longer had pain. We continued the gentle work and, after nearly nine months, he had full "normal" neck rotation

319

and flexibility. The very gentle work had succeeded where aggressive therapies failed.

In an open study of over 100 patients during the years 1999 and 2000, we found that those receiving gentle, patient bodywork (no matter what the modality) gained more benefits than those receiving assertive or aggressive work.

Practitioners, be patient and gentle with your patients diagnosed with Parkinson's disease. Patients, look for bodywork practitioners who are patient, gentle and take notice of your responses.

CHAPTER 29

BEING WELL

Lifestyle choices to stay well

Whether we are diagnosed with a chronic disorder or feel generally well, there are a number of strategies we can employ to optimise our quality of health and wellbeing. In my view, length of life is not nearly as important as quality of life, and the value we both accrue from our experience and add to the world by our being.

Gaining value

As we move along our journey of life, we have choices every day: to participate in and celebrate all the wonders of that day, or bemoan what we do not have and wish it was different. We can gain energy from the sun, or complain that it is too hot; listen to the music of rain on the roof, or wish that it would stop so we could go outside; meditate on the beauty of leaves turning red in autumn, or resent that we will need to rake them up from the ground soon. We can smile at people we meet and wish them a good day, or wonder fearfully what they are thinking about us; pick up loose paper from the footpath and put it in a bin, or whinge about litterers; discuss people who are making a positive difference in your community, or complain about the crime rate.

The way we consider our daily adventure, positively or negatively, affects the function of our immune system, inflammatory response, digestion, blood sugar, cholesterol and, of course, dopamine production.

Other daily choices include food, drink, exercise or lack of, time for meditation (or none), people with whom we associate, shows we watch on television and radio stations we listen to. Every choice impacts our health. No choice is unimportant or without consequences – positive or negative.

As a person with Parkinson's, making the right choices is critical for your recovery. In previous chapters, we have discussed almost every aspect of life, and your choices will enhance or diminish your health. Our past choices have, almost certainly, contributed to the onset of disease symptoms and/or our innate resilience. Those choices may have been made based on our knowledge at the time, and regrets are generally wasteful. However, we can and should recognise inappropriate choices from the past so that we can avoid repeating them and correct any damage they may have caused.

Once we develop great habits and good choices, those wishing to remain well will always make those same choices.

Perhaps you are well right now but have a family member with Parkinson's disease and want to reduce the likelihood of developing those symptoms. All the lifestyle choices we have discussed in previous chapters are for you. Food, drink, self-help, time for meditation and celebration, healthy associations, singing and dancing are strategies for wellness, not just "treating disease". Make the choices now and you may never need a recovery plan.

Are you the loved one or friend of a person with Parkinson's disease? Understanding the strategies and choices we have discussed throughout this book will help you to support and assist your loved one/friend to recover and maintain health. If you join them in the lifestyle choices, you will gain the bonus of improved health too.

The choices, strategies and explanations in this book are all about regaining and maintaining wellness, rather than treating disease. Wellness and illness are mutually exclusive so, if we make choices for health and wellbeing, illness will lose its place in our lives.

As a person with Parkinson's, the changes I made and the strategies I adopted more than twenty years ago are lifetime choices if I wish to remain well (as I do).[1] We cannot adopt the strategies in this book for a year or two to "cure" a disease, then revert to our old lifestyle choices. A sick lifestyle creates a sick body. A well lifestyle leads to a well life.

Case history: *Beatrice was a delightful, middle-aged woman when she presented in my clinic diagnosed with Parkinson's disease. Her life revolved around family. She had five adult children (three married and two "still looking"), seven grandchildren, and was involved in her church.*

It seemed, at first, that Beatrice had an almost ideal life, engaged and supported. However, a long conversation at that first consultation indicated some hidden stresses that had plagued her for many years. Beatrice felt that it was her responsibility to maintain the cohesion of the family, despite any conflicts between family members and/or the community. She continued to provide family dinners every week, doing most of the preparation herself. She delighted in babysitting her grandchildren, but often felt exhausted at the end of the day and wondered how she managed to continue her work the next day.

As her disease symptoms progressed, she struggled to maintain her household, family "duties" and marriage relationship. When I met her, her symptoms were at about stage 2 on the Hoehn and Yahr scale.

Her background included migration to Australia in her twenties with a great struggle to learn English, a language that never sat comfortably with her. She found it hard to express her feelings in her adopted language.

Her husband accompanied her to the consultation and, while appearing to be very pleasant and cooperative, I sensed an underlying desire to control everything and everyone. He wanted a quick result so his wife could, once again, become the compliant, busy, always-available woman he had known for 40 years.

Beatrice, reluctantly, made changes to food choices, delegated some responsibility for family dinners to older children, undertook some regular gentle exercise and agreed to try some simple meditation. She added basic supplements, the Aqua Hydration Formulas and regular Bowen therapy to her routine.

We saw moderate reduction in symptoms over six months, but her husband was impatient and not impressed with her progress.

Beatrice began a long-term homeopathic detoxification program that was gentle but effective for fragile people. Within five months, Beatrice reported to my clinic completely free from all Parkinson's disease symptoms.

I congratulated Beatrice and her husband on such a great result and advised them that the choices made during their time with me were for life. That was the last I heard from Beatrice for four years.

I was surprised to see Beatrice in my clinic after so long, displaying all the symptoms of Parkinson's disease noted at her first visit six years earlier. This time, she was accompanied by both her husband and an adult daughter.

It took very little time to establish that Beatrice and her family had considered her "cured" when she no longer had symptoms, and they had quickly reverted to old habits — reliance on Beatrice for family dinners, counselling and babysitting. Beatrice unthinkingly slipped back into old food habits with lots of wheat, dairy, sugar and coffee. Within two years, she was displaying early signs of Parkinson's disease again, so re-visited her neurologist. He said, "I told you so" and prescribed levodopa medication.

Beatrice felt embarrassed to come back and see me, as she felt she had "let me down". I explained that my opinion was unimportant, but she had really let herself down by slipping back into old habits so easily.

Once again, we commenced on the recovery pathway with food, supplements and other strategies, including detox. Progress was slow but, over nearly two years, her symptoms reduced and we were able to wean her off her levodopa drugs. Beatrice again disappeared from my life for some time.

When I saw her again, more than two years later, Beatrice's symptoms had returned. She had, again, slipped back into old habits, bowed to her family's demands, was exhausted and becoming frail. She had begun levodopa medication again and was just about to add a dopamine agonist.

I pointed out, firmly to Beatrice and her family members present, that I could not "cure" her, but regaining and maintaining wellness would require great dedication on her part and total support from her family.

Beatrice came to see me only once more about three months later. Her symptoms had not diminished, she was frail and frightened. However, nothing in her lifestyle choices, or her family's attitude had changed. The family wanted to discuss "cures" and assertive therapies, including deep brain stimulation, because they wanted the "old Beatrice" back but without making any lasting changes.

There is no "cure" for Parkinson's disease or any chronic disease. However, if we remove "illness factors" such as trauma, toxins and infections, and maintain healthy choices, we can regain and maintain wellness. This is RECOVERY.

CHAPTER 30

WHO IS IN CHARGE?

Take control and change your life

There is a recently-developed tradition in Western society to ignore wellness activities, wait until illness symptoms appear, then rely on a doctor or specialist to "fix" us. In conservative Western allopathic medicine, there is little emphasis on self-help or individual responsibility.

Over the past few years, there has been more emphasis on weight control and eating a "whole food diet", but with little real understanding of what that means and, often, quite unhealthy advice on weight-loss programs and dietary changes. We saw in Chapter 9 that the Standard American/Australian Diet (SAD) is essentially unhealthy, promoting sugar-generating foods like grains, and calcium-stripping foods like dairy.

The conflicting advice received from Western allopathic medicine practitioners and complementary/alternative medicine practitioners can be very confusing for those seeking better health, and this is compounded by the promotion of fad diets, pharmaceutical OTC drugs and supplements by celebrities and sports "heroes" who read from scripts and swell their bank accounts.

The fact is that there is no one single source of excellent health information. However, there are some principles we can follow to gain better information and take control of our lifestyle and health.

1. If a product or diet is heavily promoted by celebrities, there is, undoubtedly, a great deal of money being spent on advertising and promotion fees, and that money has to come from somewhere – either by increasing prices to ridiculous levels, or using cheaper source materials/processes to keep profit margins high. Heavily advertised products are generally best avoided unless your healthcare professional advises otherwise.

2. Standard dietary information in the Western world is usually generated by Western allopathic medically trained professionals who have not been exposed to the high-quality medical research showing the errors in established dietary advice. WAM-trained professionals I have spoken to are unaware of medical research showing the inflammatory nature of grains, the increased risk of Parkinson's disease and other chronic disorders with the consumption of animal dairy products, or the benefits of good fats like eggs, avocado and coconut oil.

3. When exploring ways to reverse or recover from a chronic illness, it is important to find the cause or aetiological pathway. If your practitioner, or a website/book, or some other source of information claims a cure or a reversal strategy without offering a rational explanation for developing that illness, that is probably not a source of information to rely on.

4. You are in charge, and the decisions on your own healthcare must make sense to you. No person, system, diet, supplement or medication can cure you or make you better. Only *you* can improve your health by adopting a range of strategies best suited to you as an individual.

When diagnosed with Parkinson's disease, you have time to think, read, discuss, explore and make decisions based on the best research available and what feels right for you. Don't be rushed into taking medication or buying very expensive supplements, simply because someone says, "You have Parkinson's disease! You must take this NOW to slow it down!" A few more days or even weeks for research and discussion will not make any difference to your symptoms.

Take your time, take control, then take positive action and get well.

CHAPTER 31

FINDING PRACTITIONERS

Creating a team

Our journey with Parkinson's disease will require a team of practitioners and supporters to help us through to the finish line where wellness awaits.

Our team may include (some or all of) a general practitioner (or PCP), neurologist, nutritionist, physiotherapist, naturopath, homeopath, herbalist, Pilates/yoga teacher, Bowen therapist, massage therapist, wife/husband/significant other, family members, friends, other people with Parkinson's on a similar journey.

When we choose a practitioner in a particular field, our range of choices may be wide or limited, depending on the discipline and our location. Sometimes it is better for our health to travel or use Skype consultations rather than remain with an unsatisfactory practitioner. My comments below are ideals. We will probably struggle to find a complete team in which every practitioner meets all criteria but, if we aim high, we are more likely to find satisfactory, supportive practitioners.

Qualities to look for

Characteristics we look for in practitioners are:
- Showing a willingness to give ample time for significant conversations about causes, treatments and plans;
- Being respectful and patient in conversation;
- Being open to contact and cooperate with other practitioners on our team;

- Showing a willingness to adjust treatments to suit our individual needs;
- Having an intention to help us develop wellness rather than treat disease;
- Remaining open to the possibility of recovery;
- Allowing us to bring ideas and questions to the consult;
- Keeping up to date with recent research and current ideas;
- Has experience in treating people with chronic disorders who are working toward wellness.

To be frank, some neurologists are arrogant and will not even consider moving beyond Western allopathic medicine. Some are bullies and assault patients with nocebo ("You *will* get worse"; "there is no cure and you *can't* help yourself"), while others will not give time for any discussion, expecting tacit obedience from patients. Where possible, move away from this type of practitioner to those who will, at least, treat you with respect and support your right to make choices that may not be totally in line with the expectations of Western allopathic medicine.

Where there is no choice of neurologist (e.g. in rural areas), you may want to limit your visits, perhaps to once each year, or travel annually to the closest city where you will have more choice.

It is often easier to find a GP/PCP who is prepared to allow you the right to make different choices and will assist with referrals to more appropriate neurologists.

Finding the right practitioners may take time and some experimentation. Several of my patients have seen three neurologists, several GP/PCP and a number of naturopaths before settling on a satisfactory team that works for them.

Complementary/alternative medicine practitioners can also be arrogant and/or closed-minded, but there is usually a greater range of choice. It is sometimes possible to have a five-minute chat with practitioners before making an appointment, or at least gain some information from their reception about the practitioner's attitude towards team work and recovery journeys.

Supportive and open-minded practitioners can enhance your journey to wellness.

Family members are a different challenge sometimes. When you read my story (Appendix 5 and/or my book *Shaky Past*[1]), you will see that I needed to "divorce" my family for a while in order to maintain a supportive environment around me. If your family is supportive, that is great! If not, and family members try to dissuade you from your recovery journey, or demand time and energy that you cannot afford while healing, reconstruct your relationship for the time needed. It is not easy but enhances healing.

Case history: *Gerald came to me in his early fifties diagnosed with idiopathic Parkinson's disease. He had significant tremor, some loss of fine motor skills and his speech was adversely affected. As he prided himself as a public speaker and master of ceremonies, his degenerating speech distressed him.*

Over the next twelve months, he made slow but significant progress. His speech became almost normal and his tremor was reduced in intensity.

During his final visit, Gerald told me he could not see me "for a while", as his wife wanted new window furnishings and they could not afford both. I tried to point out that, once he regained wellness, obtaining window furnishings would be easier, but they could probably wait for another year or so. But Gerald insisted that it was more important to make his wife happy and he would see me again when they had paid for the window furnishings and caught up financially.

I never saw Gerald again, but heard from mutual acquaintances that his health had deteriorated quite rapidly; his neurologist had prescribed heavy medication then referred Gerald for deep brain stimulation which was unsuccessful. Within four years, Gerald was ensconced in an assisted-living facility, needing help with most daily functions.

On the other hand, a supportive family is a fantastic recovery "medicine".

Case history: *Bruce was a retired businessman who was finding his Parkinson's disease symptoms quite distressing and could not increase his medication levels without exacerbated adverse effects.*

Bruce attended his first consult with me accompanied by his wife and three children who listened attentively to our discussion, asked intelligent questions, and wanted to know how they could best support Bruce on his journey.

At each subsequent visit, Bruce was supported by at least one and often two members of his family. All his family were active in helping Bruce plan his days, find appropriate therapists, and they encouraged him when he felt down.

Bruce continues to make excellent progress with this support.

You can recover on your own, but it is so much easier with a great, supportive team around you.

CHAPTER 32

DEGREES OF WELLNESS

What do you want to achieve? A reduction in your disease symptoms or real wellness?

My intention is to help you achieve total wellness. That is the aim of every strategy in this book. However, you may decide that being totally dedicated is not for you and all you want to do is reduce symptoms. That is your right. You are in control. But here is a word of warning: if you aim only to stop the disease progress and reduce symptoms, and gear your strategies around that, you will, inevitably, get worse. Only total dedication will gain wellness.

Michelangelo (1475–1564) said: "The greatest danger for most of us is not that our aim is too high and we miss it, but that it is too low and we achieve it".

Aiming for some relief from symptoms is likely to bring some success but, as time goes on and the aetiological pathways that produced those symptoms are not addressed, our health will deteriorate.

Aiming for recovery will bring relief from symptoms and, with total dedication, may make your dreams come true.

Stories of recovery

Roger

Roger was diagnosed with Parkinson's disease by a neurologist in Canberra, Australia, during May 2001. He had sought medical help for symptoms that had been developing for some time.

During 1995, he had noticed that he dribbled on the pillow during sleep. Over the ensuing six years, he progressively noticed that he developed pain in his shoulders when swimming freestyle, stiffness in his elbows and knees (bilateral), leg cramps, interrupted sleep (he would wake each night at about 2.30 am) and increasing tiredness. Roger became more concerned when he found difficulty in using a computer mouse and, six months prior to diagnosis, he developed tremors.

Following diagnosis with Parkinson's disease, his neurologist prescribed Sinemet 100/25 three times daily (300 mg levodopa daily) and gave him a normal brief prognosis – *There is no cure, there is nothing you can do, you will need more medication over time and, eventually need full-time care.* Roger felt that his neurologist displayed a lack of compassion, understanding and support. He was given no idea that he should reduce stress or look for other ways to help himself.

In June 2003, Roger came to see me when referred by one of my professional colleagues. He was concerned that his condition was deteriorating and the only help offered was more drugs. He was extremely busy in his professional life, participated in local government, endured a stressful marriage relationship, and had little time to rest or relax.

My questioning revealed a family history of degenerative disorders (although no Parkinson's disease), poor sibling relationships, low self-esteem in childhood, and a need to compensate by being "successful". I recommended a minimum of 15 minutes meditation each day, reduction of stress, dietary changes, Aqua Hydration Formulas, Bowen therapy, increased water intake, and some supplements.

Roger sent me an email in December 2003 stating that his condition was stable, he had reduced his medication, and had become president of a state-based Parkinson's disease association.

I saw Roger again nine months later, and he said that he

"feels the best he's felt in years". He had resumed playing tennis, swam three times weekly, was following all of my recommendations, was seeing a Bowen therapist each two weeks and had reduced his Sinemet to one tablet twice daily (200 mg levodopa daily). His leg cramps were now intermittent, and I suggested an increase in magnesium.

By March 2006, Roger had reduced his medication to ½ tablet twice daily (100 mg levodopa daily), was still swimming and active in local government, plus his busy professional life; he was noticing his dreams were more peaceful and felt generally pleased with his progress. On the negative side, he was experiencing tightness and tiredness in his hamstring and lower leg muscles.

I had no contact with Roger after that until 2010 when he called me to "bring me up to date". It seems that Roger slipped into some old habits after 2006. He allowed his life to become more stressful, forgot the dietary rules, let his meditation lapse, and forgot that his primary aim was to get well. His health began to deteriorate as a consequence, and Parkinson's disease symptoms increased again.

Then, after about two years, he found my *Stop Parkin' and Start Livin'* book (published 2005) and decided to re-dedicate himself to wellness. In his words, "I followed your advice to the letter," with triumphant results.

By early 2010, Roger was free from all symptoms, needed no medication, had developed a new loving relationship, maintained a sensible professional life, and become president of a national Parkinson's disease association.

I met Roger again at a lecture for people with Parkinson's disease at a country centre in Victoria (Australia) during early November 2010. He looked very well, was maintaining his good health, showed absolutely no symptoms of Parkinson's disease, and was enthusiastic about my recovery program.

Roger is not "cured" of Parkinson's disease. Through his own efforts in following a sensible, health-giving program, he has developed so much wellness in his body and mind that there is no room for illness. This is what we call RECOVERY.

Lionel

Lionel was 83 years old when he first came to see me. He had been diagnosed with idiopathic Parkinson's disease about a year earlier after a slow onset of symptoms over many years, but was also troubled with emphysema, hiatus hernia, reflux, hypertension and hypoglycaemia.

His list of prescribed medications included one levodopa drug, one anti-nausea drug, a drug for reflux, two drugs for hypertension, one antidepressant and two drugs to control the symptoms of emphysema.

Lionel's symptoms were dramatic and debilitating: he was unable to walk without support from a walking frame, but often fell even using the frame; he had significant tremor, paucity of movement and frequent freezing; his hypertension was not fully controlled in spite of the two drugs prescribed; he was nauseous most of the time and, because of that, lacked appetite; he experienced gastric reflux frequently despite drug prescriptions; he was chronically depressed despite his antidepressant drug.

After investigating his history and current circumstances, we commenced on a basic "improving health program", including changing his food choices (see earlier chapters), increasing water intake, regular moderate exercise, meditation, Aqua Hydration Formulas daily and Bowen therapy weekly.

Regular follow up appointments, each 8-10 weeks apart, showed some improvements in strength and appetite, but there seemed to be little or no progress in mobility, balance, tremor, paucity of movement or persistent nausea. Despite this, Lionel continued with his program in the hope of improving his quality of life. I was disappointed that there was not more improvement, but supported Lionel in his choice to continue with the "standard" protocol.

Exactly one year eleven months and two weeks after our first consult, Lionel's wife called me in tears. She said, "Lionel is outside walking around the back yard!"

"Why?" I asked, feeling rather puzzled and quite worried at this start to our conversation.

Her reply was simply, "Because he can!"

On that day, Lionel had suddenly felt confident in his ability to stand and walk, had left his walking frame in the living room, and started walking a circuit around his yard. This was the first time in nearly three years that he had been able to walk without support.

From then on, Lionel made good progress. His strength improved, balance and mobility continued to improve, his tremor slowly reduced (although it took another three years to disappear), his general outlook on life improved dramatically (he had gained hope of a better-quality of life) and his appetite increased. We were able to reduce his antidepressant medication (remember, most antidepressants have the possibility of exacerbating Parkinson's disease symptoms) and he increased his social activity, which brought joy to both Lionel and his wife.

However, a persistent problem was daily nausea. This did not seem to be influenced by any particular foods, so we were puzzled. Lionel found this persistent symptom distressing as it reduced his enjoyment of life. We tried herbal remedies and homeopathics without success.

After becoming frustrated with this nausea puzzle, I produced a chart of Lionel's medication including the most common adverse effects noted by each manufacturer (therefore real, not imagined by a biased investigator). Here is how it looked:

Reflux drug	nausea	weakness	depression	rash	
Nausea drug	nausea	weakness	nervousness	rash	reflux
Levodopa drug	nausea	weakness	anxiety		
Blood pressure	nausea	weakness			
Blood pressure	nausea	weakness	anxiety	rash	infection
Anti-depressant	nausea	weakness	anxiety	rash	
Emphysyma drug	nausea				
Emphysyma drug	nausea				

All his drugs had the possibility of nausea, five had the possibility of anxiety/nervousness/depression, while his nausea drug could cause reflux for which he was taking a drug that could cause nausea.

The "polypharmacy" prescription seemed illogical to me, so I wrote a letter with the above chart for Lionel to take to his doctor. I had little hope that the doctor would take notice, but felt I had to try.

Lionel's doctor was attentive and understanding, read the letter, and immediately stopped everything except levodopa (which Lionel still needed) and one blood pressure drug. The nausea reduced rapidly and, with some very low-dose herbs, disappeared entirely within three months. Most of his challenge had been drugs that had been prescribed to offset the adverse effects of other drugs. His GP was smart enough, and adventurous enough, to reduce Lionel's unnecessary drug intake (without any ill effect) and resolved a major quality of life challenge.

Eventually we were able to wean Lionel off his levodopa drug with no return of Parkinson's disease symptoms.

Over the next couple of years, I kept in touch with Lionel as his health continued to improve. My last contact was when he was 96 years old, enjoying life, active in the community, and living without any Parkinson's disease symptoms.

There are some clear lessons from Lionel's story:

- If he had not persisted against all odds for two years, he would not have made progress, and would have spent his remaining years miserable, incapacitated and nauseous. Persistence is key if we want to recover.

- Drugs are usually prescribed with our best interests in mind. However, sometimes doctors and specialists prescribe drugs without thoroughly investigating the possibility of interactions and/or accumulative adverse effects. Therefore, it is worth checking regularly with your GP to make sure your symptoms are not drug-related.

- Age is no barrier to wellness. Lionel was 83 when he started the process of recovery.

- Recovery needs our full attention and dedication. We cannot "play" at getting well. We must be fully engaged with the process and be willing to make all the changes needed to reach our goal of living without symptoms.

CHAPTER 33

STEPS TO RECOVERY

Reversing the illness process of Parkinson's disease will require your full attention and dedication. Your work, family, hobbies and life in general must all become less important than changing your daily activities, commitments and programs to focus on becoming so well that illness no longer is part of your life.

The information in the last 32 chapters may seem overwhelming, too much for you to tackle. Don't despair, here is a step-by-step guide to changing your life from an illness process to a wellness process.

1. Recognise that you have developed an illness process that has been diagnosed as a neurodegenerative disorder that cannot be "cured".

2. Understand that a "cure" is not required; many people have recovered.

3. Write down as much of your history as you can remember. Include:

    a. when you were born – any difficult social or family circumstances at the time;

    b. where you were born – any potential toxic hazards such as chemical exposure;

    c. good and bad memories of childhood – time with parents, siblings and the broader family;

    d. significant times of your life – school, achievements, losses, work successes and stressors, use of chemicals, exposure to bullying;

    e.   illnesses and accidents;

    f.   medications prescribed for any reason.

4. Use Section 2 to help decide what processes have created the symptoms diagnosed as Parkinson's disease – there are generally two or even three.

5. Where needed, use some of the processes and tests in Chapter 11 to really understand what has created these symptoms.

6. Begin your journal that will record your pathway from illness to wellness. Keep notes at least once each week.

7. You will now be able to see that you do not have a "disease" but a set of symptoms with causes that you can understand.

8. Make changes to your food intake so that you are eating only food that helps you – Chapter 13.

9. Add the basic nutritional supplements in Chapter 15 to assist health improvement.

10. Introduce the Aqua Hydration Formulas as in Chapter 19.

11. Review your exercise/activity regimen. If you have been sedentary, consult your doctor or complementary/alternative medicine practitioner about safely beginning regular exercise – high-intensity interval training, Pilates, boxing, etc. Make sure you begin an exercise program at least four days each week.

12. Speak with your doctor or complementary/alternative medicine practitioner about dealing with specific illness processes such as past traumas (Chapter 23), toxins (Chapter 25) and infections (Chapter 26).

13. Review Chapter 12-18 and add extra wellness strategies one-by-one until you are satisfied that you have included all

free and low-cost "medicines" – laughter, self-love, meditation, singing and dancing.

14. Review the company you keep – are your companions positive, happy, supportive of your choices? If not, make changes.

15. Consider bodywork, especially Bowen therapy. If you are unable to find a Bowen therapist within a one-hour drive of your home, consider craniosacral therapy or gentle massage each two to three weeks.

16. Review your healthcare team. Doctor, neurologist, complementary/alternative medicine practitioners, Bowen therapist, massage therapist, personal trainer or physiotherapist; are they all "on the same page"? Are they all open to your focus on wellness and supportive of your choices? If not, consider making changes where possible.

17. Be patient and dedicated. You have created a pathway that can lead to wellness over time. My pathway was three years, Lionel's was six years. Some have taken longer. Your journal will guide you and help you see the positive progress and what changes you may need to make to your program of wellness.

18. As you walk this pathway to wellness, review one chapter of *Rethinking Parkinson's Disease* each two weeks to make sure you are staying on track. It is easy to slip into old habits, so it is healthy and helpful to review our activities, protocols and programs regularly to ensure that we are always moving towards recovery.

SECTION 4

OTHER THINGS TO THINK ABOUT

CHAPTER 34

EVIDENCE-BASED MEDICINE

Is it really evidence-based?

Reports in major media, and commentary by conservative Western medical scientists or doctors often compare "evidence-based medicine" with "alternative medicine". The implications is that all Western allopathic medicine (WAM) is based on solid, high-quality evidence, while no "alternative medicine" (complementary/alternative medicine – CAM) has any worthwhile evidence to support it.

The truth is somewhere between these two implications.

Western allopathic medicine sets a very high standard for ideal evidence to support a drug, treatment or surgical procedure. The "gold standard" for "unfiltered information" is a double-blind randomised placebo-controlled clinical trial (DBRCT) with a large population and excellent methodology, while evidence considered to be at the top of the pyramid (the best evidence) is systematic reviews of published trials and studies.

Medical/drug control bodies in major countries (FDA in USA, TGA in Australia, and similar bodies elsewhere) purport to apply these same standards to all forms of treatment – prescribed pharmaceutical medicine and medical procedures (WAM), CAM prescriptions and procedures, and over-the-counter (OTC) medicines.

If this standard was truly applied to all treatments from all forms of medicine, we could feel safer when seeking treatment or purchasing OTC medicine. But this is far from the truth and the public is left with part truth, part silence and part lies.

Questions to answer are whether DBRCT is the best, most efficient and most accurate way to test treatments or groups of treatments, whether it is possible to conduct a systematic review when there has been little or no effort to conduct basic trials of treatments, and whether systematic reviews reflect the bias of the reviewers rather than being an unbiased view of the available research; these will be discussed a little later.

Evidence-based medicine hierarchies rank study types based on the rigour of their research methods. Different hierarchies exist for different question types, and even acknowledged experts disagree on the exact rank of information in the evidence hierarchies. The following image represents the hierarchy of evidence provided by the National Health and Medical Research Council (NHMRC) in Australia (2014).[1]

Most experts agree that the higher up the hierarchy the study

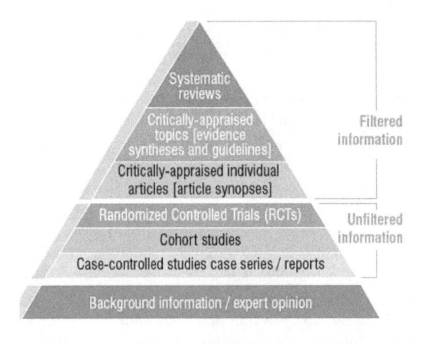

design is positioned, the more rigorous the methodology, and hence the more likely it is that the study design can minimise the effect of bias on the results of the study. In most evidence hierarchies, current, well-designed systematic reviews and meta-analyses are at the top of the pyramid, and expert opinion and anecdotal experience are at the bottom.[2]

Most major pharmaceutical drugs are supported by significant evidence for their major purpose. For instance, levodopa drugs (Sinemet, Madopar and others) are quite well understood and have been proven moderately effective and fairly safe for the treatment of idiopathic Parkinson's disease. Levodopa drugs are rarely prescribed for any other purpose.

However, some drugs are studied and trialled, and approved, for a particular purpose, then prescribed for an entirely different purpose ("off-label"), based on guesswork and conjecture. For instance, a drug used for treating cancer, and supported by evidence for this use, is often prescribed for autoimmune disorders, with no gold standard evidence supporting that off-label application.

A further challenge in these cases is severe adverse effects. When treating cancer (often a fiercely acute disease), the risk of significant adverse effects is weighed against the benefits of killing cancer cells quickly and judgements made on that basis. Autoimmune disorders, on the other hand, are generally chronic and idiopathic. While the cancer drugs are prescribed at lower doses for this purpose, the adverse effects can, and do, accumulate, causing illness and misery for patients.

Reading official drug guides highlights another challenge. Many drugs are not fully understood. Phrases such as "The mechanism of XXXX is not understood" or "the effect of XXXX on the YYYY is presumed to be ..." should cause great doubt in prescribers.[3]

Very few drugs are trialled over a long period. Trials vary from a few weeks to a year (rare). In a few cases, follow up studies have been undertaken over several years but, again, this is very rare. Adverse effects often accumulate over time so that, when a drug is declared "safe" and with "no side effects", the statements are based on a few weeks of experience. Patients may take these medicines for years and, as adverse effects accumulate, become quite ill, yet be treated for "another disease" (caused by adverse effects) with different drugs which may also create adverse effects over time.

Yet another challenge is the limited aim of any medication trial. Drugs or supplements are usually trialled to support their use for very specific purposes without necessarily answering the question of whether that purpose is valid and/or whether making changes with a particular medication will adversely affect other body systems not being observed in this study.

We have recently seen an example of the weaknesses in the current hierarchy of evidence with the news that aspirin, long prescribed at low dose as a prophylactic against cardiovascular disease (CVD), has been found to cause more disease than it prevents. A report in Australian Doctor in 2019 states that:

> Based on the totality of evidence, they found that aspirin was associated with significant reductions in cardiovascular mortality, non-fatal myocardial infarction and non-fatal stroke compared with no aspirin. The absolute risk reduction was 0.38 per cent.
>
> However, aspirin use was also linked to significant increased risks of major bleeding, intracranial bleeding and major gastrointestinal bleeding events versus no aspirin, with an absolute risk increase of 0.47 per cent.[4]

The original trials of aspirin focused only on the goal of reducing cardiovascular accidents so did not alert researchers to the dangers.

Aspirin has been prescribed for decades and is still widely prescribed/advised for prevention of cardiovascular disorders in many countries. We have no way of knowing how many people have been damaged or killed because of the limited nature of supporting evidence.

This doesn't not make aspirin bad medicine, but it does show that we need better ways to judge the efficacy and safety of treatment, especially for chronic use.

Other common examples of narrow-focused medicine that I have seen often in my clinic are patients who present for hypertension in their twenties and are prescribed an anti-hypertensive drug. Most manufactures recommend changing the medication each two years, but this rarely happens, and patients may take the same drug for twenty or more years. Over this time, the patients begin to experience anxiety or depression caused by the medication, so are prescribed an anti-anxiety or antidepressant drugs. Many manufacturers recommend that anti-anxiety and antidepressants drugs should be taken for no more than four weeks without thorough review but, all too often, I see patients who have been taking the same anxiety/depression drug for ten to twenty years with no change. A long-term adverse effect of these drugs may be tremor or twitching, somnolence, and slowed movement. When the patient presents with these symptoms, they are often diagnosed with Parkinson's disease and prescribed levodopa drugs. Levodopa may exacerbate anxiety, so the anti-anxiety drugs are increased. Levodopa may also interrupt the sleep pattern, so the patient is prescribed an anti-convulsant drug for sleep which has its own long-term adverse effects.

None of the drugs mentioned above are necessarily bad, and some are quite well studied. But there is no gold standard evidence for polypharmacy or the way these drugs are prescribed in circumstances similar to the ones I have described. Yet these circumstances are common.

Surgery is often necessary and may be lifesaving. However, much elective surgery is unnecessary and represents the "easy way out" for those who choose to rely on quick fixes rather than long-term self-help processes. More importantly, no surgical procedure has gold standard proof of efficacy or safety. The reasons for this are obvious: trials cannot be double-blind because the surgeon knows whether or not they are performing surgery. Furthermore, anatomy varies to a significant degree from person to person so each surgical procedure is, of necessity, slightly or very different from the last.

The best evidence for surgical procedures is patients who benefit from that procedure with no adverse effects. Surgical procedures must be based on necessity (e.g. removal of a tumour, or foreign body otherwise inaccessible), prospect of long-term benefits from the procedure (e.g. lifesaving, improved quality of life, pain reduction long-term), safety (e.g. no history of death or adverse effects from this procedure) and surgical competence (i.e. the surgeon has been well trained and supervised).

Evidence-based medicine has assumed a number of guises over the years since the concept was introduced and attempts to explain exactly what it means flounder in obscurity of meaning. Stories in *Medical Observer* in 2012 and 2017 seem to support the use of evidence-based medicine, but reach the conclusion that the effective application of evidence-based medicine depends on evidence-based education for evidence-based medicine. Yes, this is confusing, but discussed seriously in an online medical journal.[5]

A significant challenge that I see in all attempts to explain and support evidence-based medicine is the selection of controls in DBRCT, selection of studies to examine in meta-analyses, and the ongoing and overwhelming dominance of industry funding of research used in evidence-based medicine.

Professor John P. A. Ioannidis holds a number of prestigious posts, including Professor of Epidemiology and Population Health at Stanford University. He believes that Evidence-based Medicine (EBM) has been "hijacked" by those desiring positive outcomes to further career, status or profit.

In the *Journal of Clinical Epidemiology* 73 (2016) pages 82-86, he laments that industry dominates the medical research environment and studies often are conducted with the wrong criteria and expectations. He also believes that "Under market pressure, clinical medicine has become finance-based medicine."

Professor Ioannidis's exposition is available without charge through a link on Dr Justin Coleman's GP Sceptics Podcast.[6]

None of the comments above make Western allopathic medicine "bad medicine" or "unproven medicine", but they do mean that we must assess each treatment on its merits rather than blindly accepting that Western allopathic medicine is "evidence-based".

Complementary/alternative medicine does, in fact, have significant evidence supporting many treatments. Many herbs have been in use for thousands of years so their activity, efficacy and safety are well understood. Homeopathic medicine has been in continual use and research for over 200 years, with many excellent trials supporting its use. Over the past forty years, many DBRCT have been undertaken for single herbs or homeopathic remedies and have proven the accuracy of traditional knowledge.

The Victorian State Government (Australia) has developed a "Better Health" website to disseminate information about a wide range of health matters. On their Complementary Therapies page, there are useful and informative statements mixed with the usual platitudes and dogma. The page states:

> Some therapies or modalities are based on principles that are not recognised by conventional medicine, but have an established evidence base and have been proven to work for a limited number of health conditions.[7]

In 2014, a medical journal report estimated that the standard of proof for Western allopathic medicine and complementary/alternative medicine was about equal, and both had to rely more on clinical outcomes and traditional use for support, as good-quality DBRCT were in the minority. A more shocking admission in *The Lancet* was published in 2015.

In *The Lancet*'s April 11 edition (2015), editor-in-chief Dr Richard Horton published his own perspectives on the symposium. In what amounts to an editorial, entitled "What is medicine's 5 sigma", he wrote:

> *A lot of what is published is incorrect. I'm not allowed to say who made this remark because we were asked to observe Chatham House rules. We were also asked not to take photographs of slides. Why the paranoid concern for secrecy and non-attribution? Because this symposium on the reproducibility and reliability of biomedical research touched on one of the most sensitive issues in science today: the idea that something has gone fundamentally wrong with one of our greatest human creations. The case against science is straightforward: much of the scientific literature, perhaps half, may simply be untrue. Afflicted by studies with small sample sizes, tiny effects, invalid exploratory analyses, and flagrant conflicts of interest, together with an obsession for pursuing fashionable trends of dubious importance, science has taken a turn towards darkness. As one participant put it, poor methods get results.*[8]

Fundamental to the standard of evidence is what we expect to learn from treatment trials. DBRCT are based on one drug or treatment in isolation, and the effect on selected symptoms or criteria. However, this drug or treatment may be only one small part of an overall treatment plan for a patient. The DBRCT will give us information about the safety of the treatment in the short term, and the effect on selected symptoms. It will not give any information about the efficacy or safety of this treatment in combination with other treatments, or for particular sub-populations who may be more vulnerable to toxins or adverse effects.

Another problem facing those looking for unbiased studies or trials for medication is the fact that most drug and equipment trials (and supplement/CAM studies) are funded and/or conducted by the manufacturers. It is unreasonable to expect that companies whose sole purpose is to create profit for shareholders (which is their legitimate and expected purpose) could be completely unbiased in any assessment of their own product.

Treatment for most illnesses, particularly chronic illness, requires a multi-faceted approach, often including a number of drugs, supplements, herbals, activities, dietary changes and lifestyle adjustments. There are no possible DBRCT available for these comprehensive treatment plans.

In a few cases, excellent population studies have provided information on particular lifestyle choices or long-term use of prophylaxis, but these studies are very expensive, lack the promise of immediate profits, and so are rare.

When looking for evidence supporting various treatments for Parkinson's disease, there is a wide variety of research styles and quality. Levodopa drugs are supported by good-quality studies since the 1960s and have proven to be the drugs of choice for long-term symptom control. Long-term adverse effects of levodopa drugs were discovered during clinical use, not in DBRCT.

Evidence based medicine is the conscientious, explicit, and judicious use of current best evidence in making decisions about the care of individual patients." (from BMJ 1996).[9]

This definition from the *British Medical Journal* does not distinguish between forms or styles of medicine, but emphasises the importance of making care decisions that are right for each individual patient. That is the way it should be.

Meta-analyses and systematic reviews are at the top of the evidence pyramid, in the view of conservative medical authorities. They are considered to be relatively free from bias. But is this really the case?

A review of complementary/alternative medicine in Australia in 2015 has shown how biased these reviews can be when conducted with predetermined outcomes in mind. The reviewers claimed to have examined thousands of trials and studies but, in fact, carefully selected 176 studies conducted in Australia only (they rejected all international studies) and, from those, reviewed five systematic reviews by reading *only the abstracts*. Furthermore, none of the reviewers had any training or experience in the treatment modalities examined.[10,11]

Despite the ludicrous shortcomings of the review, national and international policy has depended on the findings that there is no evidence for the effectiveness of sixteen complementary/alternative medicine modalities in treating seventeen ailments.

This systematic review is at the top of the evidence-based medicine hierarchy, yet is patently biased, useless and misleading to the point of danger. Untrained reviewers examined five abstracts of other (possibly biased) systematic reviews and determined policy outcomes for sixteen complementary/alternative medicine modalities, seventeen ailments, thousands of practitioners and millions of patients.

We must establish better ways to judge the efficacy and safety of both Western allopathic medicine and complementary/alternative medicine treatments by working together without bias or predetermined views.

Research

Research is vital to understand how best to maintain health, prevent illness and reverse disease, but research must be focused on important matters of health rather than improving the bottom line for the drug, equipment or supplement industries.

I believe that the only way we can achieve excellence in research and unbiased evidence-based medicine knowledge is to demand that every company (national or international) that sells drugs, medical equipment, herbs or supplements gives a set percentage of their turnover (not profit) to a research body managed by an independent body controlled by the best minds in Western allopathic medicine and complementary/alternative medicine, plus traditional Chinese medicine (TCM), Ayurvedic medicine and allied health professionals who assess the benefits of each proposed research project against established criteria. This would provide billions of dollars for effective and independent research no longer dominated by the richest industry in the world, or one form of medicine that lacks tradition and holistic views.

Where studies are of food products, food producers should also be required to contribute to the cost, and outcomes must be the basis of policies around those food industries. For instance, good quality research has shown that consumption of animal dairy products (except butter and ghee) increases the risk of Parkinson's disease and other disorders significantly. Yet a number of governments spend huge amounts of money supporting an industry that makes people sick. On the other hand, despite proven benefits of growing food without chemicals, organic farmers receive little or no governmental support and may, in fact, be penalised with onerous regulations.

Studies involving large populations over many centres, looking at total "packages" – lifestyle, food, personal care, activity, social interaction – using controls of those living "normal" lives will expand knowledge without necessarily increasing profits for any industry.

For the treatment of Parkinson's disease, we need the facility to guide large numbers of diagnosed patients into exploring aetiologies, changing their lifestyle and habits, then comparing long-term outcomes with those untreated or using standard conservative Western allopathic medicine treatment only.

Evidence-based medicine is only valid when the evidence is broad-based, unbiased, created by bodies with no vested interest, focused on human health rather than symptom control, and can withstand rigorous examination over many years.

True evidence-based medicine can only be achieved with independent funding and control.

This is a utopian dream, of course, unless we ever find politicians willing to sacrifice their careers for the health of their constituents. Will this ever happen?

CHAPTER 35

WHAT DO WE NEED NOW?

Parkinson's associations around the world estimate that between seven and ten million people have been diagnosed with Parkinson's disease. This does not include those in the prodromal phase and/or undiagnosed.

This is an enormous drain on resources in treatment and care costs, and loss of expertise and productivity. Even more importantly, this represents over seven million people living with fear and misery, perhaps unnecessarily.

Parkinson's Australia commissioned Deloitte Access Economics in 2014 to prepare a report on the costs of Parkinson's disease in Australia. This report, available online,[1] estimated the annual cost of Parkinson's disease to the Australian economy at nearly 10 billion dollars! The number of people affected in Australia was estimated to be between 81,000 and 110,000. As the incidence of Parkinson's disease and the economic costs rise each year, these figures will be significantly exceeded by the time this is published.

A very interesting section of this extensive report is section 2.2 "What Causes PD?". While describing idiopathic or primary Parkinson's disease as having no known cause (section 2.1.1), the report goes on in section 2.2 to describe several possible causes, including accelerated ageing, oxidative damage, environmental toxins and genetic predisposition (for some reason indicating Alpha-synuclein as a gene instead of a protein). There are also some risk factors described, including male gender, Caucasian ancestry, herbicide/pesticide exposure, rural residence, higher intake of dietary fats (without distinguishing the type of fats), metal exposure (without detailing which metals), family history, stress, depression and head trauma (Hauser et al., 2015; NINDS 2014).[2]

Some protective factors listed include consumption of antioxidants, early-life measles infection, consumption of food and drink containing niacin and caffeine, and smoking (Hauser et al., 2015; NINDS 2014).[3] While the smoking and caffeine research have been largely discredited and niacin is proving of limited benefit, the link of better health and lower disease risk with dietary factors and lifestyle, and ways to mitigate known risks, have been almost completely ignored in the push for a "cure" or drugs to better control symptoms.

It is time to look beyond the strictures of the WAM view of one disease, one cause and one cure. In a world staggering under the burden of chronic illness, with ever-increasing rates of Parkinson's disease and related neurodegenerative disorders, we have a responsibility to put aside preconceived ideas, tunnel vision, dogmatic commercial propaganda and bigotry to fully explore all aetiological pathways leading to diagnosis with neurodegenerative disorders, including Parkinson's disease, and all rational, non-toxic strategies to reverse those processes.

Vision

We need:

- to look beyond the selfishness and self-serving paradigm of cause-disease-cure to explore a broader concept of wellness creation becoming more powerful than disease creation and maintenance;
- to embrace all forms of medicine and wellness strategies as part of a cooperative and powerful move towards a healthier and happier society.

Research

We need:

- analysis of the benefits or harm of all food groups and preparation processes on our health through life;
- cell hydration, benefits and strategies;
- extensive analysis of the aetiological pathways explored here and others that may become significant during aetiological pathway research;
- independent investigation of environmental toxins, removed from the control or influence of the manufacturers and vested interest;
- lifestyle strategies for wellness and how best to construct education campaigns to encourage the general population to live well;
- practitioner/patient relationships that help or harm;
- much more.

Leadership

We need:

- Illness has people like Michael J Fox, Clyde Campbell and Liz Cantor dedicating themselves to improving lives of those living with Parkinson's disease and ongoing research. This leadership, altruistic and with the best of intentions, is based on the premise that Parkinson's disease is a discrete and individual disease and that only Western allopathic medicine can find a "cure".
- We need people of this stature to promote the concept of wellness and to help raise funds for the research above.
- Without such leadership, we will struggle to move out of the dominance of "cure profitability" strategies.

Innovation

We need:

- a new look at evidence. The "Gold Standard" for

evidence promoted by Western allopathic medicine is a double-blind, randomised, placebo-controlled trial with a large population. However such trials are open to manipulation and abuse and, because of cost, are often short-term. Furthermore, many wellness strategies (e.g. dietary changes) do not lend themselves to such trials;

- a wide range of highly-qualified people from Western allopathic medicine and complementary/alternative medicine to develop innovative research methods that will provide realistic and reproducible results;
- new ways to interpret past and current trials that do not necessarily prove what is claimed;
- innovative ways to reach people at risk of neurodegeneration in order to alleviate the burden of disease on them, their families and society;
- innovative use of social media and public broadcasters to foster an attitude of wellness as we age instead of an expectation of illness;
- new Centres of Excellence focusing on wellness strategies and self-help strategies in place of those teaching us how to "live with illness".

Discourse

We need:

- open and respectful conversations between Western allopathic medicine and complementary/alternative medicine practitioners and researchers, exploring the contribution that all forms of medicine and research can offer to people with Parkinson's and those in the prodromal period;
- cessation of abuse and denigration of complementary/alternative medicine practitioners and researchers by Western allopathic medicine and its pharmaceutical-sponsored "support" organisations;

- a public move by Western allopathic medicine to distance itself from rambunctious anti-health campaigners mis-quoting dubious studies to denigrate complementary/alternative medicine healthcare practitioners;
- engagement of government agencies like the National Health and Medical Research Council in Australia, and similar bodies in other countries, with complementary/alternative medicine practitioners and researchers as equal partners in the work to improve the health status of all people in our society;
- a change of language to promote and focus on lifestyle and self-help strategies to promote health throughout life, rather than just treating illness or using drug therapy to prevent one illness with methods that may cause other illnesses.

Funding

Facts:

- Of all medical/health research funding, less than one per cent is spent on prevention research.
- Prevention research is largely dominated by Western allopathic medicine and so generally focuses on vaccine/drug prevention of single illnesses (often with unintended adverse effects) or outdated lifestyle/dietary strategies.
- We need funding for genuine and clinically supported lifestyle and dietary prevention strategies that is untied. Currently most funding is provided by non-pharmaceutical companies seeking to promote dietary supplement products, practitioners with particular interests or rare benefactors.
- National governments have a responsibility to enhance the health of their constituents (a responsibility most governments neglect in favour of illness treatment) and must allocate a much greater percentage of research funding

to prevention research distant from vested interest, with guidance from Western allopathic medicine and complementary/alternative medicine in equal measure.

- We urgently need Centres of Excellence focused on providing and teaching lifestyle and dietary strategies to enhance health and prevent disease. Currently all these centres are privately owned and funded by client contributions, which places access beyond all except those with a high degree of disposable income.

- All governments should allocate at least one per cent of their health/illness budget each year to prevention research and education with equal voices from Western allopathic medicine and complementary/alternative medicine. In Australia, this would mean, in 2019, 1.5 *billion dollars* spent on prevention strategies and research, ultimately yielding an ever-decreasing burden of health/ illness care on the economy. I realise that this objective is in the realm of building fairy gardens to entertain politicians in their dotage and there is no political profit or benefit in preventing illness (it is really hard to publicise something that doesn't happen). However, perhaps there are one or two altruistic politicians who will push for a much greater allocation of funds for illness preventing and life enhancement.

We CAN achieve some or all of these needs if we all focus on wellness and illness prevention, talk openly to our Western allopathic medicine and complementary/alternative medicine practitioners, politicians and business leaders. One person is a whisper, a thousand people is a murmur, 70,000 people (1 per cent of those diagnosed with Parkinson's disease) demand attention, and one million people constitute a roar that will be heard around the world. It starts with you and me.

APPENDICES

APPENDIX 1

LOW-TOXICITY LIVING

My view

The comments below on products designed for various uses are my own opinions derived from research and experience. My knowledge is confined mainly to Australia, so I have not tried to list healthy alternatives. Rather, I have attempted to warn you of the dangers of becoming too focused on sterility and appearance to the detriment of your health. Do your own research, read your alternative press, talk to your health food store proprietors and use as few personal care products as possible.

Living a low-toxicity life is essential for all those wishing to live a truly healthy life. It is *critical* for those of us who have developed any degenerative or chronic disorder. Every synthetic chemical we have contact with will have a negative effect on our physical and/or mental/emotional function. Sometimes we deliberately choose to use synthetic chemicals where we believe the benefits will outweigh the risks – for instance, when using some medications, driving our motor vehicle, flying overseas, or using antibiotics to combat a serious infection. But these circumstances need to be the exception rather than the rule.

Hints for living a low-toxicity life

Look at your work environment – if you work in an environment that exposes you to chemicals, air-conditioning of doubtful quality, light exclusively from fluoro tubes, or very high, unremitting stress, it may be time to think about a change in occupation. Yes, we may need to continue working to earn money to pay for food, clothes, education and therapies. But do we need as much money? Can we earn a reasonable living doing something less toxic while we recover? Do we ever want to go back to our toxic occupation?

Eliminate toxic chemicals from your home. Cleaning products, air fresheners, disinfectants etc., are all highly toxic – many are neurotoxic (that is why there are such strong warnings on the label). Find alternatives (look at the suggestions below) – there is always another way to do the job.

Petroleum-based chemicals are some of the most toxic in our world, and are used in many synthetic compounds such as oil-based paint, perfume, cosmetics, many cleaning products, petrol, baby oil, medicinal creams and some medications. Avoid being around petroleum-based chemicals in general, especially petrol (ask someone else to fill your tank while you stay in the car with the windows up, or better still, avoid the petrol station altogether). I use liquefied petroleum gas (LPG) in my car. This is not available in all countries but is a useful and inexpensive alternative in Australia. However, even though my vehicle is filled with a closed system (no fumes), the smell and fumes of others filling their cars with petrol at the same service station can quickly give me a headache, or some digestive disturbance. I try to fill my car during quiet times. If you use petrol and have to fill your car yourself, wear gloves (keep gardening or rubber cloves in your car), and turn your head away from the filler to avoid fumes. Always take more vitamin C on the day you fill up.

What to avoid

There are classes of chemicals commonly used in both household and personal care products that we need to avoid at all costs. Most of these are derived from petrochemicals, but some are otherwise synthesised in the laboratory. Avoid polyethylene glycol (PEG), sulfates and sulfides, sodium/ammonium laurel sulfates and sodium/ammonium laureth sulfates, ethoxylates, parabens, propylene glycol, silicones, phthalates, mineral oils, artificial colours, flavours and sweeteners. This list is not exhaustive as new chemicals are introduced each year. We don't know what most of them are, their names or composition, as manufacturing companies only need approval from a government department. They don't have to tell us what they are or what they do.

In most countries, manufacturers do have to list contents on the pack of each product (the thoroughness of this varies widely between countries). However, often the chemicals are listed by number rather than name. In this case, my policy is; *"If you can't spell it, pronounce it, understand it, or know what the number means, don't buy the product without further investigation."*

Cleaning products

Avoid using harsh cleaning products at all. First, use water (this cleans off a remarkable amount of dirt and grime with no further cleaning needed). If required, add some bicarbonate of soda, eucalyptus oil (an amazing cleaning product), white vinegar or pure, organic detergent-free "soap".

Where you are unhappy with the results of the above cleaning suggestions, ask at your health food store, organic store, or check out the "alternative press" for products that won't poison you.

There are a large number of microfibre cloths available now that clean very well without harsh chemicals. They are especially good for cleaning bathrooms, timber floors and dusting (which is very helpful for asthmatics and those with a dust allergy). Start off by buying the better quality cloths from the supermarket to see how they work. If you are as happy as I am with these moderately priced products, you won't need to spend your money on the more expensive products, or multi-level marketing products claiming spurious superiority.

If you must use a cleaning product, avoid those that contain petrochemicals, phosphates, organochlorines, synthetic fragrances and colours, or any of the chemical groups named above. Just because a product is labelled "bio-degradable" does not mean it is low-toxicity. If you do have cleaning chemicals in your home (other than those listed above as low-toxicity), get rid of them in a toxic waste disposal facility. Or, better still, get someone more robust to take them away for you.

Buy a book of old home remedies and you will have lots of ideas for low-toxicity cleaning. Many (perhaps most) "old wives" cleaning ideas work.

Avoid bleach at all costs, as it is very neurotoxic.

Here are some natural low-toxicity products that are useful in cleaning your house (and you):

Water

"Elbow grease" (muscle power)

Bi-carb soda – great for absorbing smells and is good in the bathroom and kitchen.

Vinegar (white) – good for polishing glass, tiles, metal, mirrors, ceramic surfaces and floors. It is also a good conditioner for silk and wool. If you have burned-on cooking stains on your stainless steel cookware, soak them with vinegar for several hours, then scrub. It works a treat!

Lemon juice mixed with table or sea salt makes a good abrasive scrub for chopping boards and other rugged surfaces.

Eucalyptus oil – removes stains and grease, is a mild antiseptic and an insect repellent (good for getting fleas off pets).

Cleaners made from citrus fruits (orange and lemon) – these work really well for stubborn stains.

Borax (use this sparingly) is a mildly abrasive cleaner, a water softener and an insect repellent.

Raw sea salt – a great bleach and stain remover.

Beeswax – good wood preservative and polishing agent.

A real bonus in cleaning your home in this way is that you will spend a lot less on cleaning products. I have saved hundreds of dollars over the past few years, yet my house is cleaner and nicer to live in.

Your house – more ideas

Avoid synthetic fragrances – toilet fresheners and cleaners, carpet deodorisers, room/furniture deodorisers, cleaning products with strong smells (which are not naturally derived), etc. If your toilet is really smelly then use some essential oils in a burner or use a spray bottle with eucalyptus oil diluted with water. If you can buy the citrus cleaning products, you can probably get the citrus toilet deodoriser too; it works well. Clean the bowl with a mixture of white vinegar, eucalyptus oil, psyllium husks (very little as they swell) plus water. Add a drop or two of non-toxic dishwashing liquid if you like it to foam.

Smoking is bad for everyone's health. If you smoke, stop. If you live with someone who smokes, see if you can negotiate where they can smoke (i.e. outside, or down the street) but be aware that secondary smoke is only part of the problem. Smokers have large amount of toxic gases in their clothes, so you may want to ask your smoking housemate to quit (it would be good for both of you). If possible, avoid smokers (and their clothes, cars and furniture).

A recent Senate Inquiry into air quality found that most Australian homes have poorer air quality than most factories. This is because of three reasons – 1: dust (which can contain toxic chemicals), 2: the large amount of synthetic materials we have in our houses which give off tiny amounts of Volatile Organic Compounds (VOCs or toxic gas) and 3: poor ventilation in getting dust and VOCs out of the house. Most developed countries will have similar home-toxicity challenges.

Hints for a low-toxicity house

Look at what you have on your floor. Many carpets are either synthetic, or have been treated to make them more hard-wearing and so give off large amounts of VOCs (this also applies to their underlay or rubber backing). Vinyl also gives off VOCs. The best floor coverings are wood, natural linoleum (made with linseed oil), terracotta tiles, slate, limestone, sandstone and carpet made from wool or other natural fibres (with jute or hessian underlay).

Eliminate synthetic perfumes (including most candles and incense), as these give off large amounts of VOCs. Use essential oils instead.

Paint gives off massive amounts of VOCs – never use oil-based paint (it is petroleum based as well as toxic). Water-based paint will have a lower level of VOCs. Look for low-toxicity or non-toxic paints. These are sometimes hard to find and more expensive, but worth it for your health.

Buy furniture that is made out of natural materials if you can. Plastic gives off a high rate of VOCs and should be avoided if possible. Wood, wool and leather are good.

For your towels, curtains, sheets, etc., use natural fibres. This is worth it, particularly with your bedding as you spend so much of your time wrapped up in it.

Get indoor plants – these are good at taking the toxic chemicals out of your air and replacing them with oxygen.

Dust more often, using a microfibre cloth. Keep two or three cloths discretely stored around the house so you can whisk dust away before it accumulates. It is easier to dust one room while you're there than to tackle a whole house once or twice a week.

Around the garden

Pesticides often work by either poisoning the insect or plant, or by interfering with them at a cellular level. Many are extremely neurotoxic. You don't want these products working on you as well. Use organic and permaculture practices in your garden.

Borrow a book from the library about this and you will get lots of hints about how to do things without chemicals.

Avoid having your house sprayed for pests (this includes using fly spray and flea bombs). These chemicals stay in your house for months and can make you very, very sick. When the "daddy long legs" spiders start coming back into your house, you know that you are living close to a low-toxicity life. Use Eucalyptus Oil to keep away ants (painted onto the area where they are coming in).

The best way to avoid pests in the home is to stop them coming inside the house – screens on windows and doors, don't leave stagnant water outside near your house (many pests need water to thrive and breed), and clean up sticky spills straight away (they are a magnet for ants and cockroaches).

Away from home

When you go to other people's houses for dinner, be aware that their cleaning products, food with preservatives and other chemicals added to their food and drinks, perfumes, carpet and dust may make you sick. If you do have a reaction, remember this and suggest that they come to your house next time. Really good friends will understand and accommodate your health needs. If you have friends or family who won't help you with this need to heal and stay healthy, they might need some encouragement and education, or you may need to reconsider how you relate to them.

Be aware that large shopping malls and supermarkets have large amounts of toxic gases in them. This is from the cleaning products they use, some of their tenants (nail and beauty salons) and the artificial fragrances they pump through their air-conditioning units. This does not stop you from shopping. You can shop at smaller local retailers (they will love you), spend the minimum amount of time in the larger shops or else shop online. Better still, get your partner or a friend to do the shopping!

Restaurants are a wonderful way to have a great night out. It can be even better if you asked to be seated in the non-smoking section.

In the end, there are a lot of simple things that you can do (no matter how sick you are) to live a low-toxicity life that will benefit you, your family and the environment. A good book to help you with this is *Going Organic, Your Guide to A Healthier Life* by Kris Abbey, published by New Holland (2002) and available at most bookstores.

Be gentle on yourself, don't try and do everything at once. Get rid of your household cleaning chemicals first. Then gradually work on the rest.

What we put on our body

Many people believe that the skin is an effective barrier to toxins but it is, in fact, a semipermeable membrane. That means that we can, and do, absorb many substances through our skin. What we put on our skin often passes through the skin and into the blood. From there it is carried to various organs including the brain, liver and kidneys, where it may have immediate or long-term effects. Skin absorption can be a significant source of exposure to the chemicals in personal care products, since they may be applied to the skin frequently and in large amounts. The scalp is an especially absorbent part of the body.

The skin is one of the most common routes of exposure. Many chemicals can penetrate the skin and their toxicity depends in part on how much absorption takes place. The greater the absorption, the greater the potential for a chemical to exert a toxic effect. The amount of absorption depends on the amount applied at any one time, how often we apply that substance, and the affinity of the chemical with our tissue.

Although chemicals are absorbed much more readily through damaged or abraded skin, chemicals can and do penetrate intact, healthy skin. Skin irritation is a common result of skin contact with certain chemicals but, of greater concern, these chemicals can damage many body systems, including your nervous system and brain, thus exacerbating neurodegenerative, autoimmune and chronic disease symptoms, or creating new ones.

Other routes of absorption from personal care products are ingestion (e.g. lipstick) and inhalation (e.g. talcum powder). We often swallow or inhale some ingredients of products without being aware of what is happening as we "beautify" ourselves after a shower or before a social engagement.

Essential oils

Many products claim to be "natural" because they include essential oils. While essential oils can be very useful in enhancing our environment and replacing some elements of personal care products, we must be cautious. Essential oils are very concentrated extracts of plants and, therefore, are not entirely "natural".

Some essential oils, especially those used in cosmetics, may contain residues of pesticides or other processing chemicals. Therapeutic grade (or 99 per cent pure) essential oils are the safest, but still need to be used cautiously. Remember you are at least a hundred times more sensitive to any chemical than more robust people. Essential oils may cause hypersensitivity or a neuro response if too powerful for you.

If you choose to use essential oils on your skin, always dilute them with some less concentrated, but still non-toxic oil, such as sweet almond or apricot, graded for ingestion, so that the essential oil will spread effectively without being too concentrated in any one place. They may also be diluted with pure aloe vera gel, and this can be very effective.

Natural? Safe?

Natural is not always non-toxic. Some "natural" ingredients have proven harmful effects. For example, d-limonene, found in orange peels, is a powerful solvent, has been found to be a sensitiser, and causes severe reactions in some people. Sodium lauryl sulfate, often derived from coconut, is a known skin irritant which enhances allergic response to other toxins and allergens. Sodium laureth sulfate may be contaminated with 1,4-dioxane, a carcinogen. Ammonium laurel and laureth sulfates present similar challenges.

"Natural" on a product label does not necessarily mean the product is safe to use. "Natural" may indicate that a small proportion of the product is derived from natural sources, while the remainder is petrochemical. Always read the label thoroughly. Furthermore, as indicated above, not all "natural" substances are safe; after all, snake venom is natural, but we don't want to rub it into our skin.

Your hair

Shampoo

Shampoos cause the most number of adverse reactions of all hair care products. They frequently contain harsh detergents, chemical fragrances and numerous irritating and carcinogenic compounds, including sodium lauryl sulfate/sodium laureth sulfate (irritant, can form carcinogenic nitrosamines), DEA, TEA, MEA (hormone disruptors, can release carcinogenic nitrosamines), quaternium-15, DMDM hydratoin (can release carcinogenic nitrosamines), polyethylene glycol (irritant), coal tar (carcinogenic), propylene glycol (neurotoxin, dermatitis, liver and kidney damage), and EDTA (irritant). Shampoos claiming to make your hair shinier with less work will often strip your hair over time, leaving it brittle, broken and falling.

Conditioner

Most mainstream and many "natural" conditioners rely on quaternary compounds to produce thicker, tangle-free silky hair. These compounds – benzalkonium chloride, cetrimonium bromide, quaternium 15, quaternium 18 – can be irritating to eyes and skin. Other ingredients to be aware of include carcinogenic coal tar colours (FC&C), propylene glycol, cinnamate sunscreens, and polysorbate 80 that may be contaminated with 1,4-dioxane, a carcinogen.

Again, many herbal conditioners are available that do the job well with no more cost (maybe less) and no damage to health.

Rather than buy conditioner, mix a table spoon of apple cider vinegar in one litre (2 pints) of water, soak through your hair at the end of the shower and do not wash out. The aroma will dissipate quickly and your hair will shine.

Hair colouring (permanent)

There is no safe hair colour! A study by the Harvard School of Public Health and the University of Athens Medical Schools suggested that women who use hair dyes five or more times a year have twice the risk of developing ovarian cancer. Most permanent hair dyes contain potential irritants and carcinogens like formaldehyde and ammonia. Petroleum-based coal tar derivatives and phenylenediamine cause cancer. Products containing phenylenediamine can cause blindness if the solution drips into eyes. Dr Samuel Epstein, chairman, Cancer Prevention Coalition, says the use of hair dye places women at increased risk of certain cancers, especially leukaemia, non-Hodgkin lymphoma, multiple myeloma and Hodgkin's disease. He states there is strong evidence that the use of hair colouring products accounts for up to 20 per cent of all non-Hodgkin lymphoma cases in US women, and that there is suggestive evidence these products increase breast cancer risk. Dark and black colours are particularly toxic.

Henna may be used if it is pure. The colour may vary from red to deep brown and will depend on your hair colour and texture. DO NOT use black henna as this is polluted with irritants.

Hair relaxers and straighteners

Toxic ingredients: Sodium hydroxide, calcium hydroxide, guanidine carbonate, guanidine hydroxide, thioglycolic acid, lithium hydroxide. A relaxer must be used with a neutralising shampoo and conditioner whether applied at home or in a salon. Conventional shampoos and conditioners found in hair straightening kits contain the same ingredients found in conventional shampoos and conditioners, whose health effects are shown above.

Hair styling

Aerosol and pump sprays produce fine droplets which can be inhaled deeply into lungs and transferred into your bloodstream. Inhalation of spray can also cause respiratory irritation and breathing difficulties. Hair styling products can contain TEA, DEA, MEA, FD&C colours, BHA and palmidate-O, all carcinogens. Ethoxylated alcohols, PEG compounds, and polysorbate 60 or 80 may be contaminated with 1,4-dioxane, a carcinogen. Conventional hair sprays coat hair with polyvinylpyrrolidone (PVP), a plasticiser.

Permanent waves

Chemicals in permanent wave compounds can cause eye and skin irritations, swelling of legs and feet and swelling of eyelids. These products are suspected of causing low blood sugar. Hair can become damaged and weakened, resulting in hair more susceptible to chemical and ultraviolet damage. The main ingredient in permanent waves, thioglycolic acid, is also used in chemical hair straighteners. These solutions can result in first- and third-degree burns and even hair loss. Chemical straighteners contain allergens and skin irritants like TEA, polyethelene glycol and synthetic fragrance.

Your face

Eye and face make-up

Through the ages men and women have painted their faces and bodies with colour – often with deadly results. Many substances used included lead, mercury and talcum. We now know that lead and mercury are neurotoxic and carcinogenic.

Today, most colours in conventional cosmetics are chemically synthesised from coal tar. These compounds have been shown to cause cancer in animals. Impurities like arsenic and lead in some coal tar colours have been shown to cause cancer not only when ingested, but also when applied to skin, and are very neurotoxic – therefore will exacerbate disease symptoms.

Blush

The main ingredient in most blushes is talc, a carcinogen. Colour is provided by hazardous coal tar dyes that are neurotoxic. Mineral oil, which can clog pores, and propylene glycol, a neurotoxin and skin sensitiser, are binders used to hold the formulation together. Acrylate compounds, commonly used as thickening agents, can be strong irritants.

Concealer

Concealers contain numerous irritating chemicals like propylene glycol, lanolin and paraben preservatives. These chemicals may be neurotoxic. Imidazolidinyl urea is the second most reported cause of contact dermatitis. BHA, a preservative, is a carcinogen that can be absorbed through the skin. DEA, TEA and MEA can form carcinogenic nitrosamines that are absorbed through the skin, and may be carcinogenic in themselves.

Eyeliner

Mainstream eyeliners contain carcinogenic coal tar colours, hormone-disrupting TEA, and PVP (polyvinylpyrrolidone), an allergen. Carcinogens are often also neurotoxic.

Eye shadow

Eye shadows are used for the colours they provide. However, they contain artificial colours from coal tar. Talc, a carcinogen, is the main ingredient in powdered eye shadows. Eye shadows may also contain mineral oil, a petrochemical derivative, dimethicone, a silicone oil, to make the powder stick to the eyelid, and binding ingredients like methacrylate, a strong irritant. Cream eye shadows are made with petrochemicals like paraffin and petrolatum, carcinogenic coal tar colours, and lanolin, an allergen which may contain pesticide residues. The glitter in cream eye shadows is created by adding pure aluminium, implicated in the onset of Alzheimer's disease and, perhaps, other degenerative diseases. The Consumer Agency and Ombudsman in Finland tested 49 eye shadows and found that all contained lead, cobalt, nickel, chromium and arsenic. These minerals are known neurotoxins.

Face powder

Mainstream powder products commonly contain talc, a carcinogen. Airborne talc is particularly dangerous because it can be inhaled. Other toxic ingredients include formaldehyde (carcinogenic and a sensitiser), quartenium-15 (can release formaldehyde), lanolin (irritant), imidazolidinyl urea (irritant, can release formaldehyde), MEA, TEA and DEA (hormone disruptors, can release formaldehyde) and parabens (hormone disrupters, irritants).

Foundation

Foundations are the third leading cause of contact dermatitis among cosmetics users. Because foundation is worn on the skin for many hours, products containing synthetic ingredients can cause skin problems. Mineral oil can block pores and promote cosmetic acne, while isopropyl myristate, a fatty compound, can cause blackheads. Other ingredients include propylene glycol, a neurotoxin and skin sensitiser, TEA and 2-bromo-2-nitropropane-1,3-diol which are often found together and which, combined, may cause the formation of carcinogenic nitrosamines, parabens, commonly used hormone-disrupting preservatives that may accumulate in body fat, and quaternium-15, a germicide that may break down into formaldehyde which is a carcinogen and sensitiser. Foundations include coal tar colours and synthetic fragrances. They may also contain lanolin, a common allergen.

Many foundations contain Bentonite that helps suspend water and disperse the foundation on your skin. Bentonite is believed to be carcinogenic and acts to "suffocate" your skin.

Lipstick

A woman may ingest more than four pounds (1814 grams) of lipstick in her lifetime – even more if she wears it every day. Mainstream lipsticks are composed of synthetic oils, petroleum waxes and artificial colours. Coal tar dye colours are common allergens and also carcinogenic. Lipsticks also contain amyldi-methylamino benzoic acid, ricinoleic acid, fragrance, ester gums and lanolin. Some dyes can cause photosensitivity and dermatitis.

Make-up remover

Make-up removers may contain propylene glycol (a neurotoxin), parabens (which are estrogen mimics), carcinogenic coal tar colours, DMDM hydantoin and diazolidinyl urea which release formaldehyde, polyethelene glycol and polysorbate 80 which may be contaminated with 1,4-dioxane, a carcinogen which readily penetrates skin, and fragrances.

Mascara

Conventional mascara contains petroleum distillates, shellac, acrylates (strong irritants), phenylmercuric acetate (preservative made from benzenes and mercury that can cause blisters, skin irritation and allergic reactions), parabens (hormone disrupters, allergens), quaternium-22 (preservative, allergen), quaternium-15 (eye irritant) pentaerythrityl (resin additive made from formaldehyde). Lash-extending products can contain plasticisers, like polyurethane, that cause cancer in animals, and polystyrene sulfonate which can irritate eyes and may be a hormone disruptor.

Your mouth

Mouthwash

Conventional mouthwash is alcohol-based. Products with alcohol content higher than 25 per cent can contribute to cancers of the mouth, tongue and throat when used regularly. Mouthwash can contain artificial flavours and colours, formaldehyde and sodium lauryl sulfate. Some mouthwash formulations include polysorbate 60 and polysorbate 80, which may be contaminated with 1,4-dixane, a carcinogen and fluoride which is a suspected carcinogen and may cause problems for some sensitive people.

Toothpaste

Conventional toothpastes contain artificial sweeteners like saccharin, sodium lauryl sulfate, synthetic colours and flavours, and polysorbate 80 which may be contaminated with 1,4-doxane, a carcinogen. Almost all conventional brands contain fluoride. Fluoride is linked to cancer and causes problems for some sensitive people.

Remember, any chemical that causes a sensitivity reaction, or is a known carcinogen, will affect you profoundly at cellular level, and is likely to exacerbate your disease symptoms, and may speed up the progress of the disorder.

Personal care

Avoid most deodorants and anti-perspirants – they have aluminium in them, a metal linked to Alzheimer's and breast cancer. If you keep yourself clean most of the time you don't need it anyway. Try not using it for a few days, and if you really smell – or on those hot days when we *all* smell – use a crystal deodorant that kills the bacteria that produces the smell (available from health food stores – they are more expensive than your ordinary deodorant, but will last a whole year). There are also a number of good quality deodorants that do not contain aluminium or other toxic chemicals, available from your supermarket and health food store. I have used at least three different brands, all with success. I have found that, as I improved my diet and metabolic performance, I needed deodorant much less.

Avoid make-up. You are beautiful the way you are.

Avoid mineral oil in any form and in any product. Oil on your skin prevents healthy breathing, reduces dispersal of waste products through the skin, exacerbates skin irritations and may cause rashes. The minerals may be absorbed through your skin and affect your health more profoundly.

Avoid any personal care product containing fragrances as these chemicals (even if "natural") may adversely affect you at cellular level.

What you wear

Wear natural fibres as much as possible – wool, cotton, silk, hemp. These fibres breathe better, are better for you and better for the environment. There is no chance of volatile organic compounds getting into your system from your clothes if you aren't wearing synthetic materials. Make sure you wash new clothes before wearing to reduce the chance of dye material being absorbed through your skin.

What you eat and drink

Don't drink water out of the tap!!! (unless you live in a place of peace unspoiled by human hands, or have your own rainwater tanks). The toxic chemicals that they use to treat drinking water (especially fluoride and chlorine), and the chemicals that they add to the water to preserve it (and us) are, generally speaking, bad for you. Bottles and tanks of "pure" water from the supermarket are often of doubtful quality and may, in fact, be tap water wearing an expensive label. Bottled water is expensive and not always what it seems. Most bottle water comes in soft PET plastic bottles, and is often left in the hot sun on a truck for many hours during transport; during this time, they leach DEHP, an endocrine-disrupting phthalate and probable human carcinogen into the water that you drink. ***Under no circumstances reuse a PET bottle***. If possible, install a good quality reverse osmosis water filter.

By the way, it is a good idea to use a simple osmotic filter for your tank water to remove any toxic residue collected on your roof or in the atmosphere during rainfall.

References

Colemon, John ND: ***Stop Parkin' and Start Livin'***, Michelle Anderson Publishing, Melbourne, Australia, 2005.

Victoroff, Dr Jeff: ***Saving Your Brain***; Bantam Books; Random House Australia, Milsons Point, NSW, 2002.

Coleman, Reverend Nicole: ***Low-Toxicity Living***, unpublished. Presented as an information resource by the Reverend Dr Nicole Coleman who has recovered from chronic Lyme disease.

APPENDIX 2

HEEL DETOX KIT

Low-dose schedule for sensitive patients

Continue at week 11 dose, three weeks on and one week off,
until all formulas in the Kit are consumed.

Date Remedy	wk 1	wk 2	wk 3	wk 4	wk 5	wk 6	wk 7	wk 8	wk 9	wk 10	wk 11
Nux Vomica Homaccord (NVH)	1 drop in 1+ litres water	1 drop in 1+ litres water	1 drop in 1+ litres water	*Do not take remedies for this week*	1 drop in 1+ litres water	2 drops in 1+ litres water	3 drops in 1+ litres water	*Do not take remedies for this week*	3 drops in 1+ litres water	3 drops in 1+ litres water	3 drops in 1+ litres water
Berberis (B) or Reneel (R)		1 drop in 1+ litres water with NVH	1 drop in 1+ litres water with NVH	*Do not take remedies for this week*	1 drop in 1+ litres water with NVH	2 drops in 1+ litres water	3 drops in 1+ litres water	*Do not take remedies for this week*	3 drops in 1+ litres water	3 dropsin 1+ litres water	3 drops in 1+ litres water
Lympho myosot (L)			1 drop in 1+ litres water with NVH & B	*Do not take remedies for this week*	1 drop in 1+ litres water with NVH & B	2 drops in 1+ litres water	3 drops in 1+ litres water	*Do not take remedies for this week*	3 drops in 1+ litres water	3 drops in 1+ litres water	3 drops in 1+ litres water

381

APPENDIX 3

AQUA HYDRATION FORMULAS

These may be ordered from your local health food store or online at:

https://www.returntostillness.com.au (worldwide)

https://www.hydration.net.au (worldwide)

https://www.aquas.us/ (USA)

https://aquahydration.co.uk (UK)

Taking the Aqua Hydration Formulas

Aqua Hydration Formulas should be taken in a glass of 1/3 apple juice and 2/3 pure water (e.g. spring water – not *fluoridated* water). If you have any problem with apple juice, you may use other *non-citrus* juices or plain water. Take the AM drops as soon as you get up if possible. The PM drops are preferably taken 1/2 hour or more before your evening meal.

Alternatively, the Aquas may be taken as part of a **"cocktail"** that includes some required supplement powders. The powders replace the apple juice suggested above. The "cocktail" may consist of a glass of water, plus prescribed vitamin C powder, and/or prescribed magnesium powder, and detox powders as required, plus the Aquas as prescribed.

Many practitioners suggest that the Aqua Hydration Formulas should be taken for five days each week. For people with Parkinson's, I have found they are best taken every day for the first two years, then five days per week thereafter.

Keep the Aquas away from sources of radiation such as

microwave ovens (which you should not use anyway), computers and mobile phones. Tip the bottles carefully when first using them as the rate of drip varies from bottle to bottle.

Drink at least 6 to 8 glasses of water daily to help the Aquas work effectively.

The doses below are average for moderately sensitive people diagnosed with Parkinson's disease. Work with your chosen healthcare team to adjust doses if required.

Week 1
Aqua AM 1 drop in the morning
Aqua PM 1 drop in the evening

Week 2
Aqua AM 1 drop in the morning
Aqua PM 1 drop in the evening

Week 3
Aqua AM 2 drops in the morning
Aqua PM 2 drops in the evening

Week 4
Aqua AM 3 drops in the morning
Aqua PM 3 drops in the evening

Continue at the **week 4 dose** unless advised otherwise. Should you be concerned about any symptom you think might be affected by the Aquas, please contact your health practitioner, as there are other dilution methods available to ensure that you get the most benefit with the greatest degree of comfort.

The Aquas will improve the uptake and utilisation of all other medication and supplements you are taking. Therefore, it may be necessary, from time to time, to adjust the intake of these items. **It is important to contact your health practitioner before making any adjustment to your medication dosage**.

The initial cost of the Aquas is moderate and, as each bottle lasts for eight to twelve weeks (depending on your dose), the daily cost is very small.

The Aquas are powerful, energetic medicine, which serve as a core support therapy for physical recovery from chronic disorders.

APPENDIX 4

A small sample of drugs commonly prescribed for people suffering multiple symptoms of ill health. Note how many drugs have similar potential side effects. Prescription of multiple drugs with similar side effects often increases the incidence and severity of these effects.

PHARMACEUTICAL MEDICATIONS
COMMON OR VERY COMMON ADVERSE EFFECTS

Adverse Effect / PD Drug	GIT	Tired	CNS	Dysk	Tremor	C.V.	Cramp	Weak	Pain	Conf	Anx	Dep	Dysp	Lib	Hypo
PD Drug															
Artane															
Elderpryl															
Madopar															
Parlodel															
Pergolide															
Sinemet															
NSAID															
Brufen															
Clinoril															
Indocid															
Naprosyn															
Toradol															
B.P.															
Adalat															
Betaloc															
Chlotride															
Gopten															
Inderal															
Lasix															
Moduretic															
Norvasc															
Tenormin															
Anti-Depress.															
Deptran															
Sinequan															
Tolvon															
Aurorix															
Prozac															
Zoloft															

Key

GIT = gastro intestinal disturbances

Tired = unexplained tiredness

CNS = central nervous system disturbances

Dysk = dyskinesia

Tremor = tremor/spasm

C.V. = cardiovascular problems

Cramp = cramp

Weak = unexplained weakness

Pain = pain unrelated to disorder

Conf = confusion

Anx = anxiety

Dep = depression

Dysp = dyspnea

Lib = suppressed libido

Hypo = hypotension

APPENDIX 5

MY PARKINSON'S ADVENTURE

My adventure with Parkinson's disease began at conception and continues today.

I was born in the middle of 1943 while World War II was at its peak. My father had been home on short leave nine months earlier, then went back to his Airforce post in Darwin, leaving my mother on her own with two other children to care for – my sister of four and a half who was very unwell, and my brother, just over two years old, who missed his father. Conditions were primitive – only one source of cold water in the kitchen, no hot water supply at all unless heated on the wood-fired stove which provided both cooking and heating for the whole house. My mother had to chop the wood herself, even while pregnant. There was no bathroom and an outside toilet which required my mother to bury its contents each week or so. The nearest store was a half-hour walk away down a steep hill which was also where the nearest public transport was situated. No telephone in the house, the only contact with her family being via letter or the telephone at the shop. My mother was under a great deal of stress and, undoubtedly, that affected my later health.

I did not meet my father until the end of 1945 and, as he was a stranger, I wanted nothing to do with him. He was a nice man but had no skills in bonding with a fearful child. I remained afraid of him until I was in my mid-teens, when I lost my fear but still felt estranged from him. It is a regret that, even though my father lived until 1995 (93 years old), we never found a way to really communicate and bond with each other.

Throughout my childhood I was afraid of many people, sometimes with justification. I was often subjected to emotional and physical abuse and, on at least two occasions, sexual abuse.

When I was sixteen, my parents separated and I left school to commence work at a copper mine in Tasmania. At first, I worked in their accounting office but, after a few months, I was sent to the open-cut mine itself as a time keeper (manually recording workers' times of arrival and departure, as well as tallies of ore and waste produced each shift). I enjoyed the work (it was easy), the company of older men and the freedom of earning a significant wage.

It was not enough for me, however. I wanted to learn to play trumpet, so I moved to Melbourne at eighteen years old to commence the next 40 years of stressful adventure.

Failing miserably as a trumpet player and without tertiary education, I battled my way up in the musical instrument industry, learning sales and marketing skills on the job, making mistakes and beating myself up over them, but learning to not repeat those errors. No matter how well I did in the market place (and I did well), I always felt inadequate, inferior to my better educated colleagues and awkward in executive company. I worked very long hours trying to compensate for my lack of education and perceived unworthiness, smoked heavily (I had started at nine years old after attempting suicide), began binge drinking on weekends and ate fatty, greasy, nutrition-free food too often.

I met and married Nariida in my late twenties. She was a lovely woman with some similarities in her background, so we fumbled through the first few months of our marriage, trying to make sense of our conflicting feelings, hyper-reactions to stressful situations and difficulty with intimacy.

We had two wonderful baby boys in 1972 and 1973 (just one year and two weeks apart) and, while our boys brought us enormous joy, our eldest, Damian, was fragile, and his health challenges added to our stress levels.

In April 1980, Damian was diagnosed with Acute Lymphoblastic Leukemia on his eighth birthday, so we began a frightening journey into the mysterious world of oncology and haematology, and discovered virulent opposition to any form of treatment outside the purview of Western allopathic medicine.

I had commenced naturopathic studies just before Damian's diagnosis, but had already been interested for many years. My parents, wife and children, as well as I, had been treated by naturopaths over the years in combination with treatment from Western doctors. My wife and I thought that it would be sensible to look at complementary approaches to treating our gravely ill son.

We tried many allied and complementary treatments to ease Damian's suffering while he went through the standard chemotherapy and radiation regimen recommended by the top paediatric oncologists of the day. We noted that Damian had less nausea and distress than other children receiving similar treatment, developed no opportunistic infections that seemed so common in other patients, and recovered his energy rapidly between medical treatments.

His oncologist disagreed with our view and subjected us to verbal abuse on more than one occasion. We finally decided to change hospitals and oncologists and, over the last year of Damian's life, felt much more supported as we worked with doctors to not only extend Damian's life, but to help him live well and joyfully.

Damian enjoyed over two years of remission, then suffered a testicular relapse. This was, apparently, successfully treated and we had a wonderful family holiday to Disneyland sponsored by close friends. But Damian became very unwell on the flight home and, shortly after, was diagnosed with a Central Nervous System relapse. As we were advised that there was less than one percent chance of extending his life for a few months, even with severe chemotherapy, we decided against treatment, and I had to tell Damian that he was dying. He wrote a will, gave instructions for his funeral, talked to a few special people about his death, played cricket and waterskied. He was eleven years old.

Damian died at the end of 1983. We, together with another couple whose six-year-old son was dying from leukemia, threw ourselves into the task of developing a family support charity called Very Special Kids, to help other families work through the frightening process of watching their children undergo treatment for life-threatening disorders. We felt that this would be a fitting memorial for our sons.

The medical profession thought otherwise. We were roundly abused for daring to start something new instead of raising money for research (we had already done that) or supporting grief organisations. One doctor went so far as to accuse me of child abuse and killing my child because I had provided intravenous vitamin C infusions for Damian.

After establishing Very Special Kids as a viable charity, forming a strong committee and employing an experienced Family Services Coordinator (paying her salary until other money could be raised), I left Very Special Kids to ease the levels of opposition. It is now, 35 years later, a vibrant and strong organisation supporting hundreds of families through the dark days of their child's illness. But I am not part of that, and my grief in 1985 was as if I had lost another child.

Nariida and I parted in 1989, too tired to struggle on, and I was fired from my job a few months later. I was unable to find similar work, as 1990 was a bad year for middle management in Australia. After many months of unemployment, I commenced work as an operating theatre technician at a major hospital and decided to return to my naturopathic studies.

The next three years were strange, wonderful, dreadful and very damaging to my health. I worked night shift five nights per week, commencing at around 9.30 pm and finishing at 7.15 am. I would have breakfast and a quick nap, then go to my college for lectures until 5 pm. I had another couple of hours sleep and a meal before starting work again. On weekends I did chores, studied, and tried to catch up on some sleep. Late in 1993, I changed employment to a minor management position in a different hospital, still as an operating theatre technician, but on day/afternoon shift rotations and managing sixteen other technicians over eight operating theatres. I persisted with studies at a different college that offered evening classes.

I was exhausted all the time, eating badly, smoking heavily yet had almost stopped drinking alcohol. I knew my body was suffering but was determined to complete my studies before resting.

My body had other ideas; I collapsed at work in 1995. I was unable to walk more than a few metres without festinating and falling, or simply collapsing where I stood; my speech was slurred, I stammered and was largely incoherent; I had severe tremors in my head, both arms, my right leg and internally; my fingers displayed a "pill rolling" movement; the right side of my face was frozen and I drooled; I was incontinent and constipated and I could not sleep for more than half an hour at a time.

I was referred to a professor of neurology who took a cursory glance at my referral letter, then prescribed antidepressants. I then saw several other doctors who diagnosed Parkinson's disease, so I returned to the neurologist who, after I became agitated, examined me at last and diagnosed advanced Parkinson's plus early stage Multiple System Atrophy. He offered drugs to keep me "comfortable as long as possible".

With the help of the hospital librarian, I commenced a journey of discovery, reading thousands of medical abstracts and hundreds of full studies, all about Parkinson's disease, its causes and treatments. I found nothing there to give me any hope of recovering my health, so I sought help outside of the medical profession. I worked with a homeopath, naturopath, craniosacral therapist, counsellors, and kept in touch with an open-minded western medical doctor. I tried homeopathics, supplements, herbs, body work, reiki and spiritual healing.

I was owed four weeks sick leave when I collapsed, so I sat at home for hours, reflecting on what might have caused my body to develop this dreadful disease. My father and paternal grandmother had both had Parkinson's so perhaps it was genetic, although that was not considered likely. Articles in complementary medical journals conjectured that toxic load and prolonged stress may play a role in neurodegeneration, and that gut function was critical to health. My reflections led me to realise that I had been under severe stress for most of my 52 years, had been in contact with some nasty chemicals during some of my jobs and had eaten very toxic food for a long time. Given my family history of Parkinson's and other neuro disorders (dementia and essential tremor), I may have a predisposition to express toxic triggers in this form of disease.

I determined to change as much as I could and try to regain some semblance of good health. I had to earn an income, so I needed to continue working even though the hospital environment was stressful and toxic (there are many very nasty chemicals in hospitals). I began to look at what I COULD change.

Food was an obvious starting point and, even though I struggled to prepare meals, I worked hard to introduce more vegetables and good protein into my diet.

Introducing calmness outside the work environment was another factor I could control, so I increased my meditation regimen (I had been meditating for a year before collapsing), played classical music on the radio or recordings at every opportunity, and removed myself from people who aggravated or agitated me, including members of my family.

I had stopped smoking a few months earlier and felt that was important, despite some research I had read claiming that cigarette smoking reduced the risk of Parkinson's. I felt that I needed to avoid toxins as much as I could.

With the help of practitioners and colleagues, I selected nutritional supplements that may help with energy production, remove toxic waste, support sleep and improve neural pathways.

In 1996 I read a story by Julian Baker (Bowen therapy teacher) explaining Bowen therapy. This inspired me to learn more about this lovely, gentle body work and I found that Bowen treatments helped my progress.

During that same year, I attended a lecture by Dr Jaroslav Boublik about a homeopathic product called Aqua Hydration Formulas that help to calm the hypothalamus/pituitary/adrenal axis in endurance athletes. This seemed like a missing part of my journey to better health, so I commenced using them with a promise to keep Jaroslav in touch with their effect, as the Aquas had not been used for very sick people before.

It took some trial and much error before we got the Aqua protocol right for those of us with neuro disorders, but they did become a valuable aid to my recovery. We found that, while athletes benefit from quite high doses, those with neurodegenerative disorders are generally fragile and need only very small doses; sometimes less that one drop per day. My Aqua doses averaged one drop daily.

Progress was painfully and depressingly slow. At times, I felt that I was becoming even more debilitated and often thought I had made no progress at all, notwithstanding my efforts. However, I kept a journal, despite very poor writing, and checked back each few weeks to see if I could discern any change worth noting.

One of the first changes I noticed was with night time urination. Early in my illness, I needed to urinate ten to fifteen times each night, crawling to the bathroom, trying to empty my bladder completely, then using walls for support to stagger back to bed. That, combined with pain in my shoulders, hips and head, deprived me of all but two to three hours sleep each night.

By March 1996, I noticed in my journal that I was urinating only five to seven times each night and, while it was still very difficult to walk, I could sometimes reach the bathroom without crawling. This gave me courage to keep trying.

My journal, scribbled in old diaries, was a major tool for supporting my journey towards wellness. Friends would tell me that I was "looking better" or "doing well", but I did not really believe them unless I saw evidence of progress in my journal.

Early in 1997, I decided to leave my full-time employment and become an agency technician, working in hospitals experiencing staff shortages on a casual basis. This was much less secure than full-time work as there were no sick days or holidays paid by the agency, and no guarantee that there would be work available on any given day, but it meant that, each day, I could choose to work, study or focus on my health.

I soon found that there were hospitals which presented pleasant working environments while others were largely populated with angry, mean-spirited people who treated agency staff like intruders and patients as if they were unwelcome interruptions in their day. I chose to work at the former hospitals as much as possible and avoid the stress of the latter.

Despite my journal and hopefulness, I did not really notice my recovery until a friend said that she could no longer see any Parkinson's symptoms and that I was clearly "better". I think I was afraid to admit my level of wellness, in case this somehow "spoiled it" and I collapsed again. However, she was right and, towards the middle of 1998, I found myself without any Parkinson's symptoms and regaining strength.

I was not "cured". I noticed that, if I became careless with food, or over-stressed myself with work or social activities, my hands would begin to tremor again. I also noted in my journal that reverting to old eating habits (lots of cereals, bread and/ or takeaway food) brought on fatigue, irritability and sadness. It soon became obvious that I needed to maintain a lifestyle that avoided toxins as much as possible, included lots of fresh food, exercise, meditation and, most importantly of all, self-love.

I completed my four-year Advanced Diploma of Naturopathy at the end of 1998 after nineteen years of interrupted study. My college presented me with a special prize for finishing.

I had intended to become a generalist naturopath, offering help to people with fatigue, poor digestion, skin challenges and allergies, but my first patients were those diagnosed with Parkinson's disease. This was scary as I had only my own experience to support my advice, but we worked together and those who became dedicated to a process of restoring wellness made good progress.

Over the next year, I renewed my relationships with family members, but on different terms; I made sure that I took care of myself and my interests in those relationships.

I continued to search for information about the causes of Parkinson's and better ways to reverse those causes. Conservative Parkinson's research is very focused on the damage to dopaminergic cells and ways to replace dopamine, but I found that research into neurodegeneration generally had much more to offer in terms of finding causes and ways back to health. This has been my research focus for over twenty years.

There is no "cure" for Parkinson's disease but there are ways to become well and live well with no symptoms. Since 1998, I have built a practice specialising in neurodegenerative and autoimmune disorders; I have lectured to practitioners and patients around Australia, USA, Germany, Austria and UK. I have met and married Nichol who is both the love of my life and a "research subject", as she has been diagnosed with chronic stealth infections, dysautonomia and post-concussion syndrome.

Late in 2015, I was diagnosed with stage three bowel cancer. I chose a combination of western allopathic medicine and complementary medicine with great results. I am now free from all signs of cancer.

The 25 years since my diagnosis with Parkinson's disease have taught me many important life lessons. When I am told that there is no cure and no hope, it is up to me to find a way to be well again. Once I am well, it is up to me to maintain that wellness with food, lifestyle and self-love.

I haven't climbed mountains or sailed around the world, but I have experienced great adventures. My time with Damian and the knowledge I gained from his life and death changed me and taught me about courage and determination. My adventure with Parkinson's disease taught me that hope is always valuable and we can achieve wellness with patience and determination. My adventure with cancer showed me how valuable a caring, respectful combination of western and complementary medicines can be.

Now in my late seventies, I continue to seek knowledge and delight in watching my son, Sean, blossom as a father and my grandson grow into a curious, adventurous, loving boy. Life is good.

John Coleman, August 2020

My autobiography, *Shaky Past*, is available as an ebook on Amazon.

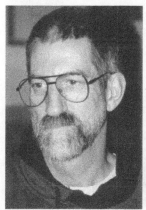 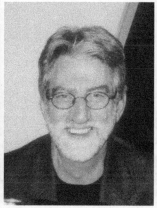 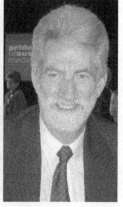

John, early 1996   John, June 2004   John, Oct 2007

GLOSSARY OF TERMS

Adipose tissue: Fat. Fat cells are called adipocytes.

Adrenal cortex: The outer part of an adrenal gland that produces aldosterone, cortisol and testosterone.

Adrenal glands: Endocrine glands placed on top of each kidney. They produce hormones – adrenaline/epinephrine, noradrenaline/norepinephrine, aldosterone, cortisol and testosterone.

Adrenal medulla: The inner, core part of an adrenal gland producing adrenaline/epinephrine and noradrenaline/norepinephrine.

Adrenaline: A hormone produced by the adrenal glands, especially under stress or in the fight/flight/freeze response.

Adrenocorticotropic Hormone (ACTH): A hormone produced by the pituitary gland in response to stimulus from the hypothalamus which triggers increased production of adrenal hormones.

Adverse Childhood Experience (ACE): Any stressful or traumatic experience before the age of 17 or 18. These experiences may cause physical or mental health challenges later in life unless addressed appropriately.

Aetiological pathway: Events or circumstances that triggers or causes a change in health status. Usually associated with ill health and identifying the reason a person displays illness symptoms.

Aldosterone: A hormone produced by the adrenal cortex.

Alkalosis: A physical imbalance where the pH of blood or tissue rises beyond a tightly controlled healthy range.

Alpha synuclein (aS): A protein produced to protect cells against infection. However, where the infection is chronic or the immune system suppressed, aS may be misfolded and become damaging to other cells.

Alpha-tocopherol: An important form of vitamin E.

ALS (Amyotrophic lateral sclerosis): Also known as Motor Neurone Disease. A neurodegenerative disorder which progressively destroys motor function.

Alzheimer's disease: a progressive brain disorder. The most common form of dementia in older people.

Ammonium sulphate: an inorganic salt with the formula $(NH_4)_2SO_4$, commonly used in fertilisers.

Anandamide: N-arachidonylethanolamine, a neurotransmitter with the formula $C_{22}H_{37}NO_2$. Cannabinoids THC and CBD partially mimic its actions in the human body by binding to anandamide receptors, CB1 and CB2.

Anecdotal evidence: Stories or anecdotes used to support an hypothesis without other supporting evidence from clinical trials, double-blind trials or other accepted scientific evidence.

Ankylosing Spondylitis: an inflammatory, autoimmune disease marked by inflammation and fusing of the spine.

Anterior olfactory nucleus: Part of the forebrain that works with other areas in processing olfactory messages (smells).

Antibiotic: Medication used to kill bacteria. Used extensively in treating bacterial infections in mammals.

Anticholinergic Drug: Medication that reduces the supply of acetylcholine. As acetylcholine is a dopamine antagonist, its reduction increases the relative amount of dopamine available.

Antioxidant: compounds in foods that scavenge and neutralise free radicals (Reactive Oxygen Species or ROS). There are also antioxidant supplements available.

Arsenic: A natural component of the earth's crust and is widely distributed throughout the environment in the air, water and land. It is highly toxic in its inorganic form. May contaminate drinking water and food irrigated with contaminated water. Smoking tobacco also exposes us to arsenic. In the past, Arsenic was used in cattle and sheep dips.

Aspartame: an artificial sweetener 200 times sweeter than cane sugar. It is also sold under the brand names of NutraSweet and Equal. It is made from phenylalanine and aspartic acid. Aspartame is an excitotoxin and may damage NMDA receptors in the brain.

Atrophy: wasting away or reduction is size and power of body tissue due to degeneration of cells.

Atypical: unusual for that group, class or process.

Axillary hair: hair under the arms.

Ayurvedic medicine: a form of herbal, lifestyle and nutrition medicine developed in India more than 3000 years ago.

Babesia: a parasite/protozoa infecting red blood cells, often carried by sanguiferous insects.

Bartonella: gram negative bacteria that are intracellular parasites generally showing preference for erythrocytes and endothelial cells in humans. May be carried by sanguiferous insects or cats ("cat scratch fever").

Biofeedback: ways of measuring autonomic activity in the body and/or gaining voluntary control over autonomic activity.

Biotoxin: toxic substance of biological origin such as mould spores or toxin produced endogenously from the breakdown of ingested substances.

Brain stem: the most primitive part of the brain connecting the cerebrum and cerebellum to the spinal cord. Critical for autonomic function.

Bristol Stool Chart/Scale: a chart/scale classifying the consistency of stools from 1 (severe constipation) to 7 (severe diarrhoea).

Building Biologist: a specially trained professional who can assess and measure the safety or dangers to health in a building (residential or commercial) and advise on strategies to remediate problems.

Carbidopa: a decarboxylase inhibitor packed with levodopa to reduce absorption of the levodopa prior to the blood-brain barrier.

Carcinogenic: causing cancer or exacerbating the process of developing cancer.

Catabolism: the breakdown of complex molecules in living organisms to form simpler ones, together with the release of energy.

Catechol-O-Methyltransferase (COMT): an enzyme that breaks down dopamine.

Centers for Disease Control (CDC): USA health/disease authority collecting data on disease rates and distribution, and developing strategies to prevent disease.

Cerebral cortex: the outer layer of the cerebrum, playing an important role in consciousness.

Challenge Test: Testing for pathogenic infections by using specific medicines (herbal or pharmaceutical) to kill a specific pathogen. The symptomatic response of the patient indicates the presence or absence of the pathogen.

Chatham House Rule: a rule or principle according to which information disclosed during a meeting may be reported by those present, but the source of that information may not be explicitly or implicitly identified.

Coeliac disease: conservatively considered a genetic autoimmune disorder caused by an adverse reaction to gluten in grains. Many Complementary/Alternative Medicine practitioners lean towards the view that Coeliac disease is, in fact, end stage gut dysfunction caused by inflammation.

Comorbidity: illness secondary to, or accompanying a primary disorder (e.g. Borrelia as primary, Bartonella as a comorbidity).

Complementary Medicine: Medicine other than conservative Western medicine used to complement or support conservative treatments.

Complementary/Alternative Medicine: Medicine that may complement or replace conservative Western medicine. Can include herbals, homeopathy, dietary advice, exercise, and many other supportive strategies.

Constipation: conservatively considered as the passing of hard, dry stools, incomplete bowel emptying or less that three bowel motions per week. In Complementary/Alternative Medicine, it is generally considered to mean less that one large bowel motion per day.

Conventional medicine: Western Allopathic Medicine including pharmaceutical drugs, surgery, medically-based dietetics and physiotherapy.

Cortex: Outer layer. E.g. Cerebral cortex or Adrenal cortex.

Corticotropin-releasing Hormone (CRH): a peptide hormone secreted by the hypothalamus in response to stress that triggers the synthesis and secretion of ACTH in the Pituitary gland.

Cortisol: a steroid hormone released by the adrenal glands in response to ACTH. Stimulates activity as part of the fight/flight/freeze response.

Cyclic AMP (cAMP): Cyclic adenosine monophosphate is a second messenger for intracellular signal induction. Involved in the regulation of glycogen, sugar and lipid metabolism.

DDT: Dichlorodiphenyltrichloroethane, developed in 1874 but commonly used as an insecticide from the late 1940s. Also extensively used in animal dips. Highly toxic.

Decarboxylase inhibiter: a chemical bound to levodopa in Parkinson's drugs to significantly reduce absorption of levodopa prior to the blood-brain barrier. Decarboxylase inhibitors cannot cross the blood-brain barrier so release levodopa into the brain.

Dietitian: a person with a degree in dietetics. This discipline looks at what foods and supplements may provide required nutrients. Dietitians do not always have an understanding of long-term effects of poorly absorbed nutrients.

Dopamine: a hormone and neurotransmitter affecting both mood and movement. Most is produced in the gastrointestinal tract and transported to the brain via the vagus nerve.

Dopamine agonist: a chemical designed to stimulate dopamine receptors in the brain.

Dopaminergic cell: a cell producing dopamine.

Double-blind-randomised-placebo-controlled trial: a formal trial of a treatment during which neither the participants or administrators know who receives the active treatment or a placebo (an inactive mimic). Patients are allocated to treatment or placebo groups by anonymous, random choice.

Dyskinesia: abnormal jerking or movement caused by Parkinson's disease medication. Occasionally occurring in late-stage Parkinson's disease unrelated to medication.

Dysregulation: an interruption to the normal regulation of a system that may have wide-ranging effects on many body functions.

Dysuria: abnormal urinary activity.

Ecstasy (MDMA): a drug that causes an increase in serotonin production and may increase brain hydration.

Efficacy: the effectiveness of a treatment or strategy.

EMF: Electromagnetic Frequencies. These may be useful or damaging.

Endogenous: produced within the body.

Endorphins: peptide hormones that have an analgesic effect.

Epinephrine: Adrenaline. Produced by the adrenal glands to stimulate activity.

Epstein Barr virus: the virus that causes mononucleosis ("mono"). Infection may be mild or very serious over a long period.

Esophagus: also spelt Oesophagus. The part of the digestive tract joining the throat and stomach.

Ethoxylates: ethoxylated alcohol is used in many industries, often to improve the mixing of water miscible and fatty substances.

Exogenous: produced outside of the body.

Familial: within the biological family.

Faraday Cage: a metal cage constructed to protect again electromagnetic frequencies such as Wi-Fi.

Fascia: jelly-like substance surrounding all internal parts of the body. Composed primarily of proteins, proteoglycans and fibrin. May become thick or "stuck" with heat, injury or illness.

FDA: USA Food and Drug Administration.

Festination: abnormal walking where steps become shorter and quicker and centre of balance moves forward until the patient needs support or may fall forward.

Fibromyalgia: inflammatory, autoimmune disorder involving pain in muscles. Often very severe or crippling.

Flower Essence: a system of medicine where parts of plants, often flowers, are infused in pure spring water then taken in drop doses under the tongue. Can help with mood and attitude.

Fluoride: an inorganic, monatomic anion. We usually use the term in speaking of mineral fluorides – calcium fluoride, sodium fluoride, sulfurhexafluoride.

Folate: 5 Methyltetrahydrofolate; an active form of folic acid.

Folic Acid: the inactive form of vitamin B9 that must be converted in the body to 5 Methyltetrahydrofolate or 5 Formyltetrahydrofolate before utilisation.

Folinic Acid: 5 Formyltetrahydrofolate; an active form of folic acid.

Formaldehyde: a colourless, irritating and odorous gas usually found in water-based solutions and used in many industrial settings. May outgas from some household and construction products.

Galen of Pergamon: a Greek physician, surgeon and philosopher. Born 130 AD, died 210 AD.

Gamma interferon: Endogenous cytokine produced by leukocytes.

Gastrointestinal tract (GIT): the tube that starts with our mouth and ends with the anus. All digestion takes place within this tube, and stools are eliminated. "Chew to poo".

Gastro-Oesophageal Reflux Disease (GORD or GERD): commonly called Reflux. This is not really a disease. Symptoms occur when the stomach pH rises and allows the Lower Oesophageal Sphincter (also known as the cardiac sphincter) to leak acidic liquid into the oesophagus causing pain, often radiating far from the local dysregulation.

Gene: basic physical and functional unit of our body. Made of DNA. Often act as "switches" or instructions to create proteins.

Gene mutation: a change in a gene causing it to malfunction. Sometimes correctable.

General Practitioner (GP): primary care medical practitioner. Usually the first medical practitioner to see a patient and may refer them to a specialist.

Ghee: clarified butter.

Gluten: a protein in many grains that is sticky. One of many inflammatory lectins in grains that act to defend the grain against predators.

Glycogen: the form in which glucose is stored in the body.

Glyphosate: a powerful herbicide. It is both carcinogenic and neurotoxic.

Guillain-Barré syndrome: a rapid-onset muscle weakness caused by autoimmune damage to peripheral nerves. Onset is often initiated following a bacterial or viral infection. Some stealth infections mimic Guillain-Barré syndrome.

Haematologist: a specialist doctor treating blood disorders.

Hair Mineral Analysis/Hair Tissue Mineral Analysis: a test of hair tissue to determine levels of helpful and toxic minerals in the body.

Heavy metal: a mineral metal of relatively high density or atomic weight. Many are toxic at low concentrations and include lead, arsenic, mercury, cadmium and, more recently, aluminium.

Helicobacter pylori (H. pylori): bacteria that may infect the digestive tract and is often implicated in GORD (reflux).

Herx: Jarische Herxheimer reaction describes the uncomfortable response when toxins released by dying pathogens overwhelm our detox/elimination pathways.

Himalayan Sea Salt: salt mined in the Himalayas resulting from the time before these mountains were formed. This salt contains over 80 useful minerals in trace quantities.

Hippocrates of Ur: a Greek physician. Born 460 BC, died 375

BC. Commonly known as the "Father of modern medicine".

Hoehn & Yahr Scale: A way of defining the severity of Parkinson's disease symptoms on a 6-step scale from 0 to 5.

Holocaust: in this context (The Holocaust), the slaughter of 6 million Jews and many millions of innocent people during World War II.

Homeopathic complex: Homeopathic medicine containing a number of different remedies to achieve a single result.

Homeopathic Medicine: a system of medicine developed by Samuel Hahnemann (Germany 1755-1843) using very dilute substances to stimulate natural body responses.

Homeopathic simplex: a single homeopathic remedy.

Homocysteine: a common amino acid in the blood. May be formed to excess when taking levodopa drugs. In healthy individuals, is converted by folate to methionine and used in the methylation detox system.

Hormone: chemical messengers in the body, formed by endocrine glands. Help to control system functions.

Hypercholesteremia: a state of health where there is excess cholesterol in the blood stream.

Hyperglycemia: an excess of sugar in the blood.

Hypochondriac: a person who worries excessively about their health.

Hypothalamus: a small organ in the base of the brain near the pituitary glad. Plays a crucial role in the fight/flight/freeze response, hydration and other important functions.

Idiopathic: of no known cause.

Immunoglobulin A: an antibody that plays a role in the immune function of mucus membranes.

Incontinence (urinary): inability to retain urine in the bladder until reaching an appropriate place for voiding, or excessive frequency of urination.

Interstitium: the fluid-filled space between cells, organs, and other (semi) solid parts of the body. Plays an important role in circulation, immune function and other activities.

Ion: an atom or molecule that has lost or gained an electron, so has an electrical charge.

Jarische Herxheimer Reaction: an illness response that occurs when pathogens are killed faster than our detoxification systems can eliminate the toxic residue resulting from the death of the pathogen. Often known as a "Herx".

K-dilution: an extreme dilution of a medicine or remedy created by the "spill and refill" method. First developed by Russian homeopath Semen Korsakov (1787-1853) who used K-dilutions to create homeopathic medicines.

Kefir: originally a fermented milk product like thin yoghurt but using a specific mesophilic symbiotic culture. May also be prepared from non-animal dairy products, fruit and vegetable juices and plain water.

Kinesiology: a method of testing muscle tension/strength to determine imbalances in the body and make corrections.

Lectins: proteins in most plants that can bind to specific sugars and cause agglutination of certain cell types. Lectins in some plants are inflammatory in the human body while others are benign.

Levodopa: the precursor to dopamine. It is converted to dopamine in the brain.

Lewy Bodies: aggregations of misfolded alpha-synuclein (aS), thought to originate in the bowel. Lewy Bodies travel to the brain via the vagus nerve and may disrupt neural function.

Liposomal: water soluble nutrients packaged with liposomes (tiny fat bubbles) to aid absorption.

Lipospheric: see liposomal.

Live Blood Analysis: a method of analysing fresh blood (drops) under a special microscope to gain an insight into the health or illness of the patient.

Lyme disease: an infection with Borrelia burgdorferi sensu stricto. Often used broadly and inaccurately to describe infections with many Borrelia species and other "co-infections". "Lyme disease" is both a specific infectious disease and a generic name given to a group of infections.

Lyme-like illness: a term sometimes used to describe infectious diseases which may mimic Lyme disease or a complex infectious disease that may include one or more species of Borrelia.

Mediterranean Diet: a term loosely used to describe common dietary choices of people living in the Mediterranean region. Often described as including whole grains, vegetables, fruit fish and oils (e.g. olive). However, there are many variations of the "Mediterranean diet".

Medulla: the inner part of an organ (e.g. kidney medulla) as distinct from the outer or cortex region.

Meta-analysis: a research process when many studies researching the same subject are gathered together and examined for quality and conclusions. An overall trend may then be described and conclusions reached on the basis of examining many independent studies.

Methylation: part of our detoxification and recycling processes when methyl groups are added to molecules to change their characteristic or action and assist many metabolic functions. Dopamine is produced from tyrosine at the end of one methylation process.

Methylenetetrahydrofolate reductase (MTHFR): an enzyme that is critical in a number of methylation processes including those involving folate.

Microbiome: a collection of bacteria which colonise various parts of our body. For example, the gut microbiome and skin microbiome.

Mitigate: to reduce the severity (e.g. mitigate symptoms)

Mitochondria: the energy-producing organelle in cells. They produce ATP energy.

Monoamine oxidase B (MAOB): an enzyme that breaks down dopamine.

Monosodium Glutamate (MSG): a flavour enhancer added to food. Health authorities class it as "generally recognised as safe", but there are indications of health hazards with its use.

Motor Neurone Disease (MND): a group of diseases in which motor neurones degenerate and die.

Multi-level Marketing (MLM): a sales device in which people choosing to sell particular products seek to recruit friends, family or associates to become "sub-sales people", thus forming a type of pyramid of untrained or semi-trained people selling product on commission. Greater commissions are generally paid to those higher on the pyramid.

Multiple Sclerosis (MS): a disorder in which myelin surrounding nerves is damaged or destroyed creating varied physical and emotional symptoms.

Multisystem Atrophy (MSA): one of the group of neurode-generative disorders sometimes known as Parkinson's plus or Parkinsonism. The aetiological pathways are the same as for Parkinson's disease.

Mycoplasma: a bacterial disorder with numerous species. The bacteria lack a cell wall around the membrane, making them resistant to antibiotics that attack the cell wall. Often a co-infection with other vector-borne infections.

Nasogastric tube: a tube passed through the nose into the stomach for introducing food or for drainage.

National Health and Medical Research Council (NHMRC): a body appointed by the Australian Government to act as the peak overseer of health and medical research. Generally strictly conservative and pharmaceutical prone in outlook and pronouncement.

Natural killer cells: a type of lymphocyte that are an important part of our innate immunity.

Neurodegenerative: describes any process that damages, degrades or kills neurones.

Neurologist: a medical specialist dealing with diseases of the nervous system.

Neurotransmitter: a chemical expressed at the end of a nerve fibre (axon) to cross the synapse (gap) and carry the nerve message to the next nerve cell or the receptor organ or tissue.

Nocebo: words or expressions that discourage belief in a positive outcome of action or treatment. For example, "there is nothing you can do to help yourself".

Non-Hodgkin's Lymphoma: cancer that originates in the lymphatic system.

Noradrenaline: a catecholamine that functions as a hormone and neurotransmitter. It is expressed from the adrenal glands

Norepinephrine: another name for noradrenaline.

Oedema: an inappropriate build-up of fluid in the body. It may occur in one place (e.g. ankles), or be more general.

Oesophagus: part of the gastrointestinal tract joining the mouth and the stomach.

Off gassing: gasses emitting from materials that are sometimes toxic.

Off-label prescription: medicine prescribed for purposes other than that for which it was researched and approved (e.g. cancer drugs used to treat arthritis and/or MS).

Oncologist: a medical specialist treating cancer.

Organelle: structures within living cells, such as mitochondria, that perform many functions.

Organophosphate: a class of organophosphorus compounds most commonly used as pesticides.

Osteoporosis: a loss of bone mass so that bones become weak and fragile.

Oxytocin: a peptide hormone and neuropeptide normally produced in the hypothalamus and released by the posterior pituitary.

Palliation: to relieve or mask symptoms without reversing them or treating the cause.

Parabens: preservatives widely used in cosmetic and pharmaceutical products.

Paralysis agitans: an early name for Parkinson's disease.

PCR (Polymerase Chain Reaction): used in molecular biology to make copies of a specific DNA segment. Tests using this method can detect infections before antibodies are present in the blood.

Peptic ulcer: ulcer inside the stomach.

Percutaneous endoscopic gastronomy (PEG): a medical procedure to pass a tube into the stomach through the abdominal wall. Often used to feed patients unable to eat or swallow.

pH: the measure of acidity or alkalinity of any substance. The scale ranges from 0 (most acidic) through 7 (neutral) to 14 (most alkaline).

Phthalates: a family of industrial chemicals use to soften PVC plastics, and as solvents in many products including cosmetics. May damage a number of human organs.

Physiotherapist: a university/college trained physical therapist working with musculoskeletal challenges and rehabilitation after injury, illness or surgery.

Placebo: a substance with no measurable therapeutic activity but which the patient believes is treating their condition.

Polypharmacy: the prescription of more than one pharmaceutical drug to one patient.

Polyphenols: micronutrients in plant foods.

POTS (Postural Orthostatic Tachycardia Syndrome): an abnormally large increase in heart rate when moving from lying to standing. May be accompanied with serious symptoms including dizziness and falls that cause injury.

Primary Care Physician (PCP): a medical doctor in public practice. Often the first therapist to see a person with an illness. Called a General Practitioner in some countries.

Prodromal (symptoms): symptoms which appear some time before a diagnosable illness is apparent.

Progressive Supranuclear Palsy (PSP): a brain disorder that affects movement and autonomic functions. Sometimes included in a group of "Parkinson's Plus" disorders.

Prophylaxis: strategies to prevent the onset of illness.

Propylene glycol: an antifreeze used by the chemical, pharmaceutical and food industries.

Proton Pump Inhibitor (PPI): medication that reduces the production of stomach acid by blocking the gastric proton pump.

Protozoa: Protozoa is an informal term for single-celled eukaryotes, either free-living or parasitic, which feed on organic matter such as other microorganisms or organic tissues and debris. Babesia and Malaria are protozoa.

Psychologist: a university-trained therapist dealing with mental and emotional challenges. Psychologists are generally not licensed to prescribe pharmaceutical medication.

Psychosomatic: disorders that are considered to be generated by the patient's thoughts and emotions rather than any identifiable cause or process.

Reactive Oxygen Species (ROS): an unstable molecule containing oxygen that easily reacts with other molecules in a cell.

Red Lead: lead oxide, coloured red, used in a number of industrial processes. Was previously used by plumbers to prevent rust.

Reflux: the regurgitation of acidic stomach contents past the lower oesophageal sphincter into the oesophagus.

Rheumatoid Arthritis: an autoimmune disorder that causes pain and swelling of the joints.

Roundup: an herbicide containing glyphosate produced by Monsanto.

Serology: the study of or diagnosis through examination of blood serum.

Serotonin: a neurotransmitter.

Shaking palsy: an early name for Parkinson's disease.

Silicones: polymers made up of chains of alternating silicone and oxygen atoms, combined with carbon and hydrogen.

Single nucleotide polymorphism (SNP): the most common type of genetic variation among people. Each SNP represents a difference in a single DNA building block, called a nucleotide.

Squalene: a hydrocarbon and a triterpene, a precursor for synthesis of animal sterols, including cholesterol and steroid hormones in the human body.

Stealth Infection: any infection in which the pathogen has the ability to "hide" from the immune system by changing form or changing antigens on the cell surface. Difficult to detect by blood test. Borrelia and Bartonella are common stealth infections.

Steroids: synthetic drugs that resemble hormones produced by the adrenal glands. Corticosteroids are often prescribed for inflammatory disorders while anabolic steroids are used to build muscle mass.

Stress: any activity which triggers release of stress hormones from the adrenal glands. Stress may be useful, neutral or damaging.

Substantia nigra pars compacta: part of the substantia nigra, located in the mid brain, formed by dopaminergic cells. These cells have an indirect influence on fine motor movement.

Sulfates: complex chemicals that form when sulphuric acid reacts with another chemical.

Sulphides: inorganic anions of sulphur used in the manufacture of many inorganic products, including pesticides.

Supplement (nutritional): a refined or synthesised nutrient prepared as tablet, capsule or powder for consumption to increase ingestion of that nutrient.

Syndrome: a group of symptoms that consistently occur together, but not necessarily defined as a disease.

Systematic review: summarises the results of available carefully designed healthcare studies (controlled trials) and provides a high level of evidence on the effectiveness of healthcare interventions.

Tachycardia: a heart rate that exceeds the normal resting rate. Often defined as over 100 BPM at rest.

Tannins: astringent, polyphenolic biomolecules found in some foods, particularly teas (from Camelia sinensis) and dry wines. May be useful as antioxidants and antimicrobials but are also dehydrating and may be carcinogenic in high doses.

T-cells: a type of lymphocyte critical for our immune response.

Testosterone: an anabolic steroid hormone expressed from the adrenal glands. The predominant male hormone which drives the development of male sexual characteristics.

TGA: Therapeutic Goods Administration (Australia). The peak approval body in Australia for the release and use of pharmaceutical drugs, medical devices, nutritional supplements, herbs and other Complementary/Alternative Medicine.

Thalidomide: an immunomodulatory drug used to treat certain cancers. From 1954 to 1961, Thalidomide was marketed as a mild anti-nausea/sedative drug for pregnant women. However, in 1962, it was revealed that it could cause very severe birth defects and it is estimated that up to 100,000 babies worldwide were affected, most dying at or before birth. 10,000 babies were born with limb defects. Approximately 3000 "Thalidomide Babies" are still alive today.

Tight junction: the joining of cells in epithelial tissue, particularly the lining of our gastrointestinal tube. Tight junctions prevent the transfer of large molecules between the gut and interstitium. If tight junctions become loose or expand, inappropriate molecules may transfer and cause irritation, inflammation, or more serious dysfunction.

Tinnitus: a physical condition, experienced as noises or ringing in the ears or head when no such external physical noise is present.

Traditional Chinese medicine: a style of medicine using herbs, diet, exercise, lifestyle and other modalities developed by Chinese physicians over many thousands of years.

Transdermal: passing through the dermis (skin).

Trauma: an event or circumstance that is shocking to the victim, participant or observer.

Vagus nerve: the tenth cranial nerve that controls autonomic function in the torso. Transfers neurotransmitters and aS from the gut to the brain.

Western Allopathic Medicine: Interventionist medicine developed in the Western world during the 19th Century and beyond. It relies heavily on combating symptom expression using pharmaceutical or surgical intervention based on mechanical or technological assessment of the patient.

Wilson's disease: a rare genetic disorder that causes accumulation of copper in the body to toxic levels.

Yoghurt: food produced by bacterial fermentation of milk. Traditionally made from animal milk, it may also be made from plant-based milk products (e.g. coconut).

ENDNOTES

1: I USED TO HAVE PARKINSON'S DISEASE

1   "Diagnosis – Rating Scales", https://parkinsonsdisease.net/
diagnosis/rating-scales-staging/

2   Coleman, John C: *Stop Parkin' and Start Livin': Reversing the symptoms
of Parkinson's disease*, Michelle Anderson publishing, 2005.

3   Coleman, John C: Shaky Past, *Return To Stillness*/TB Books,
2012.

4   ibid.

5   Small, Terry: "Brain Bulletin #47 – The Science
of Hope", https://www.terrysmall.com/blog/
brain-bulletin-47-the-science-of-hope

2: WHAT IS PARKINSON'S DISEASE?

1   World Health Organisation (WHO) Constitution.

2   Scully, Jackie Leach: "View Point: What is a disease?", EMBO
Reports VOL 5 (7) 2004

3   ibid.

4   ibid.

5   University of Pittsburgh Schools of the Health Sciences:
"Key to Parkinson's disease neurodegeneration found."
ScienceDaily. ScienceDaily, 8 June 2016. www.sciencedaily.com/
releases/2016/06/160608154030.htm

6   Clouston, Dr Paul: "New Thoughts on the Pathogenesis
of Parkinson's Disease", Stand By Me, 2015, https://
www.parkinsonsnsw.org.au/wp-content/uploads/2015/06/
SBM_Winter_2015_final-web.pdf

7   ibid.

8   Ribeiro, Marta: "11 Facts About Parkinson's Disease
     You May Not Know", https://parkinsonsnewstoday.
     com/2017/08/03/11-facts-parkinsons-may-not-know/

3: A BRIEF HISTORY OF PARKINSON'S DISEASE AND ITS TREATMENT

1   Parkinson's Disease Information: "Parkinson's disease History",
     http://www.parkinsons.org/parkinsons-history.html, accessed
     December 2018.

2   ibid.

3   Newman, Tim, reviewed by Gregory, Philip, PharmD,
     MS: "Penicillin: How do penicillins work?", https://www.
     bellevernonarea.net/cms/lib/PA01001262/Centricity/Domain/298/
     Penicillin%20Reading.pdf

4   Parkinson, James: "An Essay on the Shaking Palsy",
     first published as monograph by Sherwood, Seely and
     Jones, London, 1817; republished with original wording
     and punctuation in Journal of Neuropsychiatry Clinical
     Neuroscience 14:2, Spring 2002. https://neuro.psychiatryonline.
     org/doi/10.1176/jnp.14.2.223

5   Goetz, Christopher G.: "The History of Parkinson's Disease:
     Early Clinical Descriptions and Neurological Therapies", Cold
     Spring Harbor Perspectives in Medicine 2011; 1(1):a008862,
     https://www.ncbi.nlm.nih.gov/pmc/articles/PMC3234454/

6   University of California PD Center; "Parkinson's Disease
     Medications: Patient Edition", copyright The Regents of
     the University of California 2014, https://pdcenter.ucsf.edu/
     parkinsons-disease-medications

7   The Science of Parkinson's, Plain English information about
     the research being conducted on Parkinson's: "The Agony
     and the Ecstasy", July 27, 2017, https://scienceofparkinsons.
     com/2017/07/27/the-agony-and-the-ecstasy/

4: WESTERN ALLOPATHIC TREATMENT OF PARKINSON'S DISEASE

1   Jie-Qiong, Li, Tan Lan and Yu Jin-Tai; "The role of the LRRK2 gen in Parkinsonism", Li et al., Molecular Neurodegeneration 2014, 9:47, https://www.ncbi.nlm.nih.gov/pmc/articles/PMC4246469/

2   Centers for Disease Control and Prevention: Adverse Childhood Experiences (ACEs), https://www.cdc.gov/violenceprevention/childabuseandneglect/acestudy/index.html, 19 March 2019.

3   Schrag A, Y. Ben Schlomo, N. Quinn: "How valid is the clinical diagnosis of Parkinson's disease in the community?" J Neurol Neurosurg Psychiatry 2002; 73:529-534.

4   Scott, Sophie (medical reporter, ABC, Australia): "Calls to scrap diagnosis of 'Parkinson's disease', with one in four misdiagnosed", ABC News, updated Mon 21 Nov 2016, 3:05 pm.

5   Clements, Joanne: "Doctors thought I had Parkinson's for nearly a decade – they were wrong", Parkinson's Life Perspectives: 29 September 2016; https://parkinsonslife.eu/parkinsons-misdiagnosis-joanne-clements/

6   Shrourou, Alina, BSc (ed), review: "Experts highlight emerging evidence of impending Parkinson's disease pandemic", https://www.news-medical.net/news/20200405/Experts-highlight-the-impact-of-COVID-19-pandemic-on-patients-with-Parkinsone28099s-disease.aspx

7   Alcalay, RN, MD, MSc , et al.: "The Association between Mediterranean Diet Adherence and Parkinson's Disease", NIH Public Access, Author Manuscript; Movement Disorders 2012 May; 27(6): 771-774. Doi: 10.1002/mds.24918. https://onlinelibrary.wiley.com/doi/abs/10.1002/mds.24918

5: COMPLEMENTARY/ALTERNATIVE MEDICINE APPROACHES TO PARKINSON'S DISEASE – AN OVERVIEW

1   Hechtman, Leah, PhD (Cand), MSciMed (RHHG), BHSc, ND:

Clinical Naturopathic Medicine; Elsevier 2018.

2   Coleman, John C, ND: *Shaky Past,* Return To Stillness/TB
     Books, 2012.

6: CAUSES AND DEVELOPMENT OF PARKINSON'S DISEASE

1   Lipton, Bruce H. PhD: *The Biology of Belief*, Mountain of Love/
     Elite Books, Santa Rosa, CA 95404, USA 2005.

2   Jie-Qiong, Li, Tan Lan and Yu Jin-Tai; *The role of the LRRK2 gen
     in Parkinsonism*; Li et al., Molecular Neurodegeneration 2014,
     9:47.

7: WHAT CAUSES PARKINSON'S?

1   Lipton, Bruce H. PhD: The Biology of Belief, Mountain of
     Love/Elite Books, Santa Rosa, CA 95404, USA 2005.

2   Ji, Sayer: The Dark Side of Wheat, page 4.

3   Editors of Encyclopedia Britannica: "Single nucleotide
     polymorphism", updated by Kara Rogers, 2019.

4   US National library of Medicine: "What are single nucleotide
     polymorphisms (SNPs)?", https://ghr.nlm.nih.gov/primer/
     genomicresearch/snp; 2019.

5   Genetics Home Reference: https://ghr.nlm.gov/condition/
     parkinson-disease, March 19, 2019.

6   ibid.

8: THE TRAUMA PATHWAY

1   Oxford Dictionary definition of trauma: https://
     en.oxforddictionaries.com/definition/trauma

2   Sidran Institute: Resources, for Survivors and Loved Ones,
     https://www.sidran.org/wp-content/uploads/2019/04/What-Is-
     Psychological-Trauma.pdf

3   Merriam Webster: definition of "stress", https://www.merriam-
     webster.com/dictionary/stress

4   Victoroff, Dr Jeff: *Saving Your Brain*, Bantam Books (Random
     House Australia), Milsons Point, NSW, Australia, 2002.

5   McEwan, Professor Bruce: interview by Dr Norman Swan on ABC Radio National "The Health Report", 10 January 2005, downloaded from ABC website 11 January 2005. "Study finds link between upper GI infections and protein implicated in Parkinson's disease", http://www.news-medical.net/news/20170628/Study-finds-link-between-upper-GI-infections-and-protein-implicated-in-Parkinsone28099s-disease.aspx, June 28 2017.

6   ibid.

7   ibid.

8   Centers for Disease Control and Prevention: Adverse Childhood Experiences (ACEs), https://www.cdc.gov/violenceprevention/childabuseandneglect/acestudy/index.html?CDC_AA_refVal=https per cent3A per cent2F per cent2Fwww.cdc.gov per cent2Fviolenceprevention per cent2Facestudy per cent2Findex.html, 19 March 2019.

9   ibid.

10   ibid.

11   ibid.

12   ibid.

13   ibid..

14   ibid..

9: THE ENVIRONMENTAL TOXIN PATHWAY

1   Harmon, Katherine: "Humans feasting on grains for at least 100,000 years", Scientific American, December 17, 2009.

2   Gibbons Ann: "The Evolution of Diet", National Geographic, https://www.nationalgeographic.com/foodfeatures/evolution-of-diet/

3   Ji, Sayer: *The Dark Side of Wheat*, page 4.

4   Gutierrez, David: "Dairy Consumption Increases Parkinson's Risk in Men"; http://www.naturalnews.com/z022463_dairy_Parkinsons_risk.html

5   Walia, Arjun: "A Massive New Study Shows How A Cow's Milk Does NOT Do The Body Good"; http://thespiritscience. net/2015/09/12/a-massive-new-study-shows-how-a-cows-milk-does-not-do-the-body-good/, September 12, 2015.

6   Hyman, Mark MD: "Dairy: 6 Reasons You Should Avoid It at all Costs"; https://drhyman.com/blog/2010/06/24/ dairy-6-reasons-you-should-avoid-it-at-all-costs-2.

7   Goldschmidt Vivian: "ALERT: New Study Confirms Dairy Harms Bones"; https://saveourbones.com/alert-new-study-confirms-dairy-harms-bones/; December 2018.

8   Mercola, Dr Joseph: "Aspartame – By Far the Most Dangerous Substance Added to Most Foods Today", , https://articles. mercola.com/sites/articles/archive/2011/11/06/aspartame-most-dangerous-substance-added-to-food.aspx

9   University Health News staff: "Aspartame Side Effects: Recent Research Confirms Reasons for Concern", https:// universityhealthnews.com/daily/nutrition/aspartame-side-effects-recent-research-confirms-reasons-for-concern/

10   Lillis, Charlotte, reviewed by Katherine Marengo LDN, RD: "What are the side effects of aspartame?" https://www. medicalnewstoday.com/articles/322266.php

11   "Aspartame Being Re-Branded as AminoSweet: The Next Chapter in Aspartame's Dangerous History", https://realfarmacy. com/fda-aspartame-name-change/

12   Alcohol and Drug Foundation (Australia): "Caffeine", https://adf. org.au/drug-facts/caffeine/

13   Klotz, Katrin, et al.: "The Health Effects of Aluminum Exposure", Medicine, Deutsches Arzteblatt International 2017; 114: 653-9

14   Exley, C: "The toxicity of aluminium in humans", The Birchall Centre, https://www.sciencedirect.com/science/article/pii/ S1286011516000023?via per cent3Dihub

15   Fergus, Alex: "Glyphosate: The Weed Killer Found In Our Food & Water", https://www.alexfergus.com/blog

16   Fergus, Alex; "Why You Need To Eat Organic", https://www.alexfergus.com/blog

17   Agriculture Victoria (Australia): "Spraying, spray drift and off-target damage", http://agriculture.vic.gov.au/agriculture/farm-management

18   Nancarrow, Tom, ABC Rural: "Spray drift towards SA vineyards prompts calls for crackdown on crop spraying 'recklessness'", https://www.abc.net.au/news/rural/2018-02-28/calls-for-crackdown-on-spray-drift-amid-rise-in-sa-reports/9490130

19   "PPI use linked to chronic kidney damage even without acute disease", http://www.medicalobserver.com.au/medical-news/gastroenterology/ppi-use-linked-to-chronic-kidney-damage-even-without-acute-disease

20   Kresser Chris: "Eight More Reasons to Avoid Proton Pump Inhibitors", https://kresserinstitute.com/eight-reasons-avoid-proton-pump-inhibitors/

10: THE INFECTION PATHWAY

1   Wang, Guiqing, Alie P van Dam, Ira Schwartz, Jacob Dankert: "Molecular Typing of Borrelia burgdorferi Senu Lato: Taxonomic, Epidemiological, and Clinical Implications", http://www.ncbi.nih.gov/pmc/articles/PMC88929/

2   ibid.

3   ibid.

4   Horowitz MD, Richard I: *Why Can't I Get Better? – Solving the Mystery of Lyme and Chronic Disease*, St. Martin's Press, New York, 2013.

5   ibid.

6   ibid.

7   McFadzean, N.D. Nicola: *Lyme Disease in Australia*, BioMed Publishing Group, South Lake Tahoe, CA, USA, 2012.

8   Buhner, Stephen Harrod: *Healing Lyme*; Raven Press, Silver City, NM, USA, 2005.

9   Horowitz, op. cit.

10 ibid.

11 Carnahan, Dr Jill and Dr Sandeep Gupta: "Mast Cells and Mold Illness" Transcription of a webinar held on 21 September 2017. www.moldillnessmadesimple.pdf

12 Horowitz, op. cit.

13 ibid.

11: FINDING THE AETIOLOGICAL PATHWAY

1   Horowitz MD, Richard I: *Why Can't I Get Better? – Solving the Mystery of Lyme and Chronic Disease*, St. Martin's Press, New York, 2013.

13: FOOD, HELPFUL AND HARMFUL

1   Raloff, Janet;: *"Reevaluating Eggs' Cholesterol Risks"*; https://www.sciencenews.org/blog/food-thought/reevaluating-eggs-cholesterol-risks; May 2, 2006.

2   UHN Staff: "Cholesterol in Eggs, Facts Replace Common Myths and Prove Eggs' Many Benefits"; https://universityhealthnews.com/daily/heart-health, Aug 10, 2018.

3   Blesso, Christopher N, Maria Luz Fernandez: "Dietary Cholesterol, Serum Lipids, and Heart Disease: Are Eggs Working for or Against You?"; Nutrients 2018, 10, 426; doi: 10.3390/nu10040426; www.mdpi.com/journal/nutrients

4   Bullet Proof Staff: "The Complete Bulletproof Guide to Gluten and Grains", https://blog.bulletproof.com; 2018.

5   Gutierrez, David: "Dairy Consumption Increases Parkinson's Risk in Men"; naturalnews.com, January 7, 2008.

6   Walia, Arjun: "A Massive New Study Shows How A Cow's Milk Does NOT Do The Body Good", http://thesprirtscience.net/2015/09/12/, September 12, 2015.

7   Whiteman, Honor: "Low-fat dairy intake may raise Parkinson's risk", https://www.medicalnewstoday.com/articles/317834.php, Thursday 8 June 2017.

8   "12 Reasons to Stop Drinking Cow's Milk", https://www.peta.
     org/living/food/ 2018.

9   ibid.

10   Gutierrez, David: "Dairy Consumption Increases Parkinson's
     Risk in Men"; naturalnews.com, January 7, 2008.

11   Whiteman, Honor: "Low-fat dairy intake may raise Parkinson's
     risk", https://www.medicalnewstoday.com/articles/317834.php,
     Thursday 8 June 2017.

12   Mercola, Dr Joseph: "Aspartame – By Far the Most Dangerous
     Substance Added to Most Foods Today", https://articles.mercola.
     com/sites/articles/archive/2011/11/06/

13   Lopes, Jose Marques, PhD: "Study Links Smoking,
     Reduced Parkinson's Risk, But Comes with Caveat";
     Parkinsonsnewstoday.com/2018/11/28.

14   Godwin-Austen, RB, PNP N Lee, MG Marmot, GM Stern:
     "Smoking and Parkinson's disease", Journal of Neurology,
     Neurosurgery, and Psychiatry 1982;45:577-581.

15   Celentano, Joanne Curran PhD: "Where do Eggs Fit in a Heart-
     healthy Diet?", Am J, Lifestyle Med. 2009; 3(4):274-278.

14: DETOXING

1   Agriculture Victoria: "Spraying, spray drift and off-target
     damage", http://agriculture.vic.gov.au/agriculture/farm-
     management/chemicaluse, 2017.

2   Fergus, Alex: "Glyphosate: The Weed Killer Found In Our Food
     & Water", https://alexfergus.com/blog/, 2018.

15: BASIC NUTRITIONAL SUPPLEMENTS

1   Saul, Andrew W: "Hidden in Plain Sight: The Pioneering Work
     of Frederick Rober T Klenner, M.D."; J Orthomolecular Med,
     2007. Vol 22, No 1, p 31-38.

2   Klenner, Frederick R, MD, FCCP: "Observations On the Dose
     and Administration of Ascorbic Acid When Employed Beyond
     the Range Of A Vitamin In Human Pathology", Journal of

Applied Nutrition Vol 23, No's 3 & 4, Winter 1971.

3   Coleman, John C: *Measure of Love – The Story of a Boy and the Founding of Very Special Kids*, unpublished.

4   Slutsky, Inna et al.: "Enhancement of Learning and Memory by Elevating Brain Magnesium", Neuron 65, 165-177, January 28, 2010 © Elsevier Inc.

5   Grober, Uwe et al.: "Myth or Reality – Transdermal Magnesium?"; Nutrients. 2017 Aug: 9(8): 813; PMCID: PMC5579607; PMID: 28788060.

6   Jelinek, Professor George: *Overcoming Multiple Sclerosis – an evidence-based guide to recovery*, Allen & Unwin, 2010.

7   Prasad, Hari and Rao Rajini: "Amyloid clearance defect in ApoE4 astrocytes is reversed by epigenetic correction of endosomal pH", PNAS vol 115 no. 28, 2018.

8   "PPI use linked to chronic kidney damage even without acute disease", http://www.medicalobserver.com.au/medical-news/ gastroenterology/ppi-use-linked-to-chronic-kidney-damage-even-without-acute-disease

9   *MIMS Annual 2018*; UBM Medica Australia Pty Ltd, St Leonards, NSW Australia.

16. ACTIVITY

1   Yeager, Selene: "Why Cycling May be the Best Way to Handle Parkinson's", https://www.bicycling.com/news/g20011415/-16/

17. ENGAGE WITH HEALTHY PEOPLE AND DEVELOP A HEALTHY MINDSET

1   Case histories taken from clinical notes between 2001 and 2018.

18. LAUGH, LOVE AND MEDITATE

1   Marjama-Lyons, Jill, MD: *What Your Doctor May Not Tell You About Parkinson's Disease*, Warner Books, New York, USA, 2003.

2   Flanagan, Dr Gael Crystal and Dr Patrick: "Laughter – Still the Best Medicine", www.heylady.com/rbc/laughter.htm, downloaded

25 January 2005.

3   Doskoch, Peter: "Happily Ever Laughter", *Psychology Today*, July/August 1996.

4   Welch, Susan: "The Best Medicine"; Sunday *Herald Sun*, January 30, 2005, Melbourne, Australia.

5   Doskoch, Peter: op. cit.

6   Welch, Susan: op. cit.

7   Borge, Victor: "Quotations By Subject", The Quotations Page, www.quotationspage.com, downloaded 30 January 2005.

8   Dietrich, A,WF McDaniel: "Endocannabinoids and exercise"; Br J Sports Med 2004;38:536-541. Doi: 10.1136/bjsm.2004.011718.

9   Sparling PB, A Giuffrida, D Piomelli, L Rosskopf, A Dietrich: "Exercise activates the endocannabinoid system", PMID: 14625449, DOI: x10.1097/01.wnr0000097048.56589.47.

19. HYDRATION

1   Boublik, Dr Jaroslav: "Natural Health Supplement Guide – What Is Hydration?", https://www.hydration.net.au/publications/

2   Coleman, John C: *Shaky Past*, Return To Stillness/TB Books, 2012.

3   Coleman John C: *Stop Parkin' and Start Livin': Reversing the symptoms of Parkinson's disease*, Michelle Anderson Publishing, 2005.

20. MITIGATING SYMPTOMS, WAM AND CAM

1   Gonzalez-Usigli, Hector A.: *Parkinson's Disease*, MSD Manual Professional Version, Merck Sharp and Dohme Corp., Kenilworth, NJ, USA 2019.

2   Parkinson's Australia: "Information Sheet", www.parkinsons.org.au, 2019.

3   McCance Kathryn L, Sue E Huether: *Pathophysiology – The Biologic Basis for Disease in Adults and Children*, The C. V. Mosby Company, 1990.

4 Iansek Robert: "Parkinson's disease: Practical approach to treatment", Current Therapeutics, October 1995.

5 Marjama-Lyons MD, J and Mary J Shomon: *What Your Doctor May Not Tell You About Parkinson's Disease*, Warner Books, New York, USA, 2003.

6 The Conversation: "What we know and suspect about the causes of Parkinson's disease", http://www.medicalobserver.com.au/medical-news/what-we-know-and-suspect-about-the-causes-of-parkinsons-disease

7 Evans, Dr Andrew H, FRACP, MD: Letter to John Coleman 16 July 2012.

8 Hechtman, Leah: *"Foundations of Clinical Naturopathic Medicine – Second Edition"*, Elsevier Australia, Chatswood, Australia,15 October 2018.

9 *MIMS Annual 2018*: UBM Medica Australia Pty Ltd, St Leonards, NSW Australia.

10 ibid.

11 ibid.

12 ibid.

13 ibid.

21. BODYWORK

1 Coleman, John, C: *Shaky Past*, Return To Stillness/TB Books, 2012.

2 ibid.

3 Baker, Julian: "Less is more", International Journal of Alternative and Complementary Medicine, Vol 14 No 12, December 1996, pp 16-18.

4 Stammers, Glen: "The Bowen Technique", WellBeing Magazine, International Edition, No 65, pp. 88-89.

5 Oyston, Eleanor: *A Simple Explanation of the Science of Bowen therapy*, unpublished, 2004.

6 ibid.

7   ibid.

8   Baker, Julian: "Less is more", International Journal of Alternative and Complementary Medicine, Vol 14 No 12, December 1996, pp 16-18.

9   Morling Greg: "Parkinson's disease and massage therapy", International Journal of Alternative and Complementary Medicine, Vol 16 No 3, March 1998, pp. 24-25.

10   Chaitow Leon: "Energy and bodywork", International Journal of Alternative and Complementary Medicine, Vol 15 No 8, August 1997, pp. 28-32.

11   Chaitow Leon: "Muscular influences on cranial dysfunction", International Journal of Alternative and Complementary Medicine, Vol 16 No 1, January 1998, pp. 30-32.

12   Chaitow Leon: op. cit., pp. 31-33

13   ibid.

14   Australian Feldenkrais Guild Inc.: *Feldenkrais*, a training brochure.

15   ibid.

16   ibid.

17   ibid.

18   ibid.

19   This definition was suggested by Dr. Alfred Flechas of Ocala, Florida, https://www.alexandertechnique.com/at/

20   The Complete Guide to the Alexander Technique, https://www.alexandertechnique.com/at/

21   ibid.

22. COMORBIDITIES AND CONFLICTING TREATMENTS

1   General reference and inspiration: Turner, Kelly A. PhD: Radical Remission: Harper One, New York, USA, 2014.

23. REVERSING THE TRAUMA/STRESS PATHWAY

1   MIMS Annual 2018: UBM Medica Australia Pty Ltd, St

Leonards, NSW Australia.

2   Edwards Scott: "Dancing and the Brain", On The Brain Newsletter, Harvard Mahoney Neuroscience Institute, https:// neuro.hms.harvard.edu/harvard-mahoney-neurosceince-institute

3   Bergland, Christopher: "Why Is Dancing So Good for Your Brain?", https://www.psychologytoday.com/au/blog/the-athletes/way/201310/

24. FOR PRACTITIONERS

1   Burrows Graham D: "Depressive Disorders", Disease Index, E-MIMS, February 2001.

25. REVERSING THE TOXIN PATHWAY

1   Atlay, Kemal: "The science is in: aspirin for CVD primary prevention is out", *Australian Doctor*, 23 January, 2019.

2   Juderon Associates: "Societal vs Individual Risk of Death in Australia", 2017.

3   Moran, Rick: "Medical Errors now the 3rd leading cause of death in the US", American Thinker, http://americanthinker.com/blog/2016/05/

4   Waking Science: "Fluoride Officially Classified a Neurotoxin in World's Most Prestigious Medical Journal", http://wakingscience.com/2016/02/

5   McFadden Christopher: "How Does a Faraday Cage Work", https://interestingengineering.com/how-does-a-faraday-cage-work

6   Charlton Karen: "Explainer: what is scurvy and is it making a comeback?", The Conversation, 2016, http://theconversation.com

7   Unknown author: "Scurvy returns to Australia due to poor diet", mydr.com.au/nutrition-weight/

8   8. Levy MD, JD, Thomas, E: *Primal Panacea*, MedFox Publishing, USA, 2011.

9   Slutsky, Inna et al.: "Enhancement of Learning and Memory by

Elevating Brain Magnesium", Neuron 65, 165-77, January 28, 2010.

26. REVERSING THE INFECTION PATHWAY

1   Horowitz MD, Richard I: *Why Can't I Get Better? – Solving the Mystery of Lyme and Chronic Disease*, St Martin's Press, USA, 2013.

2   Buhner, Stephen Harrod: *Healing Lyme*, Raven Press, USA, 2005.

3   McFadzean ND, Nicola: *Lyme Disease in Australia*, BioMed Publishing Group, USA, 2012.

4   Horowitz MD, Richard I: op.cit.

5   ibid.

27. CAN WAM AND CAM CO-EXIST IN ONE PATIENT?

1   Case histories taken from clinical notes between 2001 and 2018.

28. STRATEGIES TO AVOID

1   Goldman, Rena and Rachel Nagelberg, medically reviewed by Natalie Butler, RD, LD: "Alkaline Water: Benefits and Risks", https://healthline.com/health/food-nutrition/alkaline-water, 2018.

2   Unnamed authors: "Deaths from Marijuana vs. 17 FDA-Approved Drugs (Jan. 1, 1997 to June 30, 2005)", https://medicalmarijuana.procon.org/view.resource.php?resourceID=000145

3   Bass BSc, Kate: "New Research defines impact of cannabis on health", http://www.news-medical.net/news/201701113, 2017.

4   Unknown author: "How CBD Works", https://www.projectcbd.org/how-cbd-works

5   Jelinek, Professor George: *Overcoming multiple sclerosis – an evidence-based guide to recovery*, Allen & Unwin, 2010.

6   Oyston, Eleanor: *A Simple Explanation of the Science of Bowen therapy*, unpublished: 2004.

29. BEING WELL

1   Coleman, John C: *Shaky Past*, Return To Stillness/TB Books, 2012.

30. FINDING PRACTITIONERS

1   Coleman, John C: *Shaky Past*, Return To Stillness/TB Books, 2012.

34. EVIDENCE-BASED MEDICINE

1   National Health and Medical Research Council (2009): "NHMRC Levels of Evidence and Grades for Recommendations for Developers of Clinical Practice Guidelines", retrieved 2 July, 2014 from: https://www.nhmrc.gov. au/_files_nhmrc/file/guidelines/developers/nhmrc_levels_grades_ evidence_120423.pdf

2   Hoffman, T, S Bennett, & C Del Mar (2013): *Evidence-Based Practice: Across the Health Professions* (2nd ed.), Chatswood, NSW: Elsevier.

3   *MIMS Annual 2018*, UBM Medica Australia Pty Ltd, St Leonards, NSW, Australia.

4   Atlay, Kemal: *"The science is in: aspirin for CVD primary prevention is out"*, Australian Doctor, 23 January, 2019.

5   https://www.medicalobserver.com.au/medical-news/psychiatry/ evidence-based-medicine?pri= This Update explores the efficacy of evidence-based medicine in clinical practice. It is by Professor Chris Del Mar, MD, FRACGP and Associate Professor Tammy Hoffmann, PhD, BOccThy (Hons), 2012.

6   Ioannidis John PA: "Evidence-based medicine has been hijacked: a report to David Sackett", https://drjustincoleman. com/2017/01/17/gp-sceptics-pod7-ebm-hijacked/

7   Victorian Government: "Complementary Therapies", https:// www.betterhealth.vic.gov.au/health/conditionsandtreatments/ complementary-therapies?fbclid=IwAR2bJlBcAmjM1LuOU80TsFFl TnNosJsdZO4LITXH9cMxVV2rJg2gwEb1JRE

8   Ross Gil: "Science Publication Is Hopelessly Compromised, Say Journal Editors", https://www.acsh.org/news/2015/05/19/science-publication-is-hopelessly-compromised-say-journal-editors Gyles, Carlton: "Skeptical of medical reports?". The Canadian Vetinary Journal, CVJ VOL 56/OCTOBER 2015.

9   David L Sackett, William M C Rosenberg, J A Muir Gray, R Brian Haynes, W Scott Richardson: "Evidence based medicine: what it is and what it isn't", BMJ 1996; 312:71

10 Your Health Your Choice: "Procedural irregularities", (discussion of the NHMRC review of Homeopathic Medicine), http://www.nhmrchomeopathy.com/procedural.html

11 Your Health Your Choice: "NHMRC under scrutiny in the Senate – Full ad accurate answers not provided", https://www.yourhealthyourchoice.com.au/news-features/nhmrc-under-scrutiny-in-the-senate-full-and-accurate-answers-not-provided/#gf_1

35. WHAT DO WE NEED NOW?

1   Parkinson's Australia Inc: "Living with Parkinson's disease – An updated economic analysis 2014", Deloitte, August 2015, available as PDF download from: https://www.parkinsonsvic.org.au/about-us/media-release/cost-of-Parkinsons/

2   ibid.

3   ibid.

INDEX

medication 247-52, 341

Medicine Tree Organo LiverGall Tone 277

meditation 22, 27, 80, 159-66, 176-7, 223-4, 233, 322, 342, 395

Mediterranean diet 7, 23, 56, 156

mercury 69, 91, 104, 253-4, 269, 375

methylation 270

milk 58, 106, 107-8, 122

mindset 151-58

mineralocorticoids 43

mirror talk 232-3

mitochondria 25, 26

Modified Activated Clinoptilolite (MAC) 271, 277

monosodium glutamate (MSG) 69

mood swings 46

motor neurone disease (MND) *see* amyotrophic lateral sclerosis (ALS)

mould 90, 267

MSIDS 76-81, 88, 279

MTHFR 134

Mucuna puriens 318

Multiple Sclerosis (MS) 59, 72, 74, 84, 280

Multisystem Atrophy (MSA) 19, 20, 84, 198, 280, 391

muscle atrophy 46

Mycoplasma 72, 286, 297

N

National Health and Medical Research Council (Australia) 346, 361

niacin 358

nocebo 23, 330

noradrenaline 43

norepinephrine *see* noradrenaline

O

oil pulling 273-4

osteoporosis 46, 58, 314

P

Parkinson, Dr James 16

Parkinson's disease 84, 391
   associations 4, 6, 21, 357
   causes 31-94, 158, 175, 244, 357
     definition 11
     diagnosis 18, 19-20, 66, 215, 222, 288, 302
     genetic 20, 33, 35-6, 392
     history 14-18
     idiopathic 20, 357
     process 11
     stages 3, 144
     treatment 21-4

Pasteur, Dr Louis 9

PD Warrior 155

perfume 263-4, 364

personal care products 257-64

PET plastic 379-80

phototherapy *see* light therapy

Pilates 26, 146, 149, 150, 329, 341

placebo 17, 360

polypharmacy 20, 66, 86, 338, 349

polytoxicity 70

post-traumatic stress disorder (PTSD) 42

potassium 44, 46

postural hypotension 190-1

POTS 190-1, 220

probiotic 138-9, 183

Progressive Supranuclear Palsy (PSP) 19, 20, 33, 84

protein 104, 105, 115, 118, 121, 168

Proton Pump Inhibitor (PPI) 9, 67, 141, 142, 189, 214

CPSIA information can be obtained
at www.ICGtesting.com
Printed in the USA
LVHW091135031120
670570LV00004B/380